AF758100

Diagnosis and Management of Marfan Syndrome

Anne H. Child
Editor

Diagnosis and Management of Marfan Syndrome

Springer

Editor
Anne H. Child, MD, FRCP
Cardiovascular and Cell Sciences Research Institute
St George's, University of London
London
UK

ISBN 978-1-4471-5441-9 ISBN 978-1-4471-5442-6 (eBook)
DOI 10.1007/978-1-4471-5442-6

Library of Congress Control Number: 2016934597

© Springer-Verlag London 2016
This work is subject to copyright. All rights are reserved by the Publisher, whether the whole or part of the material is concerned, specifically the rights of translation, reprinting, reuse of illustrations, recitation, broadcasting, reproduction on microfilms or in any other physical way, and transmission or information storage and retrieval, electronic adaptation, computer software, or by similar or dissimilar methodology now known or hereafter developed.
The use of general descriptive names, registered names, trademarks, service marks, etc. in this publication does not imply, even in the absence of a specific statement, that such names are exempt from the relevant protective laws and regulations and therefore free for general use.
The publisher, the authors and the editors are safe to assume that the advice and information in this book are believed to be true and accurate at the date of publication. Neither the publisher nor the authors or the editors give a warranty, express or implied, with respect to the material contained herein or for any errors or omissions that may have been made.

Printed on acid-free paper

This Springer imprint is published by Springer Nature
The registered company is Springer-Verlag London Ltd.

This book is dedicated to all those with Marfan syndrome – past, present and future – who teach us how to care for them, and inspire our research efforts
To all my colleagues internationally, whose unceasing efforts to improve our understanding of Marfan syndrome in all its ramifications have been willingly shared to speed progress
To my family, especially my husband, Dr. Geoffrey V Child, who have supported me in all my endeavours
To my students, who carry on the battle against disease
And in memory of Professor F Clarke Fraser who first introduced me to the rewarding field of genetic research

Preface

The Marfan Trust has become increasingly active over the past few years. Our support network has grown and we have engaged with many more people through events and fundraising activities. Our website and social media are becoming central in explaining what the charity is doing and how our Marfan patient community and supporters are engaging with us and one another. The Trustees held their strategy meeting early in 2015 to determine the charity's direction and goals over the next few years. The outcome is published on our website. Our three key objectives remain: medical research as a high priority; producing educational literature and raising awareness; and support and guidance provided for our patient community. We are growing as a charity, providing top quality research in our designated laboratory, education, awareness and support in the UK and beyond.

The AIMS (Aortic Irbesartan in Marfan Syndrome) Trial, continuing until 2018, is one of a number of international trials comparing beta-blocker therapy with losartan or irbesartan therapy. This UK trial, co-funded by the Marfan Trust and the British Heart Foundation, is a main priority. With 21 participating Marfan syndrome clinics around the UK, this trial has provided an opportunity for Marfan syndrome patients to have local diagnosis and support. Additional research is undertaken in our laboratory into overlapping syndromes such as ectopia lentis and scoliosis, and translational research, which will ultimately benefit patients through improved clarification of diagnosis and the utilisation of results to develop resources for medical professionals and education. One example of this is our new paediatric guide, formulated from research incorporated into our children's database. We have provided funding support to recruit a number of medical and bioscience students to undertake research work. This has assisted our resident researchers and also introduced a new generation of future medical and scientific professionals to genetics and Marfan syndrome in particular.

Knowledge is everything and the first step to knowledge is awareness. We provide a February Awareness Month over various media platforms. Family Fun Days are held twice yearly and permit families to share problems and solutions. Our updated literature is now available. We are particularly targeting general practitioners in the UK, where there seems to be a lack of awareness and understanding of Marfan syndrome.

This present textbook has been eagerly awaited. It reports new research funded by the Marfan Trust. We are most grateful to the authors for sharing their knowledge, and we know that increased awareness and improved care of Marfan syndrome patients will result. We cannot thank you all enough.

W: www.marfantrust.org

E: marfantrust@sgul.ac.uk

F: Facebook/marfantrustcharity

Marfan Trust

Supporting Research into Marfan Syndrome

Patrons: Sir Magdi Yacoub FRCS, Mr Anthony Latter MA and Lady Maryanna Tavener

Registered Charity No: 328070

Marfan Trust
London, UK

Les Tippin

Contents

Contributors

Jose Antonio Aragon-Martin, PhD Sonalee Laboratory, Cardiovascular and Cell Sciences Research Institute, St George's, University of London, London, UK

Aman Chandra, MRCSEd, FRCOphth, PhD Department of Ophthalmology, Southend University Hospital, Southend-on-Sea, Essex, SSO ORY, UK

David G. Charteris, MD, FRCS, FRCOphth Vitreo-Retinal Unit, Moorfields Eye Hospital, London, UK

Nicholas J. Cheshire, MD, FRCS(Eng), FRCS(Ed) Department of Surgery, Imperial College London, London, UK

Department of Surgery, Royal Brompton and Harefield Aortic Centre, London, UK

Anne H. Child, MD, FRCP Cardiovascular and Cell Sciences Research Institute, St George's, University of London, London, UK

Bethan Davies, MBBS Royal Sussex County Hospital, Brighton, UK

Anthony L. Estrera Department of Cardiothoracic and Vascular Surgery, Memorial Hermann Heart and Vascular Institute, University of Texas, Austin, TX, USA

Sabiha Gati, MBBS, MRCP Cardiovascular and Cell Sciences Research Institute, St George's, University of London, London, UK

Rodney Grahame, CBE, MD, FRCP, FACP Rheumatology Unit, Hospital of St John and St Elizabeth, London, UK

Nanjundappa S. Harshavardhana, MS, Dip SICOT, EBOT Department of Spinal Surgery, Twin Cities Spine Center, Minneapolis, MN, USA

Ali Hasan, MBBS, FRCS Clinical Operations Director, Vitality UK, London, UK

Ee Ling Heng, MBBS, BSc, MRCP NIHR Cardiovascular Biomedical Research Unit, Royal Brompton and Harefield NHS Foundation Trust and Imperial College London, London, UK

Lucy N. Hyde, BDS Marfan Trust, Cardiovascular and Cell Sciences Research Institute, St George's, University of London, London, UK

Yukiko Isekame, MB Cardiovascular and Cell Sciences Research Institute, St George's, University of London, London, UK

Corrine Jabs, MD, FRCS-C Department of Obstetrics and Gynecology, Regina Qu'Appelle Health Region, Regina, Saskatchewan, Canada

Marjan Jahangiri, FRCS(CTh) Department of Cardiothoracic Surgery, St George's Hospital, London, UK

Timothy L. Jones, PhD, FRCS(SN) Academic Neurosurgery Unit, St George's, University of London, London, UK

Rosemary J. Keer, MSc, MCSP, MACP Department of Hypermobility Unit, Hospital of St John & St Elizabeth, London, UK

Anna Marciniak, PhD, MRCP Department of Cardiology, St George's Hospital, London, UK

Raad H. Mohiaddin, FRCR, FRCP, FESC, PhD NIHR Cardiovascular Biomedical Research Unit, Royal Brompton and Harefield NHS Foundation Trust and Imperial College London, London, UK

Mohammed H.H. Noordeen, MA, BM, MCh Ortho, FRCS(Tr&Orth) Department of Trauma and Orthopaedic Surgery, Spinal Deformity Unit (SDU), Royal National Orthopaedic Hospital, London, UK

Marios C. Papadopoulos, MD, FRCS(SN) Academic Neurosurgery Unit, St George's, University of London, London, UK

J. Poloniecki, MSc, DPhil Population Health Research Institute, St George's, University of London, London, UK

Ulrich Rosendahl Department of Surgery, Royal Brompton and Harefield Aortic Centre, London, UK

Joanna Rowntree Cardiovascular and Cell Sciences Research Institute, St George's, University of London, London, UK

Diane L. Rust, MJF, LCIF Chairman, Marfan Association UK, Courtmoor, Fleet Hants, UK

Hazim J. Safi Department of Cardiothoracic and Vascular Surgery, Memorial Hermann Heart & Vascular Institute, University of Texas, Austin, TX, USA

Karen Sage, BSc, MSc, GC Department of Preimplantation Genetic Diagnosis, The Bridge Centre, London Fertility Clinic, London, UK

Benedict Scoones, BSc, MBBS Norfolk and Norwich University Hospital, Norwich, UK

Rajan Sharma, BSc(Hons), MBBS, MRCP(UK), MD Department of Cardiology, St George's Hospital, London, UK

Anita K. Simonds, MD, FRCP NIHR Respiratory Biomedical Research Unit, Royal Brompton & Harefield NHS Foundation Trust, London, UK

Graham Stuart, MBChB, MSc, FRCP, FRCPCH Congenital Heart Disease Centre, Bristol Royal Hospital for Children, Bristol, UK

Les Tippin, OBE Chairman, Marfan Trust, St George's, University of London, London, UK

Fiona Walker, BM(Hons), FRCP, FESC Barts Heart Centre, St Bartholomew's Hospital, London, UK

Ruwan A. Weerakkody, PhD Department of Surgery, Imperial College London, London, UK

Don B. Wijetunge[†]**, MBBS(Ceylon), FRCS(Ed), FFAEM** Formerly of Department of Accident and Emergency Medicine, St George's Hospital, London, UK

Pouya Youssefi, BSc (Hons), MBBS, MRCS(Eng) Department of Cardiothoracic Surgery, St George's Hospital, London, UK

[†]Author was deceased at the time of publication

Introduction

1

Anne H. Child

Rare or Common?

Marfan syndrome is generally thought to be rare, but clinicians who have seen how the gene expression can shade into normality in affected members of a family, suspect that its overall frequency could be underestimated, as a recent collaborative publication states [1]. The fact that the syndrome presents in many different ways may also hinder its recognition. Marfan syndrome patients may first be referred to any one of a number of specialists. Each doctor is likely to be familiar with a particular aspect of the syndrome, but less familiar with its other features. The aim of this guide is to pool the knowledge available from different experienced specialists, and to make it available to the many clinicians likely to encounter a patient with this condition.

Co-ordinated Care

Who should care for the Marfan syndrome patient? I believe the answer is that we should all do so. Whoever first suspects the diagnosis should pursue the question until it is either proved or disproved, and should consider what other specialist opinions might be required. All patients should be referred for genetic counselling, both to help with diagnosis, and to identify other affected family members, as well as provide guidance about the risk to future children. Each patient is best cared for by a team, led by one co-ordinating physician who is familiar with all aspects of the condition. This is likely to be a geneticist or cardiologist. The rise of aortopathy

A.H. Child, MD, FRCP
Cardiovascular and Cell Sciences Research Institute,
St George's, University of London, London, UK
e-mail: achild@sgul.ac.uk

© Springer-Verlag London 2016

A.H. Child (ed.), *Diagnosis and Management of Marfan Syndrome*,
DOI 10.1007/978-1-4471-5442-6_1

diagnostic and follow-up clinics is to be applauded. As a result, patients can be referred locally rather than having to travel long distances for management.

International Collaboration and Patient Support

National and international patient support group networks have been set up, and active research is being undertaken into the cause, early diagnosis, treatment, and prevention of Marfan syndrome. A summary of diagnosis and management is provided in Chap. 2, Table 2.2. Subsequent chapters show that the management of this condition can be much improved by wider knowledge of its principal features, most of which can now be effectively treated, resulting in more normal lifespan [2]. The discovery that the underlying connective tissue defect in Marfan syndrome results from a primary deficiency of fibrillin-1 has led to attempts at more fundamental methods of prevention and treatment, such as the international trials of losartan and irbesartan aimed at preserving the aortic media [3].

First Gene for Familial TAAD

International collaborative groups aimed at discovering new genes and new treatments are proving effective [3]. Marfan syndrome has led the way in this field of Familial Thoracic Aortic Aneurysm and Dissection (FTAAD), and clinicians experienced in managing this condition will be called upon to manage many similar genetically-determined aneurysms in future [4].

References

1. Arslan-Kirchner M, Arbustini E, Boileau C, et al. Clinical utility gene card for: marfan syndrome type 1 and related phenotypes [FBN1]. Eur J Hum Genet. 2010;18(9): doi: 10.1038/ejhg.2010.42.
2. Pyeritz RE. Marfan syndrome: 30 years of research equals 30 years of additional life expectancy. Heart. 2009;95(3):173–5.
3. Pitcher A, Emberson J, Lacro RV, et al. Design and rationale of a prospective, collaborative meta-analysis of all randomized controlled trials of angiotensin receptor antagonists in Marfan syndrome, based on individual patient data: a report from the Marfan Treatment Trialists' Collaboration. Am Heart J. 2015;169(5):605–12.
4. Milewicz DM, Regalado E. Thoracic aortic aneurysms and aortic dissections. www.ncbi.nlm.nih.gov/books/NBK1120/.

2 Diagnosis and Management (Summary)

Anne H. Child

In my personal experience, when a patient, whether child or adult, is referred with the possibility of a diagnosis of Marfan syndrome, they are assessed after echocardiogram, from a cardiovascular genetic point of view using the following approach.

Taking the Family History

A three or four generation family history is obtained wherever possible, remembering that 25 % of patients are the result of a new mutation, while 75 % have inherited the condition from one parent or the other. Each patient is asked to bring already existing snapshots of siblings, parents and offspring so that if dominant inheritance is present, it can be tracked through photographs. Operative reports and death certificates may have to be obtained. Manifestations of early onset eye, heart or skeletal problems are sought (Table 2.1). Ages and causes of death of close relatives are recorded.

Physical Examination

Careful examination of the patient for any sign of connective tissue disorder is undertaken. Our examination sheet is shown in Fig. 2.1. The examination is performed starting from the head down. The joint hypermobility score is that of Beighton [1] and any value of 5 or greater should be considered abnormal. In addition, small joint hypermobility of fingers and toes should be taken into account. This may be racial (Africans, Indians, Arabs, Spaniards) [1, 2] and should be discounted

A.H. Child, MD, FRCP
Cardiovascular and Cell Sciences Research Institute,
St George's, University of London, London, UK
e-mail: achild@sgul.ac.uk

© Springer-Verlag London 2016

A.H. Child (ed.), *Diagnosis and Management of Marfan Syndrome*,
DOI 10.1007/978-1-4471-5442-6_2

Table 2.1 Salient features of the Marfan syndrome

Physical/skeletal: Tall, thin physique with long limbs, spinal curvature, flattening of chest (with pigeon or funnel deformity)
Cardiovascular: Dilation of ascending (and sometimes descending) aorta, incompetence of aortic (and sometimes mitral) valve, dissection and/or rupture of aorta
Ocular: Dislocation of lens, myopia and refraction problems (often unstable), detachment of retina, glaucoma
Dental: High-arched narrow palate, crowding of teeth
Genetic: Inheritance by boys or girls from either parent (50 % risk of any child of affected parent having Marfan syndrome); 25 % cases sporadic (new mutation)
Variability: In severity and pattern of features affected

if it is racial. Joint contractures should also be noted. Particular attention should be paid to skin, since it contains all of the connective tissue elements found in the aortic wall. Is it thin (anterior chest wall), stretchy (side of neck), or striated, especially in the lumbar area? Horizontal striae in the lumbar area are usually found in Marfan syndrome. Vertical striae on the buttocks suggest joint hypermobility syndrome (Ehlers Danlos Type III).

If the patient is a child, physical examination should be placed in the middle column of the examination form, with father's and mother's examinations placed either side. In this way, common features shared with either parent can be highlighted. Often a tall slim pubertal hypermobile child may simply result from the genetic combination of joint hypermobility from one parent, and tall stature from the other parent, in the presence of a normal echocardiogram in the child. Demonstrating shared features indicates that the child is not affected with a new condition, but simply a new combination of family genes from both sides. But it must be considered that a Marfan syndrome child may be born into a family which has hypermobility.

A differential diagnosis includes many conditions and we must not overdiagnose Marfan syndrome. The commonest condition mistaken for Marfan syndrome is undoubtedly Ehlers Danlos syndrome Type III (joint hypermobility syndrome). Rare conditions include rarely congenital contractural arachodactyly [3], and overgrowth syndromes, for example Sotos syndrome [4]. Another common overlap syndrome is Ectopia Lentis as an isolated problem [5]. If the echocardiogram is normal, and a parent is affected with dislocated lenses, then this may still be due to mild fibrillin-1 deficiency, often with a mutation in the first 15 exons of the gene [6]. If the child with Ectopia Lentis is the only one in the family and parents are related (consanguineous), this is most likely an autosomal recessive type of Ectopia Lentis due to ADAMTSL4, ADAMTS18, or other gene [5]. Adolescent idiopathic scoliosis can also be inherited dominantly, and is now being shown to be due to separate genes [7].

Suspected cases under the age of two should have plasma amino acid analysis in the absence of pyridoxine supplementation to rule out the diagnosis of homocystinuria, since failure to treat may lead to mental retardation [8].

Name:			
Date:			
Date of birth:			
Age:			
Weight:			
Height:			
Arm span:			
Upper/lower segment ratio:			
Thin?			
Eye findings:			
Antimongoloid slant:			
Head shape:			
Palate:			
Teeth:			
Ears:			
Hearing:			
Facial appearance:			
Chest: lordosis / kyphosis:			
Scoliosis:			
Pigeon breast:			
Pectus excavatum:			
Other: (nipples, sulcus, barrel chest, etc.)			
Heart: murmur:			
Arrhythmia:			
Blood pressure:			
Hernia:			
Skin: Soft:			
Thin:			
Hyperextensible:			
Scars: Spread:			
Papyraceous:			
Keloid:			
Striae: Lumbar:			
Elsewhere:			
Bruising: easy:			
Arachnodactyly:			
Medications:			

		Lf	Th	El	Kn	Bk			Lf	Th	El	Kn	Bk			Lf	Th	El	Kn	Bk	
Joints: Hypermobile (hands, elbows, knees, back)	L							L							L						
	R						9	R						9	R						9

Hypermobile fingers (small joints):			
Feet: Size:			
Flat feet:			
Pronated ankles:			
Hammer toes:			
Hypermobile toes:			
Joints general: painful:			
Stiff:			
Swollen:			

Fig. 2.1 Physical examination form

Diagnostic Pathway

The diagnostic features for Marfan syndrome have been presented and updated [9]. However, this highly detailed classification of findings is difficult to remember, and a simple guideline is that the patient must have classical severe findings in two out of three systems (eyes, heart, skeleton) in order to make a clinical diagnosis, or in the presence of a dominant family history, one system involvement. We have created a diagnostic pathway to make the clinical classification easier (Figs. 2.2 and 2.3). For a detailed summary of the minor features considered, please see the revised Ghent criteria [10].

Fibrillin-1 Mutation Screen

Most importantly, this condition is no longer just a clinical diagnosis. Because it is very variable with reduced penetrance, a mutation screen including MLPA should be performed in any questionable case. The cost of this is fully justified, since other tests such as a scan for dural ectasia, or repeated echocardiograms, very quickly add up to the same sum. Also, the psychological damage of bringing an unaffected patient back on an annual basis for echocardiography must be considered. Such patients can become hypochondriacal through repeated examinations. It is much more professional to do a simple test which will rule out the condition with 97 % accuracy.

Timetable of Care

In Table 2.2 you will find an overview of management. Table 2.3 is a timetable of care which could be filed by the general practitioner in the notes so that the patient is referred for specialist care at key points in their life.

Endocarditis Prophylaxis

Recent summaries of best care for Marfan syndrome patients abound [11–13]. One point of difference is whether patients require antibiotic therapy for dental or other minor surgery. Because cases of endocarditis have occurred following dental work, this should be considered as seriously as minor surgery, and the patient covered adequately with antibiotic before treatment and after treatment. Any patient who has had heart surgery should have antibiotic therapy. This is because Marfan syndrome patients have weak connective tissue which cannot resist infection normally. Any bacterial or even viral infection can invade rapidly and may prove life-threatening.

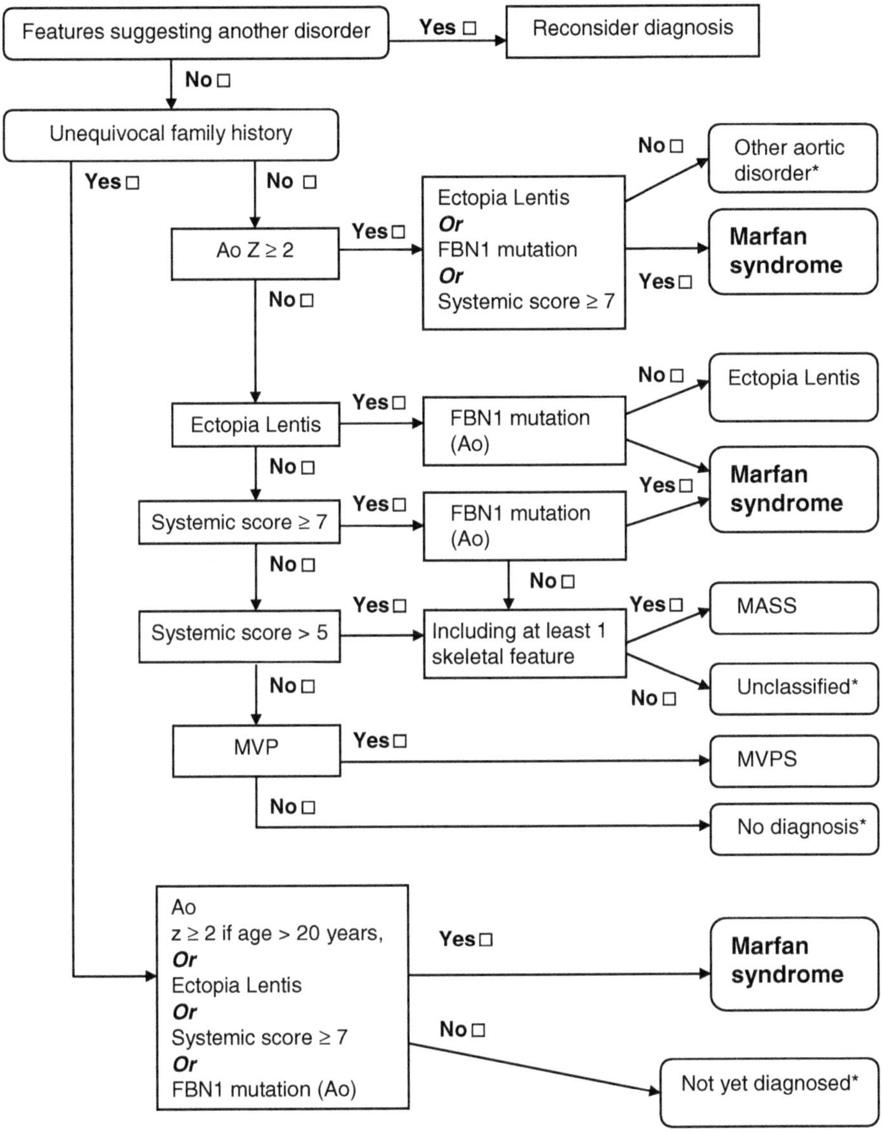

Fig. 2.2 Diagnostic flow diagram for adults over 20 years of age (Diagnostic flow diagram courtesy of Dr John Dean, Consultant Geneticist, Aberdeen Clinical Genetics Centre, Foresterhill, AB24 2ZN, UK, based on Loeys et al. [10]). Note: FBN1 mutation (*Ao*) refers to any mutation already reported in the literature affecting heart or aorta in Marfan syndrome

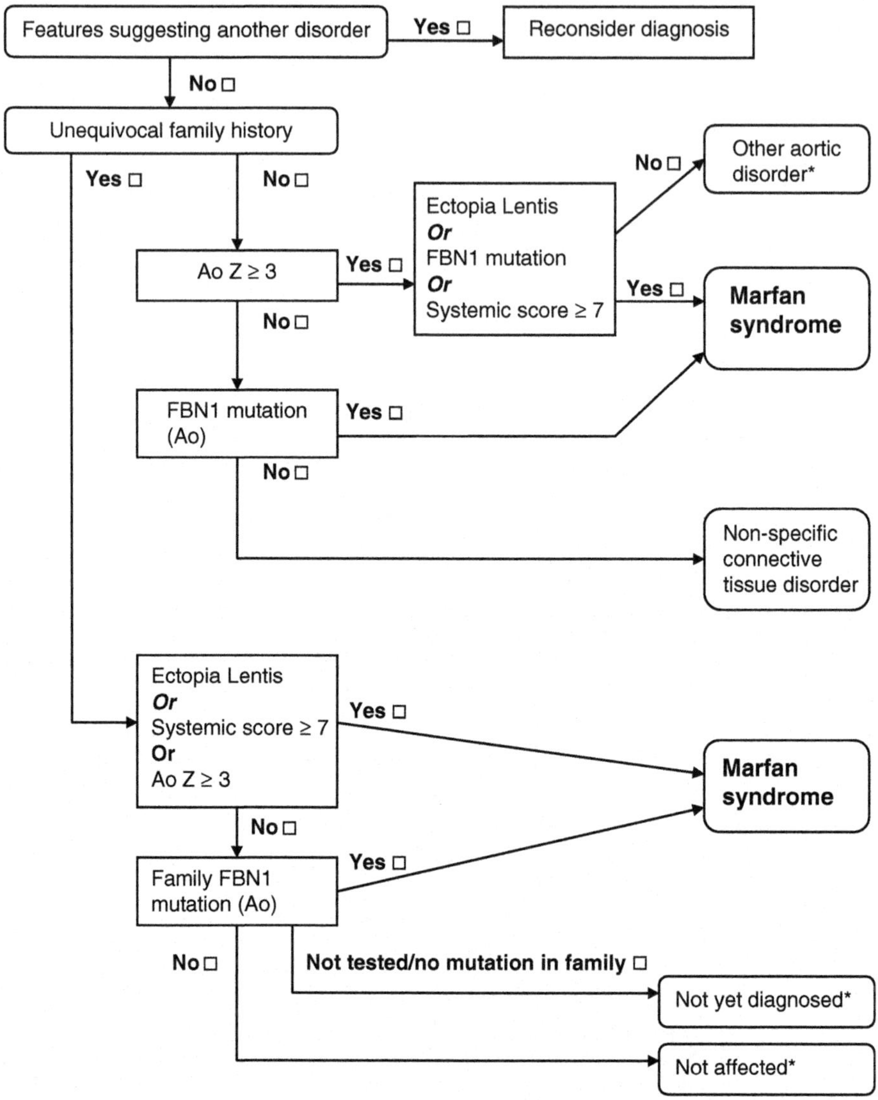

Fig. 2.3 Diagnostic flow diagram for children under 20 years of age. This algorithm for diagnosis in people less than 20 years of age is based on the suggestions for the diagnosis of young people made in the Revised Nosology [10]: Young people (<20 years) with no family history, systemic score <7, aortic root z<3 and no FBN1 mutation may be diagnosed "non-specific connective tissue disorder" and followed up until adult. The category "potential Marfan Syndrome" discussed in the revised nosology is subsumed within "Marfan syndrome" in this algorithm. * Not formally part of the Revised Nosology (Note: FBN1 mutation (*Ao*) refers to any mutation already reported in the literature affecting heart or aorta in Marfan syndrome)

Table 2.2 Overview of management

Regular examination by one co-ordinating physician
Periodical multidisciplinary evaluation:
Ophthalmological – between birth and 6 months; annually thereafter
Orthopaedic – scoliosis, pectus deformity, flat feet, to age 20
Cardiovascular – new-born; every 2 years to age 11; annually thereafter
Genetic counselling – at first diagnosis, and again with partner
Periodic ECG and echocardiogram, focusing on dysrhythmias, mitral valve prolapse and aortic root dilation
Chest radiograph, focusing on apical blebs – tall pubertal males at greatest risk of pneumothorax
CT or MRI scan of entire aorta – baseline assessment in all adults and periodically in patients with aneurysm or dissection – annually after aortic surgery
Endocarditis prophylaxis during dental care involving bleeding, and surgery
Beta-adrenergic blockade and/or ARB, e.g. irbesartan
Restriction of strenuous activities, especially contact sports and isometric exercises, e.g. Weightlifting
Consider prophylactic surgical replacement of ascending aorta at 4.5–5.0 cm dilatation (or earlier if a family history of dissection/rupture is present)
Life-long regular monitoring of all unreplaced aortic segments and heart

Aortic Surgery

Secondly, the exact timing for cardiac surgery is debatable. The patient could be referred, due to the low mortality risk in experienced cardiac surgeon's hands, at sinus of Valsalva diameter between 4.5 and 4.8 cm, but because of possible delay in making an operative date, the patient should not be left until the aortic root is 5 cm. In some families, with documented dissection at aortic root diameter below 4.5 cm, the patient should be referred even earlier, at approximately 4.2 cm.

Any aortic root diameter over 4 cm is considered abnormal. Aortic root diameter does not depend on the excessive height of the patient in this regard.

Prediction of Severity

Patients with new mutations are at higher risk of early cardiac disease than familial cases. This is because familial cases survive to reproduce, or they would not be familial; whereas new mutation cases are unknown entities, and usually represent a more severe disease model.

To some degree, genotype-phenotype correlation is helpful in predicting long-term prognosis [14, 15]. Each mutation behaves uniquely in each family, thus the family history, with dates of dissection and death, or of lens dislocation or other complication, may be very helpful in predicting severity of disease. An international genotype-phenotype database has been set up for clinicians to consult [16].

Table 2.3 Timetable of care

	Newborn	Pre-school	Pubertal years	Adulthood
Cardiac	Echocardiography 'Echo' parents if first affected child	Repeat 'echo' and/or ARB Beta-blockers if 'cardiac' family	Repeat 'echo' every 1–2 years Restriction of strenuous exercise and contact sports	Regular 'echo' Pre-, intra- and postpartum echos for females. Avoid pregnancy if aortic root >4.2 cm
Ocular	Examine for dislocated lenses, strabismus	Glasses if required	Advice about glaucoma if dislocated lenses	See regularly if ocular problems. If none, see only when necessary
Skeletal	Measure length Look for high palate, and arachnodactyly	Check for scoliosis, flat feet	Stop scoliosis check at age 18	Joint pain, early osteoarthritis require NSAIDs
Lung		Asthma frequent problem	Age 18 – chest X-ray for blebs, fibrosis. Pneumothorax 11 %	Avoid smoking contribution to emphysema and bronchiectasis
Genetic	Counsel parents about the 50:50 risk in subsequent pregnancy if one parent is affected (75 % of cases). Prenatal diagnosis? PGD? AID? Ovum/sperm donation? Adoption?	Why am I different?	Explain inheritance and variability, offer counselling session with partner, when should I tell boy/girl friend?	
Psycho-social	Help family handle guilt, grief, anger	Anger, coping with teasing	Career advice	Diagnosis after marriage – acceptance counselling. Pre- and post-cardiac operation counselling

Familial Thoracic Ascending Aortic Aneurysm and Dissection (FTAAD)

In recent years, many genes other than fibrillin-1 which can produce FTAAD have been described [17]. Most of these patients do not look marfanoid, and so the diagnosis can be very puzzling. Nonetheless, a first screen of fibrillin-1 could then be followed by a screening panel of the commonest TAAD genes. If no cause is found, the DNA sample should be stored for future research.

References

1. Grahame R, Bird HA, Child A. The revised (Beighton, 1998) criteria for diagnosis of benign joint hypermobility syndrome (BJHS). J Rheumatol. 2000;27:1777–9.
2. Beighton PH, Solomon I, Soskoline CI. Articular mobility in the African population. Ann Rheum Dis. 1973;32:413–7.

3. Takeda N, Morita H, Fujita D, et al. Congenital contractural arachnodactyly complicated with aortic dilatation and dissection: case report and review of literature. Am J Med Genet A. 2015;167A:2382–7.
4. Türkmen S, Şahin S, Koçer N, et al. Neuroimaging and clinical characterization of Sotos syndrome. Genet Couns. 2015;26(1):1–12.
5. Chandra A, Patel D, Aragon-Martin JA, et al. The revised Ghent nosology; reclassifying isolated ectopia lentis. Clin Genet. 2015;87(3):284–7.
6. Zhang L, Lai YH, Capasso JE, et al. Early onset ectopia lentis due to a FBN1 mutation with non-penetrance. Am J Med Genet A. 2015;167(6):1365–8. doi:10.1002/ajmg.a.37035.
7. Patten SA, Margaritte-Jeannin P, Moldovan F, et al. Functional variants of POC5 identified in patients with idiopathic scoliosis. J Clin Invest. 2015;125(3):1124–8.
8. Hafidi Z, Berradi S, Handor H, et al. Atypical presentation of ectopia lentis in homocystinuria. J Pediatr. 2015;166(4):1091.
9. von Kodolitsch Y, De Backer J, Schüler H, et al. Perspectives on the revised Ghent criteria for the diagnosis of Marfan syndrome. Appl Clin Genet. 2015;8:137–55.
10. Loeys BL, Dietz HC, Braverman AC, et al. The revised Ghent nosology for the Marfan syndrome. J Med Genet. 2010;47(7):476–85.
11. Hiratzka LF, Bakris GL, Beckman JA, et al. 2010 ACCF/AHA/AATS/ACR/ASA/SCA/SCAI/SIR/STS/SVM Guidelines for the diagnosis and management of patients with thoracic aortic disease. J Am Coll Cardiol. 2010;55(14):e27–129.
12. National Marfan Foundation. www.marfan.org/resources/professionals/management.
13. Erbel R, Aboyans V, Boileau C, et al. 2014 ESC guidelines on the diagnosis and treatment of aortic diseases the task force for the diagnosis and treatment of aortic diseases of the European Society of Cardiology (ESC). Eur Heart J. 2014;35:2873–926.
14. Faivre L, Collod-Beroud G, Loeys BL, et al. Effect of mutation type and location on clinical outcome in 1,013 probands with Marfan syndrome or related phenotypes and FBN1 mutations: an international study. Am J Hum Genet. 2007;81(3):454–66.
15. Faivre L, Masurel-Paulet A, Collod-Beroud G, et al. Clinical and molecular study of 320 children with Marfan syndrome and related type I fibrillinopathies in a series of 1009 probands with pathogenic FBN1 mutations. Pediatrics. 2009;123(1):391–8.
16. Collod-Beroud G, Le Bourdelles S, Ades L, et al. The UMD-FBN1 mutations database. Hum Mutat. 2003;22:199–208. www.umd.be/FBN1/.
17. Milewicz DM, Regalado E. Thoracic aortic aneurysms and aortic dissections. www.ncbi.nlm.nih.gov/books/NBK1120/.

Diagnosis and Management of Acute Complications Associated with Marfan Syndrome: Pitfalls in the Emergency Setting

3

Don B. Wijetunge† and Anne H. Child

Introduction

The complications of Marfan syndrome (MFS), which may present as medical emergencies, are well recognised [1–3] and include aortic dissection/rupture, pneumothorax, retinal detachment, lens dislocation and joint dislocation. The optimum management of these complications has also been well described. Some of the above-mentioned complications are life-threatening, the most notorious being aortic dissection. If this condition is undiagnosed the early mortality is 1 % per each hour delay [4, 5]. The outcome is proportional to the time spent in making the diagnosis and moving the patient from the Emergency Department to the operating room. Unfortunately establishing the diagnosis of aortic dissection/rupture in the Emergency Department proves difficult, leading to avoidable mortality and morbidity. We have attempted in this chapter to highlight some of the pitfalls in the diagnosis. Our objective is that these complications will be recognised in a timely manner so that patients are moved to the appropriate facility with the least possible delay.

Chest Pain in a Young Adult with Known or Suspected MFS

If an MFS patient presents with chest pain, the first and the only diagnosis to consider at the beginning is aortic dissection or rupture. Only when this life-threatening condition is excluded is one free to consider other possibilities.

† Deceased

D.B. Wijetunge, MBBS(Ceylon), FRCS(Ed), FFAEM
Formerly of Department of Accident and Emergency Medicine, St George's Hospital, London, UK

A.H. Child, MD, FRCP (✉)
Cardiovascular and Cell Sciences Research Institute,
St George's, University of London, London, UK
e-mail: achild@sgul.ac.uk

© Springer-Verlag London 2016

A.H. Child (ed.), *Diagnosis and Management of Marfan Syndrome*,
DOI 10.1007/978-1-4471-5442-6_3

Aortic Dissection

Acute dissection of the thoracic aorta is a life-threatening situation and carries a high mortality if definitive care is delayed. If untreated the mortality rate is 28 % within 24 h, 50 % in 48 h, 70 % within 1 week and 90 % or more within months [6, 7]. Marfan syndrome is a predisposing factor for aortic dissection. If a patient with known or suspected Marfan syndrome presents to the Emergency Department with chest pain, the diagnosis should be acute dissection of the aorta until proven otherwise. Such an attitude will make it imperative for us to consider the probability of the condition, thus avoiding the catastrophic situation where these patients are sent home with an alternative diagnosis.

It is important to recognise that 50 % of aortic dissections in women younger than 40 occur during pregnancy [8].

Presenting Symptoms and Signs in Aortic Dissection

In aortic dissection the mechanism for all the symptoms and signs are:

1. Dissection/rupture of the aorta.
2. Compression of adjoining structures by the expanding aorta.
3. Ischaemia caused by occlusion of the branches of the aorta.

The common presenting symptoms are as follows:

Chest pain. The pain is severe and sudden in onset. The maximum pain is at the onset. Patients often describe the pain as cutting, searing, ripping, or tearing. It is commonly retrosternal and interscapular and may be felt both above and below the diaphragm. A common characteristic of aortic dissection pain is midline truncal pain, but aortic chest pain may be atypical. Chest pain is the commonest symptom which could be due to cardiovascular, pulmonary, gastrointestinal, neurological or musculoskeletal causes. A high degree of suspicion in this special group of patients will lead to the diagnosis being made expeditiously.

Gastrointestinal symptoms. Abdominal pain can be the presenting complaint. This may be due to acute mesenteric ischaemia due to occlusion of the superior mesenteric vessels. One of the clues in this situation is pain, which is totally out of proportion to the abdominal findings.

Shortness of breath. Patients with acute dissection may present with acute shortness of breath, which could mimic asthma. This is due to acute pulmonary oedema from sudden onset of severe aortic insufficiency. The other causes are compression of trachea from the expanding ascending aorta. In Marfan syndrome the diagnosis to be considered with these symptoms are first aortic dissection and then spontaneous pneumothorax.

Fainting episode. About 5 % of all patients with aortic dissection present with a history of a syncopal attack [9]. Causes for this vary from cardiac tamponade to hypovolaemia to conduction disorders of the heart. Again, in Marfan syndrome patients one should think of the worst case situation, which is aortic dissection.

Neurological complaints. About 20 % of patients with aortic dissection may present with a neurological symptom or we may elicit a neurological sign. The commonest cause of these symptoms is ischaemia of the spinal cord due to spinal artery occlusion or else cerebral vessel occlusion.

Clinical Signs in Aortic Dissection

Patients with acute aortic dissection may show a wide variety of signs. It is not uncommon, however, for there to be few clinical signs. Some clinical signs are very non-specific and some may clearly indicate the diagnosis. Possible signs include:

General signs – Anxious patient, diaphoresis, pale, raised pulse rate, raised respiratory rate, mottled extremities.

Cardiovascular – Hypotensive, normotensive, hypertensive, pulsus paradoxus, wide pulse pressure, aortic regurgitation murmur, muffled heart sounds (pericardial tamponade), asymmetrical pulses.

Head and neck – Horner's syndrome, vocal cord irritation or paralysis.

Respiratory system – Decreased breath sounds, basal crepitations, wheezing.

Central nervous system – Altered level of consciousness, hemiplegia, and paraplegia.

Investigations

Bearing in mind the high and time-dependent mortality of aortic dissection one should ask the question as to how suspicious are you of aortic dissection? If the suspicion is high then very early consultation with the local cardiothoracic surgeons is essential.

The most important adjunct to making the correct diagnosis is a high degree of suspicion. If according to the clinical information, the probability of dissection is high or moderate, the objective will be to transfer the patient to a cardiothoracic surgical centre. The other group of patients in whom the diagnosis of aortic dissection is considered to be a low probability should rapidly undergo diagnostic procedures to rule out the possibility.

ECG may mislead one through showing ischaemic changes or may be relatively normal. Chest x-ray can also be misleadingly normal. It is said that the chest x-ray will show one or more features of aortic dissection in 80 % of the cases of aortic dissection [10], but nonetheless in practice the chest x-ray may be easily passed as normal and provide dangerously false reassurance. Radiological features suggesting aortic dissection/rupture are: widened mediastinum, depression of the left main bronchus, small basal effusion, oesophagus shifted to the right (seen when a nasogastric tube is inserted before the x-ray), and a left-sided pleural cap.

Case History A supine chest x-ray of 26 year old female presenting to A & E with severe chest pain was normal. ECG showed ischaemic changes. The chest x-ray was initially used to exclude a dissection and diagnosis of acute myocardial infarct was made. Forty-five minutes later dissection was considered and confirmed by CT.

The other diagnostic tests available are aortography, computed tomography (CT), magnetic resonance imaging (MRI), transthoracic echocardiography (TTE) and transoesophageal echocardiography (TOE). It has to be recognised that excessive delays in awaiting investigation could do more harm to the patient. In this situation one has to weigh the risks to the patient and benefits carefully, in close early consultation with the local cardiothoracic surgeons, at any hour of the day or night.

Aortography is not as sensitive as believed earlier. In a study in 1989 its sensitivity and specificity were judged to be 88 % and 94 % respectively [11]. The sensitivity of CT is similar to that of aortography with values for sensitivity ranging from 83 to 90 %. Specificity ranges from 90 to 100 % [10, 12, 13]. A study in 1993 concluded that sensitivity and specificity of MRI could be 95 % and 100 % respectively [14, 15].

Even though TTE can give a rapid bedside diagnosis it has a low sensitivity of 60–80 % and low specificity of 60–90 % [10, 11, 14]. However, TOE has a high sensitivity of 95–100 % and specificity ranges from 70 to 95 % [9, 10, 13, 16].

Transfer of the Patient to the Regional Cardiothoracic Centre

It is very common for this group of patients to be transferred urgently from the initial receiving hospital to regional cardiothoracic centres.

The process of transfer has to be properly planned and then executed accurately and speedily. Transporting ill patients between hospitals is hazardous and adds to the patient morbidity and mortality. Seriously ill patients do not easily tolerate lifting, tipping, or any sudden abrupt movement. Sudden acceleration and deceleration is associated with potentiation of cardiovascular instability. It is observed that during transfer there is deterioration of oxygenation in seriously ill patients. Every hospital department which moves patients (inter hospital or intra hospital) should have a transfer checklist which has to be completed before moving the patient. This checklist is normally structured in three main parts: (1) Preparation for the transfer (administrative aspects); (2) Preparation of equipment, drugs and personnel; (3) Preparation of the patient. Prior to transfer of the patient, it is important to ensure the patient is stable and will remain stable throughout the journey. The patient should be accompanied by the most appropriate, experienced medical personnel. Specifically in this group of patients, if the patient is hypertensive, it is necessary for the blood pressure to be reduced. If the patient is hypertensive one has to bring down the pressure carefully by using a nitroprusside infusion to maintain the blood pressure around 90 mm of Hg to 100 mmHg. A beta-blocker given intravenously will reduce the velocity of the ventricular contraction thus helping to contain the dissection. All these patients should have adequate analgesia in the intravenous form.

Pneumothorax

Spontaneous pneumothorax is more common in Marfan syndrome patients than in the general population [17, 18]. This should be excluded early in the investigation of an MFS patient with chest pain or unexplained breathlessness by doing an erect PA chest x-ray. If confirmed, the management will be as for any spontaneous pneumothorax. If it is small and the patient is asymptomatic one can manage expectantly. However, if the patient is symptomatic the pneumothorax should be aspirated.

Endocarditis

Marfan syndrome patients have an increased risk of endocarditis compared to the general population [19, 20]. This applies to MFS patients in whom no cardiac lesion has been demonstrated as well as those more obviously at risk through implants or known mitral valve disease. In the emergency care setting this is relevant both in terms of diagnosis of unexplained symptoms, and during treatment, when the need to follow up-to-date guidelines for antimicrobial prophylaxis is important [21].

General Anaesthesia

It is known that general anaesthesia in Marfan syndrome patients carries an increased morbidity and mortality risk [22]. These risks include cardiac and pulmonary complications, and difficult endotracheal intubation. In addition to consideration of antimicrobial prophylaxis for Marfan syndrome patients during procedures under general anaesthetic in the emergency care setting, the need for an experienced anaesthetist is therefore emphasised.

Visual Disturbance in a Patient with Marfan Syndrome

The propensity of patients with Marfan syndrome to develop important ocular complications is quite high. These complications are best treated early in their development. Early consultation with the ophthalmologists is essential to achieve good outcomes. Wakita et al. evaluated the ocular complications associated with Marfan syndrome and listed them in order of frequency of the incidence and their findings are as shown below [23].

1. Dislocation of the lens 72.6 %.
2. Retinal detachment 36.4 %.
3. Glaucoma 15.2 %.

Lens Dislocation

Lends dislocation is the most common ocular abnormality in MFS, affecting 60–80 %. In the majority of cases it is present before 10 years of age. Ectopia lentis refers to a subluxated lens and may occur in Marfan syndrome. Once the lens has become displaced enough, it is no longer able to focus light and monocular diplopia or blurred vision occurs. Dislocation into the vitreous can occur in these conditions as well as in trauma. If increased intraocular pressure (IOP) occurs in the setting of a dislocated lens, a vitrectomy and lens removal are necessary to save the eye. Acutely, medication to lower the IOP can be used. Early referral to an ophthalmologist is important to ensure optimum outcome.

Retinal Detachment

Detachment of the retina is a well-recognised complication in MFS. The incidence of retinal detachment in aphakic eyes (16 %) is higher than in the phakic group (9 %) [23]. In order to get good results, early recognition of the condition and referral are very important.

Summary

Patients with Marfan syndrome can suddenly develop life- or vision-threatening complications. Aortic dissection is a life-threatening condition and if recognised early and referred in time the outcome remains return to normal life. Similarly, eye complications associated with Marfan syndrome should be referred to specialists early to avoid permanent visual impairment.

References

1. Beighton P, editor. MKusick's heritable disorders of connective tissue. 5th ed. St Louis: CV Mosby Company; 1993.
2. Pyeritz RE. The Marfan syndrome. In: Royce PM, Steinmann B, editors. Connective tissue and its heritable disorders: molecular, genetic and medical aspects. New York: Wiley-Liss; 1993. p. 437–68.
3. Murdoch JL, Walker BA, et al. Causes of death in the Marfan syndrome. N Engl J Med. 1972;13:804–8.
4. Hirst Jr AE, Johns Jr VJ, Kime Jr SW. Dissecting aneurysms of the aorta: a review of 505 cases. Medicine. 1958;37:217–79.
5. Anagnosopoulous CE, Manakavalan KSP, Kittle CF. Aortic dissections and dissecting aneurysms. Am J Cardiol. 1972;30:263–73.
6. Bourland MD. Aortic dissection. In: Rosen P, Barkin R, Braen GR, et al., editors. Emergency medicine concepts and clinical practice. 3rd ed. St Louis: CV Mosby; 1992. p. 1384.
7. Fielman JA. Thoracic and abdominal aortic aneurysms. In: Tintinalli JE, Krome RL, Ruiz E, editors. Emergency medicine: a comprehensive study guide. St Louis: Mosby; 1992. p. 247.

8. Da Sancis RW, Doroghazi RM, et al. Aortic dissection. N Engl J Med. 1987;317(17):1060–7.
9. Zappa MJ, Harwood-Nuss A. Recognition and management of aortic dissection and thoracic aortic aneurysm. Emerg Med Rep. 1993;14(1):3–4.
10. Treasure T, Raphael MJ. Investigation of suspected dissection of the thoracic aorta. Lancet. 1991;338:490–5.
11. Erbel R, Daniel W, Visser C, et al. Echocardiography in the diagnosis of aortic dissection. Lancet. 1989;1:457–61.
12. Cigarroa JE, Isselbacher EM, DeSantis RW, et al. Diagnostic imaging in the evaluation of suspected aortic dissection. N Engl J Med. 1993;328:35–43.
13. Morgan JM, Oldershaw PJ, Gray HH. Use of computed tomographic scanning and aortography in the diagnosis of acute aortic dissection of the thoracic aorta. Br Heart J. 1990;64:261–5.
14. Nienaber CA, Kodolitch Y, Nichplas V, et al. The diagnosis of thoracic dissection by non-invasive imaging procedures. N Engl J Med. 1993;328:1–9.
15. Panting JR, Norell MS, Baker C, Nicholson AA. Feasibility, accuracy and safety or magnetic resonance imaging in acute aortic dissection. Clin Radiol. 1995;50:455–8.
16. Simpson IA, De Belder MA, Camm JA, Pumphrey CW. Cardiovascular manifestations of Marfan syndrome: improved evaluation by transoesophageal echocardiography. Br Heart J. 1993;69:104–8.
17. Hall JR, Pyeritz RE, Dudgeon MDG, Haller A. Pneumothorax in the Marfan syndrome. Ann Thorac Surg. 1984;37:500–5.
18. Wood J, Bellamy D, Child A, Citron KM. Pulmonary disease in patients with Marfan syndrome. Thorax. 1984;39:780–4.
19. Wunsch CM, Steinmetz EF, Fisch C. Marfan syndrome and subacute bacterial endocarditis. Am J Cardiol. 1965;15:102–6.
20. Bowers D, Lim DW. Subacute bacterial endocarditis and Marfan syndrome. Can Med Assoc J. 1962;86:455–8.
21. Prevention of endocarditis. *British National Formulary*. No 28 and subsequent editions. London: Brtish Medical Association.
22. Verghese C. Anaesthesia in Marfan syndrome. Anaesthesia. 1984;39:917–22.
23. Wakita M, Ryu E, Nakayasu K, et al. Statistical analysis of Marfan syndrome. Acta Societatis Opthalmologicae Japonicae. 1989;93(6):682–90.

Infantile and Neonatal Marfan Syndrome

4

Anne H. Child

Marfan syndrome may be diagnosed clinically at any time of life, with those most severely affected attracting medical attention in infancy (the first year of life) or even at birth (neonatal Marfan syndrome). Sometimes affected infants are from affected families that are already aware that they carry the Marfan gene, but most often, infants are affected as a result of a new mutation of the fibrillin-1 gene. Early recognition of the correct diagnosis can aid medical and surgical management, and genetic counselling.

Infantile Marfan Syndrome

A review of infants diagnosed in the first 3 months of life indicates that they may be recognised by the following features in at least 2 of 3 major systems (eyes, heart, skeleton). Other systems may be involved such as the lungs [1] and the central nervous system [2, 3]. Typically, the baby will be long and thin with a long head and face (dolichocephaly), wise "old man" facial appearance with large deep-set eyes, large corneas and dislocated lenses, large soft ears, high arched palate, small chin, loose joints, arachnodactyly (long spidery fingers), contractures of fingers and large joints, flat feet and anterior chest deformity. Additional features may include blue "whites" of the eye, down-slanting eyes (antimongoloid slant), retinal detachment, low-set ears, partial cleft palate, dislocated hip, inguinal hernia, overlapping toes, in turned or out turned feet, poor muscle tone (floppiness) and very thin muscles [4].

During the first 3 months of life, heart murmurs are heard in 45 % of affected infants, and echocardiography reveals abnormalities in 70 % of infants, including mitral valve prolapse, aortic or mitral regurgitation and aortic root dilatation.

A.H. Child, MD, FRCP
Cardiovascular and Cell Sciences Research Institute, St George's, University of London, London, UK
e-mail: achild@sgul.ac.uk

© Springer-Verlag London 2016

A.H. Child (ed.), *Diagnosis and Management of Marfan Syndrome*,
DOI 10.1007/978-1-4471-5442-6_4

Structural defects of the aortic valve and atrial and ventricular septa should be ruled out. Cardiac function ranges from normal to poor, with a tendency to worsen. Each infant is unique and must be monitored closely (at least every 3 months) during the first year so that medical or surgical treatment for dilating aortic roots, leaking mitral or tricuspid valve, or poor ventricular function may be offered at the earliest moment [5]. Atenolol (1 mg per kg) is indicated for children with aortic dilatation two standard deviations greater than the mean full body surface area. Repair or replacement of a leaking valve, with antibiotic treatment to prevent infective endocarditis may be indicated. Infants with severe heart disease understandably have a significant mortality risk of approximately 15 % in the first year of life [4]. Familial cases have a better long term outlook, generally following the family pattern of involvement.

Overlapping Conditions

Homocystinuria and Beals syndrome (congenital contractural arachnodactyly) should be ruled out. Beals syndrome infants have mutations in the gene for fibrillin-2. These infants have no major eye problems, tend to have crumpled ears and more severe scoliosis. Heart involvement tends to be less, with non-progressive dilation of the aortic root, but occasional structural cardiac defects [6].

To date, intelligence does not seem to be affected in infantile Marfan syndrome or Beals syndrome, whereas mental retardation can occur in untreated homocystinuria.

Neonatal Marfan Syndrome

Neonatal Marfan syndrome represents the most severe end of the clinical spectrum of Marfan syndrome [7]. The cardiovascular features are severe with early dilatation of the aortic root, pronounced atrial ventricular valve dysfunction and congestive heart failure [8–10]. Death usually occurs in the first years of life, most often within the first 12 months, but careful timely medical and surgical management can prolong lifespan. This condition is characterised by several features rare in classical Marfan syndrome such as crumpled ears, contractures, loose skin and prominent forehead. To date, the majority of reported cases of neonatal Marfan syndrome have been sporadic [11], with mutations occurring in a relatively short region of the gene between exons 24–32, usually in calcium binding EGF-like sequences, a region critical for microfibril assembly [12]. Electron microscopy of the fibrillin strands for neonatal Marfan syndrome patients reveals that the patients seem to make "beads only" – the beads are not strung together in the usual necklace-like pattern, and so do not contribute to the elastic strength of tissues. This helps to explain why these babies are so severely affected in every system.

Progeroid facial features and lipodystrophy are associated with mutations at the 3′ end of the fibrillin-1 gene [13, 14].

Diagram of FBN1 gene indicating region where neonatal Marfan syndrome mutations are usually found (exons 24-32)

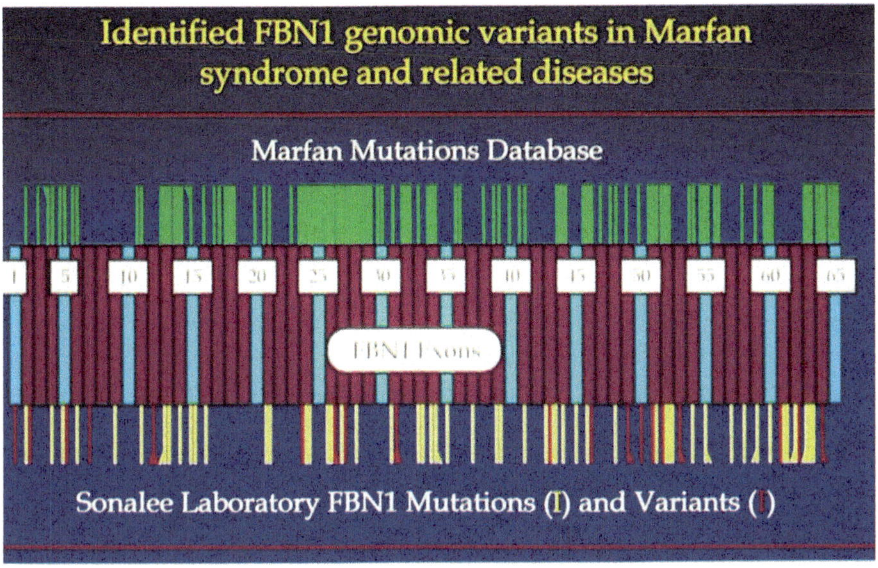

Counselling

If the neonate or infant has a new mutation in the FBN1 gene, parents need to know that this could happen to any couple (population incidence is 1 in 3300 [15]) and is not the result of anything they did, or did not do, before or during the pregnancy. Each individual has approximately 20,000 genes, and carries on average three significant mutations, but usually these mutations are not in important genes, and so do not cause disease. A child with Marfan syndrome has a change in an important gene and therefore does not make fibrillin-1 which therefore cannot participate in strengthening the connective tissue, including the aortic wall.

No couple has as yet been reported to have two affected children when both parents are normal [16]. The risk of having a further child with Marfan syndrome is virtually the same as for any other couple (1 in 3300) – a negligible risk.

To reassure anxious parents in a further pregnancy, foetal normality could be confirmed by amniocentesis or chorionic villus biopsy, or mutation analysis of cord blood at the time of birth. Foetal echocardiography at 20 weeks of pregnancy together with limb length measurements should be offered and the new baby examined carefully at birth including echocardiography and ophthalmology.

Unaffected children of the couple do not bear a risk of passing on the condition. Therapy for severely affected children is available. Medical and surgical treatment can help to prevent progression of the disease, but cannot reverse the organ involvement already present at birth.

Parents should remember that their affected infant is their baby first, and has Marfan syndrome as a secondary feature. Physical development will be delayed somewhat, but mental and physical stimulation should be provided to match the child's ability. Quiet pursuits, physiotherapy exercises, and play in a small supervised nursery school are recommended. Grandparents and other family members can help by spending time with the child, and this would be greatly appreciated by the parents, for whom caring for the child will be a demanding task. The infant should participate in family outings and holidays, which may have to be somewhat restricted. Short air flights are possible, but parents should check with the physician responsible for overseeing their child's care before travelling abroad. If the child has respiratory distress on the ground, oxygen should be available during the flight. If a chest x-ray has revealed emphysema or bullae in the lung, then sudden changes of air pressure, for example during mountain climbing, are not recommended as pneumothorax may result. Antibiotics should be packed for travel in case of lung or ear infection, and a doctor's letter summarising care for the infant should accompany the family in case of illness while abroad, necessitating hospitalisation.

References

1. Domingues R, Weisgaru RA, Santamaria M. Pulmonary hyperinflation and emphysema in infants with Marfan syndrome. Pediatr Radiol. 1987;17:365–9.
2. Vasu V, Child AH, Modi N, Rutherford M, Cowan F. Neonatal Marfan. BMJ Case Rep. 2011. pii:bcr0620114328. doi: 10.1136/bcr.06.2011.4328.
3. Barnett CP, Wilson GJ, Chiasson DA, Gross GJ, Hinek A, Hawkins C, Chitayat D. Central nervous system abnormalities in two cases with neonatal Marfan syndrome with novel mutations in the fibrillin-1 gene. Am J Med Genet A. 2010;152A(9):2409–12. doi:10.1002/ajmg.a.33406. No Abstract available.
4. Morse RP, Rockenmacher S, Pyeritz R, et al. Diagnosis and management of infantile Marfan syndrome. Paediatrics. 1990;86(6):888–95.
5. Amado M, Colado MA, Ferreira R, Lourenço T. Neonatal Marfan syndrome: a successful early multidisciplinary approach. BMJ Case Rep. 2014. Pii: bcr2013202438. doi:10.1136/bcr-2013-202438.
6. Meena JP, Gupta A, Mishra D, Juneja M. Beals-Hecht syndrome (congenital contractural arachnodactyly) with additional craniospinal abnormality: a case report. J Pediatr Orthop B. 2014;24(3):226–9.
7. Booms P, Cisler J, Mathews KR, Godfrey M, Tiecke F, Kaufmann UC, Vetter U, Hage-Meier F, Robinson PN. Novel exon skipping mutation in the fibrillin-1 gene: two 'hot spots' for the neonatal Marfan syndrome. Clin Genet. 1999;55:110–7.
8. Geva T, Sander SP, Diogenes MS, et al. Two-dimensional and Doppler echocardiographic and pathologic characteristics of the infantile Marfan syndrome. Am J Cardiol. 1990;65(18):1230–7.
9. Buntix IM, Willems PJ, Spitaels SE, et al. Neonatal Marfan syndrome with congenital arachnodactyly, flexion contractures, and severe cardiac valve insufficiency. J Med Genet. 1991;28(4):267–73.
10. Bresters D, Nikkels PG, Meijboom EJ, et al. Clinical, pathological and molecular genetic findings in a case of neonatal Marfan syndrome. Acta Paediatr. 1999;88(1):98–101.

11. Pees C, Michel-Behnke I, Hagl M, Laccone F. Detection of 15 novel mutations in 52 children from 40 families with the Marfan or Loeys-Dietz syndrome and phenotype-genotype correlations. Clin Genet. 2014;86(6):552–7. doi:10.1111/cge12314. Epub 2013 Dec 4.
12. Kielty CM, Phillips J, Child AH, et al. Fibrillin secretion and microfibril assembly by Marfan dermal fibroblasts. Matrix Biol. 1994;14:141–99.
13. Horn D, Robinson PN. Progeroid facial features and lipodystrophy associated with a novel splice site mutation in the final intron of the FBN1 gene. Am J Med Genet A. 2011;155A(4):721–4. doi:10.1002/ajmg.a.33905. Epub 2011 Mar 15.
14. Jaoquinet A, Verloes A, Callewaert B, Coremans C, Coucke P, de Paepe A, Kornak U, Lebrun F, Lombet J, Piérard GE, Robinson PN, Symoens S, Van Maldergem L, Debray FG. Neonatal progeroid variant of Marfan syndrome with congenital lipodystrophy results from mutations at the 3' end of FBN1 gene. Eur J Med Genet. 2014;57(5):230–4. doi:10.1016/j.ejmg.2014.02.012. Epub 2014 Mar 6.
15. Arslan-Kirchner M, Arbustini E, Boileau C, Child A, Collod-Beroud G, De Paepe A, Epplen J, Jondeau G, Loeys B, Faivre L. Clinical utility gene card for: Marfan syndrome type 1 and related phenotypes [FBN1]. Eur J Hum Genet. 2010; doi:10.1038/ejhg.2010.42.18(9)
16. Sípek Jr A, Grodecká L, Baxová A, Cibulková P, Dvořáková M, Mazurová S, Magner M, Zeman J, Honzík T, Freiberger T. Novel FBN1 gene mutation and maternal germinal mosaicism as the cause of neonatal form of Marfan syndrome. Am J Med Genet. 2014;164A(6):1559–64. doi:10.1002/ajmg.a.36480. Epub 2014 Mar 25.

The Child with Marfan Syndrome: A Paediatric Cardiology Approach

5

Graham Stuart

Introduction

In 1886 the French paediatrician, Professor Antoine Marfan, published the description of a 5 year old girl with an unusual combination of musculoskeletal abnormalities which subsequently became known as Marfan syndrome [1]. In recent years exciting advances in our understanding of the pathogenesis of Marfan syndrome have led to a rational approach to diagnosis and management in the child. The purpose of this chapter is to discuss the role of the paediatric cardiologist in the management of the child and adolescent with Marfan syndrome with particular emphasis on pitfalls in diagnosis and areas of controversy in management. A pragmatic approach to treatment in the child with Marfan syndrome will also be given in light of new developments in drug therapy and, in particular, developments in modulation of the TGF-beta pathway.

Diagnosis of Marfan Syndrome

Frequently, Marfan syndrome is not diagnosed until adolescence or adulthood. However, with improved understanding of the value of early diagnosis, it is becoming increasingly common for children to be referred for assessment. Assessment of the child suspected of Marfan syndrome requires a team approach and ideally this should be in a specialist, multidisciplinary clinic (Table 5.1). This has the benefit of concentrating medical expertise, facilitating research and reducing the number of clinics the family have to attend. An interested paediatric cardiologist is an essential member of the multidisciplinary team. Internationally-accepted diagnostic criteria

G. Stuart, MBChB, MSc, FRCP FRCPCH
Congenital Heart Disease Centre, Bristol Royal Hospital for Children,
Upper Maudlin Street, Bristol BS2 8BJ, UK
e-mail: graham.stuart@nhs.net

© Springer-Verlag London 2016

A.H. Child (ed.), *Diagnosis and Management of Marfan Syndrome*,
DOI 10.1007/978-1-4471-5442-6_5

Table 5.1 'Ideal' multidisciplinary clinic for children with Marfan syndrome

Specialist	Role
Clinical geneticist/genetics counsellor	Co-ordinator of clinic with responsibility for genetic counselling, coordination of molecular genetic studies. Family studies. Exclusion of similar/overlapping syndromes. Should be assisted by genetics nurse/counsellor
General paediatrician	Assessment of growth velocity, joint symptoms, pulmonary pathology. Assessment of scoliosis. Liaison with school medical service. Advice about sports, exercise, career options. Lifestyle advice. Referral to orthopaedic surgeon and paediatric endocrinologist if appropriate
Orthopaedic surgeon	Assessment of spinal curvature, foot deformities, joint dislocation
Ophthalmologist	Regular slit lamp assessment. Management of lens dislocation, myopia, retinal problems
Paediatric cardiology clinical nurse specialist	Liaison with school medical service and teachers, advice on lifestyle. Initiation of transition process from paediatric to adult cardiology services
Paediatric cardiologist	Monitoring of aortic root dilatation. Assessment of mitral and pulmonary valve dysfunction and arrhythmias. Liaison with adult cardiologist/adult congenital heart disease specialist during adolescence

for Marfan syndrome have been published (the "revised Ghent nosology") and are summarised elsewhere [2]. The definitive diagnosis of Marfan syndrome requires a combination of aortic root dilation with ectopia lentis or a known pathogenic Fibrillin 1 (FBN1) mutation or an indicative score created from systemic features such as pectus carinatum, dural ectasia or a positive wrist and thumb sign. Cardiovascular abnormalities are often asymptomatic and careful assessment of the cardiovascular system is essential for both diagnosis and follow-up. The paediatric cardiologist may be involved in diagnosis and management at any stage from fetal life to adolescence (Table 5.2).

Prenatal Diagnosis

Two approaches to prenatal diagnosis are possible. Standard ultrasonic measurements of skeletal length have been used but are insensitive and non-specific. Genetic familial mutation detection can be provided through chorionic villus biopsy at 11 weeks gestation. Genetic linkage studies can be also carried out in families with more than one affected member. Fetal echocardiography can be performed from 16 to 18 weeks gestation and the aortic root compared with growth centiles in the normal fetus. There are no data on growth of the aortic root in the fetus with Marfan syndrome. Fetal echocardiographic diagnosis of Marfan syndrome has been reported but only in a severely affected fetus [4].

Table 5.2 Cardiac abnormalities in infants with Marfan syndrome

Structure	Abnormality	Frequency (%)	Comments/pathology
Mitral valve	Mitral valve prolapse	73/76 (96 %)	Mitral and tricuspid valves exhibited elongation of chordae tendinae with myxomatous thickening of valve leaflets
	Mitral regurgitation	64/76 (84 %)	
Tricuspid valve	Tricuspid valve prolapse	28/51 (55 %)	Severe heart failure was often associated with mitral/tricuspid regurgitation (7/9 patients)
	Tricuspid regurgitation	18/60 (30 %)	
Aortic valve and root	Root dilatation	71/81 (88 %)	The aortic root had a 'cloverleaf' appearance in parasternal short-axis view on echocardiography
	Aortic regurgitation	17/60 (28 %)	
Pulmonary valve/root	Pulmonary root dilatation/regurgitation	3/7 (43 %)	

Adapted from Geva et al. [3]

Diagnosis in the Infant

A rare type of severe infantile Marfan syndrome exists [3,5]. This is discussed in detail elsewhere in this textbook. Most are sporadic mutations associated with a specific fibrillin deletion (exons 24–32). Severe cardiac problems are common at birth including mitral and tricuspid regurgitation [3] (Table 5.2). Other typical features include contractures, dolichocephaly, high arched palate, micrognathia, hyperextensible joints, pes planus, chest deformity, megalocornea, dislocated lenses and characteristic facies "like an old man" [3]. Heart failure in infantile Marfan syndrome is common and cardiac surgery, in particular to the atrioventricular valves, may be necessary in early childhood. Most familial cases present at an older age, have a milder presentation and are more difficult to detect during infancy.

Diagnosis in the Child

The published diagnostic criteria have limitations in children [2]. For example, it is inappropriate to perform a CT scan to confirm dural ectasia or protrusion acetabula (systemic features) in an asymptomatic child. Moreover, the growing child with Marfan syndrome has an evolving phenotype [6]. Stheneur and colleagues reviewed this phenotypic evolution in 259 children with a FBN1 mutation who fulfilled the modified Ghent criteria [7] (Table 5.3). Ectopia lentis and aortic dilatation were the best discriminating features although height >3.3 standard deviations above the mean was also a useful guide for the non-specialist [7]. Thus, although some children with Marfan syndrome fulfill the diagnostic criteria in infancy, others may not do so until adolescence. Children with overlapping syndromes, connective tissue disorders or even constitutional tall stature may also be referred for assessment (e.g.

Table 5.3 Phenotype evolution in children with Marfan syndrome (Stheneur et al. [7])

Abnormality	Age group 0–6 years (%)	Age group 15–17 years (%)
Pectus deformity	43	62
Hypermobility	67	47
Pes planus	73	65
Ectopia lentis	66	72
Aortic root dilatation[a]	75	80

[a]This study population were all treated with betablocker therapy

Ehlers Danlos syndrome, familial annuloaortic ectasia, mitral valve prolapse syndrome). In a large multicentre study of 320 children with Marfan syndrome and related type 1 fibrillinopathies, only 56 % could be classified as having Marfan syndrome by internationally recognised clinical criteria although this increased to 85 % of child probands after molecular studies [8]. The authors concluded that the diagnostic criteria for Marfan syndrome had poor applicability in childhood. They emphasised the need for follow-up monitoring in cases where there is strong clinical suspicion of Marfan syndrome and recognised that the discovery of a FBN1 mutation can be a useful adjunct to diagnosis [8].

In our paediatric clinic four diagnostic terms are used;

- not Marfan syndrome,
- possible Marfan syndrome
- probable Marfan syndrome
- definite Marfan syndrome.

The term 'definite' Marfan syndrome is used where the modified Ghent criteria are fulfilled. 'Probable' Marfan syndrome is used where several characteristic features are present and overlapping syndromes have been excluded but the diagnostic criteria have not been fulfilled. These children are followed up as if they had Marfan syndrome. The Fibrillin-1 gene screen is strongly advised to guide management. The term 'possible' Marfan syndrome is used where children are at 50 % genetic risk and have some clinical features. They are reviewed infrequently (at 5, 10 ,13, 16 years old) until the diagnosis is confirmed or refuted. The most common features of Marfan syndrome in children are shown in Fig. 5.1.

Types of Cardiac Dysfunction in the Child

Although cardiac abnormalities are common in the child with Marfan syndrome most have no cardiovascular symptoms (Table 5.4). Chest pain is relatively common but is usually musculoskeletal. The most common abnormalities are asymptomatic mitral regurgitation, mitral valve prolapse and aortic root dilatation. Aortic root dilatation can accelerate during childhood and occasionally

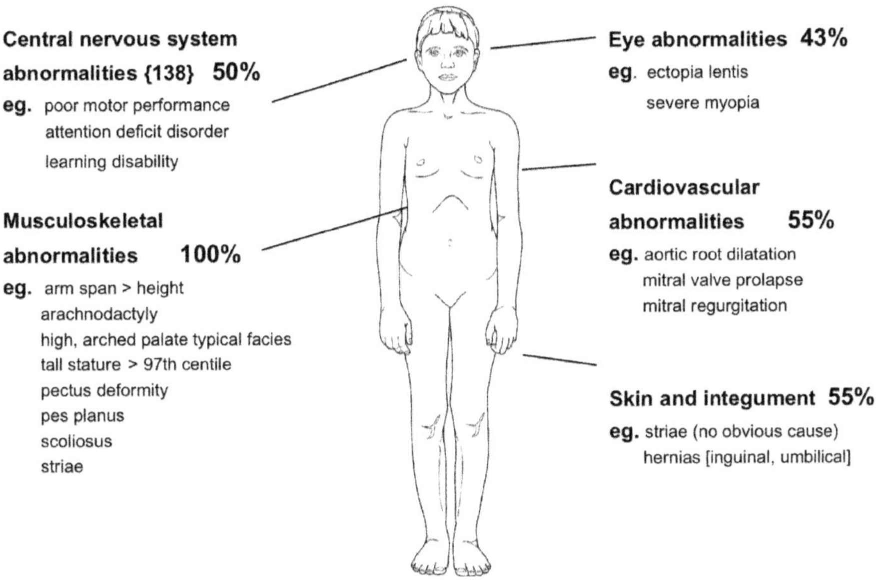

Fig. 5.1 Abnormal features in children with Marfan syndrome (Figure is adapted from Stuart [9])

prophylactic root replacement is indicated to prevent aortic dissection. Other cardiovascular abnormalities include pulmonary artery dilatation, tricuspid valve prolapse and left ventricular diastolic. The cardiac features in the child have been described in detail elsewhere [13]. Arrhythmias are an under-recognised source of symptoms and morbidity in the child with Marfan syndrome [14].

Mechanism of Cardiovascular Dysfunction

Marfan syndrome is associated with an abnormality in the structural protein fibrillin. This is discussed in detail in Chap. 22. Fibrillin-containing microfibrils are found throughout the cardiovascular system and act as a "scaffold" which orientates elastin deposition [15]. This occurs early in development implying that cardiovascular abnormalities are present at birth. The abnormal elastin deposition results in increased stiffness of blood vessels, in particular the aorta [16]. Endothelial dysfunction has also been reported which results in selective impairment of flow-mediated dilatation of the great arteries [17]. Recently, there has been considerable research linking elevation in tissue levels of the cytokine Transforming-Growth Factor beta (TGFβ) to the phenotypic changes observed in Marfan syndrome. Elevated levels of this cytokine lead to downstream changes in elastin homeostasis and microfibril function. This discovery has led to new therapeutic possibilities where the prime target is to act on the TGFβ pathway.

Table 5.4 Cardiac abnormalities in children with Marfan syndrome

Author	Sex		Number in study	Clinical features % murmurs			Echocardiographic features %			Abnormal CVS %	Comments
	Male	Female		Click	MR	AR	MVP/MR	AR	ARD		
Phornphutkul [10]	NA	NA	36	33	47	11	NA	NA	NA	61	No echocardiographic assessment available
El Habbal [11]	NA	NA	186	NA	NA	NA	25	NA	100	100	Serious CVS complications occurred in 4.3 %. All developed aortic dilatation during follow up. 14 % had additional congenital heart disease (BAV 18, TOF 2, ASD 5, WPW 1)
Geva [6]	4	21	25	84	44	20	100	28	80	100	5 (25 %) had an aortic aneurysm. 5 deaths during follow up
Stuart [12]	26	26	52	23	23	6	25	13	83	83	Figures refer to abnormal findings at referral. Study represents results of a screening project for Marfan syndrome in childhood
Stheneur [7]	205	183	389	NA	NA	NA	72.3 (51.7)	NA	80	80	ARD was defined using >2Standard deviations above norm for body surface area. MVP was higher in probands (72.3) than non-probands

Abbreviations: *BAV* bicuspid aortic valve, *TOF* Tetralogy of Fallot, *ASD* atrial septal defect, *WPW* Wolf-Parkinson-White syndrome, *MR* mitral regurgitation, *AR* aortic regurgitation, *NA* data not available

Cardiovascular Risk Stratification

Not all children with Marfan syndrome have the same risk of progressive, life threatening cardiovascular disease. Most families carry a unique mutation and individual risk estimation is necessary. Probands tend to have more severe phenotypic manifestations [7]. Other factors associated with the development of serious cardiovascular disease include family history of aortic dissection, mitral and aortic regurgitation at presentation, rapid rate of aortic root dilatation, generalised (not localised) aortic dilatation, spontaneous mutations, systemic hypertension, gross fibrillin abnormalities on biopsy, diagnosis in early childhood, infantile-type Marfan syndrome and aortic root greater than 50 mm [18]. An aortic root measurement of >50 mm in an adult is an indication for elective aortic root replacement although dissection can occur below this level, and root replacement should be considered if there are additional risk factors or a rapid rate of dilatation [18]. The indication for surgery in the growing child is discussed below. In most studies, sporadic cases and children diagnosed below 10 years old have a worse cardiovascular prognosis. To some extent this may reflect the earlier presentation of children with more severe abnormalities of fibrillin.

Management of Marfan Syndrome in the Child

Proposals for health supervision of the child with Marfan syndrome were published recently by the American Academy of Paediatrics [19]. This includes recommendations for assessment of growth, eye and lung manifestations, psychosocial issues, exercise participation and transition to adult services. Regular clinical assessment of the cardiovascular system is recommended throughout childhood.

Clinical Assessment

Most children with Marfan syndrome have no cardiovascular symptoms but palpitations and chest pain occur and may be associated with mitral valve prolapse. The cardiovascular history should include a detailed family history. In particular, a family history of cardiovascular complications should be sought as this is a risk factor for the child and may also influence the family reaction to the diagnosis of Marfan syndrome. Cardiovascular examination should include auscultation for murmurs of valve regurgitation and mid or early systolic clicks. Blood pressure should be measured. In the child and adolescent the cardiovascular examination is often normal but this does not exclude significant cardiovascular pathology.

Echocardiography

High quality echocardiography is the mainstay of cardiovascular assessment in the child with Marfan syndrome. This should include an assessment of ventricular systolic function (right and left) and the function of all four valves. Diastolic function should be assessed as it may be impaired and this can occur independent of aortic dilatation [20]. Measurement of the ascending aorta at the level of the aortic sinus and sinotubular junction should be plotted against body surface area and compared with normal centiles [19]. This is of particular importance in the growing child where a sequential comparison of aortic root growth in comparison to somatic growth is essential to establish the presence and progression of aortic dilatation. Although aortic root measurement >2 standard deviations (SD) above the norm for body surface area are often used, Stheneur proposed that measurements >3 SD are of more value in diagnosis as 16 % of non-Marfan children referred for assessment in their Marfan clinic had an aortic root >2 SD using the Roman centiles [7,21]. It is essential for an identical and reproducible technique to be used for measuring the aortic root on each occasion. Serial measurements of aortic diameter can be used to identify a low-risk subgroup who are less likely to require aortic surgery or dissect. ulmonary artery dilatation may be present and should be assessed. Transoesophageal echocardiography is useful in older children with a poor echocardiographic window but is seldom necessary in the young child. The frequency of measurement is debated but most authors recommend an annual echocardiogram in children with definite Marfan syndrome and more frequent assessment if there is significant aortic dilatation or aortic regurgitation. Although aortic dilatation is present in the majority of children with Marfan syndrome, the presence of normal aortic dimensions in childhood does not preclude progressive aortic dilatation in adult life and regular echocardiographic assessment should continue after transfer to the adult cardiologist.

Electrocardiography (ECG)

Electrocardiographic abnormalities are common in children with Marfan syndrome. Partial right bundle branch block is common but other abnormalities occur including supraventricular and ventricular premature beats and arrhythmias [22]. In one study 33 % of children were found to have ventricular arrhythmias on extended monitoring and this was not always associated with valve dysfunction [14]. An ambulatory ECG should be recorded in children with palpitations or chest pain which does not have an obvious musculoskeletal origin.

Other Investigations

Most children with Marfan syndrome do not require additional cardiovascular investigations. Occasionally an electrophysiology study is helpful in children with palpitations and episodes of collapse. Lung function assessment may also be indicated if there is a marked sternal anomaly as this can compromise cardiac function and may be complicated by bronchial hyperreactivity. Magnetic resonance imaging is a useful alternative to transoesophageal echocardiography and allows the assessment of aortic stiffness. This can be of particular value if there is a severe sternal abnormality which makes reproducible measurement of the ascending aorta difficult or if there is difficulty visualizing the descending aorta.

Medical Therapy

Beta blockers have been used for many years in Marfan syndrome to try to prevent aortic dissection. In theory, a reduction in the force of left ventricular ejection (dP/dT) should reduce the risk of dissection and this has been shown in non-Marfan dissection and animal models. In 1994 Shores published a randomised study of the effect of β-blockade in adolescents and young adults with Marfan syndrome [23]. Seventy patients were followed up for approximately 10 years and were randomised to β-blockers (propranolol) or control. The treated group had a slower rate of aortic dilatation and a reduced rate of complications including aortic regurgitation, cardiac surgery, aortic dissection and death. Moreover, the 2 deaths in the control group were probably due to an arrhythmia and not dissection, suggesting propranolol might have a protective antiarrhythmic function. Propranolol was not effective in every patient, however, and the high dose (mean 212 mg/day) caused significant side-effects in 30 %.

The routine use of betablockers in Marfan syndrome has been questioned in recent years with contradictory evidence of efficacy in different patient subgroups [24]. Thus, atenolol does not improve aortic distensibility and stiffness in all children and, in some adults, aortic stiffness actually increases after β-blockade. Alternative drugs including ace-inhibitors and calcium antagonists have been tried but their long-term efficacy is unproven [24]. Recently, there has been considerable interest in the use of angiotensin-receptor blockade in the prevention of aortic complications in Marfan syndrome. This is discussed in detail by Loeys [25]. Angiotensin receptor blockade is thought to act via modulation of expression of the cytokine transforming-growth factor Beta (TGFβ). In a small retrospective study of young children with aortopathy who had not responded to standard therapy, angiotensin-receptor blockade was found to slow the progression of aortic root dilatation [26]. Similarly, Pees demonstrated that monotherapy with losartan reduced aortic dilatation in a small, unselected group of children and adolescents with Marfan syndrome with the suggestion that efficacy was improved when therapy was started at a younger age and patients were treated for longer periods [27]. However, in a much larger cohort of 608 children and young adults (6 months to 25 years of age; mean 11.5 years) randomised to atenolol or losartan, there was no difference in reduction of aortic root Z scores, aortic dissection rates, or the need for aortic root surgery over a 3 year period [28]. Thus, at present, the evidence suggests that children with Marfan syndrome may develop less aortic dilatation when treated with an angiotensin receptor blocker but the relative merits of betablockade and angiotensin converting enzyme blockade remain unclear. On the basis of current evidence, it would seem prudent to treat children with beta-blockers if they have definite Marfan syndrome and known risk factors for dissection and to have a low threshold for adding an angiotensin-receptor blocker if the betablocker is not tolerated, if there is progressive aortic root dilatation despite beta-blockade or if the child is perceived to have a high risk of dissection on the basis of phenotype, genotype or family history. However, the optimum dose and preparation of both drugs are unknown. Furthermore, where there is a contraindication to betablockers (for example, asthma) or where betablockers are not tolerated due to side-effects, angiotensin-receptor blockers should be used. Further research may inform this exciting area of medical therapy.

Cardiothoracic Surgery

In older children with severe pectus excavatum cardiopulmonary performance can improve after sternal repair. The usual indication for cardiac surgery, however, is rapid aortic dilatation or dissection. Occasionally mitral or aortic valve repair or replacement is also necessary but this is seldom required in childhood except in the most severe phenotypes. Surgical morbidity and mortality have steadily improved in recent years largely due to elective surgery (composite graft with coronary reimplantation) being carried out prior to dissection. Root replacement with preservation of the aortic leaflets has also been described thus avoiding the need for lifelong anticoagulation. The long-term results of valve sparing root replacement in children with Marfan syndrome are unknown but it has been suggested that the aortic remodelling technique (Yacoub) should be avoided due to the high rate of reoperation [29].

The precise timing of aortic root surgery in the child is unclear but in our unit we consider aortic root size >45–50 mm or rapid acceleration of root growth (>97th centile for body surface area) despite medical therapy indications for surgery. If there is a family history of dissection and the aortic valve is competent, valve-sparing surgery may be considered at a lower level (40–45 mm at sinus of Valsalva).

Risk Modification and Lifestyle

It is essential to balance the normal needs of the growing child with the benefit of early diagnosis and treatment of Marfan syndrome. Many children will have witnessed the death of a relative with Marfan syndrome and this, together with an embarrassment about body image, may cause considerable distress and resentment. In many families, the reassurance of a clear diagnosis with regular monitoring is itself of considerable value. Advice on exercise and school activities should be given. Children with significant aortic root dilatation should avoid contact sports but it is important to maintain reasonable fitness. Ideally, children with Marfan syndrome should be given a formal exercise prescription to include at least 60 minutes of total aerobic activity per day. This does not need to be intense exercise and can be the equivalent of brisk walking. From an early age parents should be advised to guide their children towards leisure activities which can be continued even if cardiac complications develop. Advice on avoidance of cigarette smoking, good dental hygiene and antibiotic prophylaxis against endocarditis should be given. Dietary advice to encourage a Mediterranean-type diet (high in fruit, fibre and vegetables) should be given due to the long-term benefits this can have on endothelial function. The process of transition and patient (as opposed to parent) education should start in the early teenage years. The natural rebellion of the teenage years can be particularly difficult and it is important teenagers are given the opportunity to discuss their worries when not accompanied by their parents. Contraception and the risks of pregnancy should be discussed and a clear referral pattern developed which allows transfer to the adult cardiologist when the teenager feels ready.

Conclusion

An interested and dedicated paediatric cardiologist is essential for the management of the child with Marfan syndrome. It is important to try to minimise cardiovascular risk factors and in particular to monitor the development of aortic root dilatation. At the same time it is essential to be sensitive to the emotional needs of the growing child and adolescent. Regular, systematic assessment balanced with encouragement and reassurance are the cornerstones of management.

References

1. Marfan AB. Un cas de deformation congenitale des quatre membres, plus prononce aux extremetes, characterise par l'allongement des os avec un certain degre d'amincissement. Bull Mem Soc Hop (Paris). 1896;13:220–6.
2. Loeys BL, et al. The revised Ghent nosology for the Marfan syndrome. J Med Genet. 2010;47(7):476–85.
3. Geva T, et al. Two-dimensional and Doppler echocardiographic and pathologic characteristics of the infantile Marfan syndrome. Am J Cardiol. 1990;65(18):1230–7.
4. Lopes LM, et al. Echocardiographic diagnosis of fetal Marfan syndrome at 34 weeks' gestation. Prenat Diagn. 1995;15(2):183–5.
5. Morse RP, et al. Diagnosis and management of infantile Marfan syndrome. Pediatrics. 1990;86(6):888–95.
6. Geva T, Hegesh J, Frand M. The clinical course and echocardiographic features of Marfan's syndrome in childhood. Am J Dis Child. 1987;141(11):1179–82.
7. Stheneur C, et al. Study of phenotype evolution during childhood in Marfan syndrome to improve clinical recognition. Genet Med. 2014;16(3):246–50.
8. Faivre L, et al. Clinical and molecular study of 320 children with Marfan syndrome and related type I fibrillinopathies in a series of 1009 probands with pathogenic FBN1 mutations. Pediatrics. 2009;123(1):391–8.
9. Stuart AG. The paediatric cardiologist and Marfan syndrome. In: Child AH, Briggs MJ, editors. The Marfan syndrome. A clinical guide. London: British Heart Foundation; 2002. p. 16–23.
10. Phornphutkul C, Rosenthal A, Nadas AS. Cardiac manifestations of Marfan syndrome in infancy and childhood. Circulation. 1973;47(3):587–96.
11. el Habbal MH. Cardiovascular manifestations of Marfan's syndrome in the young. Am Heart J. 1992;123(3):752–7.
12. Stuart AG, Davies S. Welsh paediatric surveillance system report: Marfan syndrome. Cardiff: Welsh Office; 1997.

13. Stuart AG, Williams A. Marfan's syndrome and the heart. Arch Dis Child. 2007;92(4):351–6.
14. Chen S, et al. Ventricular dysrhythmias in children with Marfan's syndrome. Am J Dis Child. 1985;139(3):273–6.
15. Adams JN, et al. Aortic distensibility and stiffness index measured by magnetic resonance imaging in patients with Marfan's syndrome. Br Heart J. 1995;73(3):265–9.
16. Hirata K, et al. The Marfan syndrome: abnormal aortic elastic properties. J Am Coll Cardiol. 1991;18(1):57–63.
17. Wilson DG, et al. Endothelial function in Marfan syndrome: selective impairment of flow-mediated vasodilation. Circulation. 1999;99(7):909–15.
18. Keane MG, Pyeritz RE. Medical management of Marfan syndrome. Circulation. 2008;117(21):2802–13.
19. Tinkle BT, Saal HM, Committee on Genetics. Health supervision for children with Marfan syndrome. Pediatrics. 2013;132(4):e1059–72.
20. Das BB, Taylor AL, Yetman AT. Left ventricular diastolic dysfunction in children and young adults with Marfan syndrome. Pediatr Cardiol. 2006;27(2):256–8.
21. Roman MJ, et al. Two-dimensional echocardiographic aortic root dimensions in normal children and adults. Am J Cardiol. 1989;64(8):507–12.
22. Wilson DG, et al. Electrocardiographic abnormalities in the child with Marfan syndrome. Eur J Paediatr. 1996;155:730.
23. Shores J, et al. Progression of aortic dilatation and the benefit of long-term beta-adrenergic blockade in Marfan's syndrome. N Engl J Med. 1994;330(19):1335–41.
24. Williams A, et al. Medical treatment of Marfan syndrome: a time for change. Heart. 2008;94(4):414–21.
25. Loeys BL. Angiotensin receptor blockers: a panacea for Marfan syndrome and related disorders? Drug Discov Today. 2015;20(2):262–6.
26. Brooke BS, et al. Angiotensin II blockade and aortic-root dilation in Marfan's syndrome. N Engl J Med. 2008;358(26):2787–95.
27. Pees C, et al. Usefulness of losartan on the size of the ascending aorta in an unselected cohort of children, adolescents, and young adults with Marfan syndrome. Am J Cardiol. 2013;112(9):1477–83.
28. Lacro RV, Dietz HC, Mahony L. Atenolol versus Losartan in Marfan's syndrome. N Engl J Med. 2015;372(10):980–1.
29. Patel ND, et al. Valve-sparing aortic root replacement in children: intermediate-term results. Interact Cardiovasc Thorac Surg. 2011;12(3):415–9; discussion 419.

6 Cardiac Management

Yukiko Isekame and Sabiha Gati

Marfan syndrome (MFS) is a disease in which connective tissue becomes weak because of genetic mutation, resulting in aortic dilatation, aneurysm, dissection, aortic regurgitation and mitral valve prolapse.

Epidemiology

MFS is inherited in an autosomal dominant mode, caused by mutations in the FBN1 gene which encodes fibrillin-1. Seventy-five percent of all patients inherit the condition from one affected parent; 25 % are affected as the result of a new mutation. The population incidence is 2–3 per 10,000 [1].

Marfan syndrome autosomal dominant inheritance was described in 1931, due to abnormal fibrillin-1 protein found in 1990, encoded by FBN1 gene as reported in 1991 [2].

In Marfan syndrome patients, most of the primary causes of death are due to cardiovascular manifestations, especially aortic dissection and rupture. According to Taiwanese research, aortic dissection is the most deadly complication. This occurs in 9.7 %, and 61 % of patients who dissect are male. The average mortality after dissection is 10.6 % [3].

Y. Isekame, MB (✉) • S. Gati, MBBS, MRCP
Cardiovascular and Cell Sciences Research Institute,
St George's, University of London, London, UK
e-mail: yukiko.isekame@gmail.com; sabihagati@yahoo.co.uk

© Springer-Verlag London 2016

A.H. Child (ed.), *Diagnosis and Management of Marfan Syndrome*,
DOI 10.1007/978-1-4471-5442-6_6

Cardiovascular Manifestations

The main cardiovascular manifestations are aortic dilatation and mitral valve prolapse. Tricuspid regurgitation (TR), pulmonary artery dilatation, ventricular arrhythmia, and cardiomyopathy which causes ventricular dilatation also occur. FBN1 is a matrix glycoprotein and the major constituent of extracellular matrix (ECM) microfibrils composing elastic fibre. Abnormal microfibrils are made, and the resultant fibroelastic fibres are weak. Abnormal fibrillin cannot inhibit TGFβ activation and signaling. This causes excessive TGF-β signaling and thereby ECM degradation, apoptosis and inflammation are activated. This causes aneurysm or dissection [4] (Fig. 6.1).

Aorta and Aortic Valve

Aortic dilatation or aneurysms are caused by cystic medial necrosis, in which the medial layer of the aorta demonstrates few cells and lacunar appearance. Most aortic dilatation in patients with MFS starts from sinus of Valsalva, and this occurs in 60–80 % adult MFS. There are some reasons why dilatation starts from aortic root; the first reason is that higher elastic fibre including fibrillin is thought to be contained there, the second reason is continual force from left ventricular cyclic torsion applied to wall of aortic root [5].

If the dilatation tears, aortic dissection occurs, and if dissection involves coronary artery, myocardial infarction may also occur. Aortic root dilatation causes aortic regurgitation with central jet because of annulus dilatation. Syndromic thoracic aortic aneurysm (TAA) growth rate is variable. Average speed of TAA growth in patients with MFS is 0.5–1.0 mm per year. In comparison, average speed of TAA growth in patients with Loeys-Dietz syndrome which is also one of the connective tissue disorders is more than 10 mm per year [6]. Aortic dilatation/dissection are major criteria in revised Ghent criteria [7].

Figure 6.2 is about ascending/descending aorta and normal size in healthy people. Aortic size is strongly affected by body surface area, weight, age, and sex. For estimation of aorta, we use Z score taking into account these factors [8, 9]. When the aorta dilates, risk for aortic dissection/rupture becomes higher. Aortic diameter is used for monitoring, but it is influenced by body surface area (BSA), so Z score which is adjusted to BSA and age is used [7].

According to ESC guidelines, the growth speed of aneurysm occurring in ascending aorta is 1 mm per year. On the other hand, the growth speed of aneurysm occurring in thoracic descending aorta is 3 mm per year in general population. In case of patients with Marfan syndrome, the growth speed of distal descending aorta is 0.58 ± 0.5 mm per year after undertaking aortic dissection surgery [6].

Distal Aorta

Although sudden death from aortic dissection is decreasing due to improved aortic monitoring and elective aortic root surgery, some patients need to undertake surgery

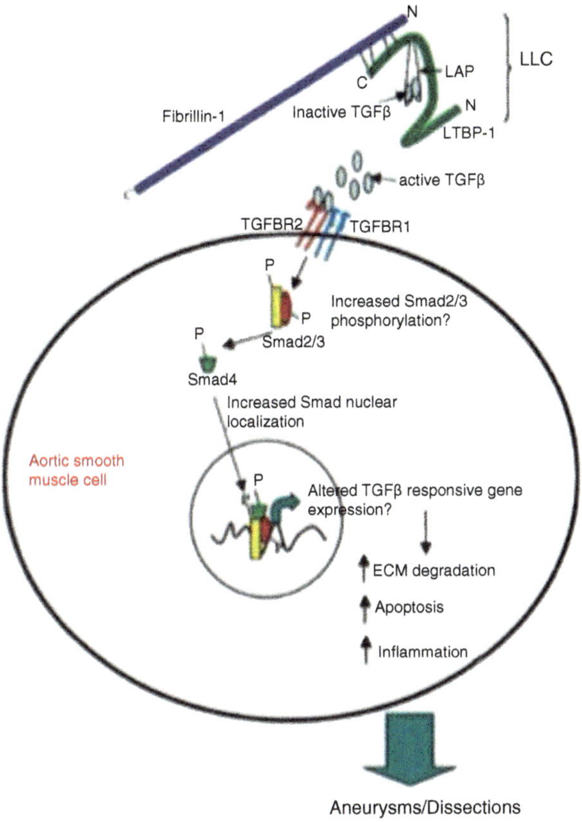

Fig. 6.1 A potential molecular pathway of dysregulation of TGFβ leading to aneurysms and dissections. Transforming growth factor β (TGFβ) is secreted in a biologically inactive form and stored in the extracellular matrix in a complex termed the large latent TGFβ complex (LLD), consisting of a TGFβ homodimer associated with the latency-associated peptide (LAP), and the latent TGFβ binding protein-1 (LTBP-1). Dysregulated TGFβ signaling results from mutations in fibrillin-1, TGFBR1, or TGFBR1, leading to altered transcription of TGFβ-responsive genes, and ultimately resulting in degenerative changes in the vessel wall leading to aneurysms and dissections [4]

for distal aorta after aortic root surgery [10]. After elective aortic root surgery, dilatation of the distal aorta is more common than before [11].

Careful monitoring of the entire aorta is important even though the aortic root is repaired. Ischemia of mesenteric and femoral artery have been seen with abdominal dissection [12].

Aortic dissection is defined as disruption of the medial aortic layer provoked by intramural bleeding, resulting in separation of the aortic wall layers and subsequent formation of a true lumen and a false lumen with or without communication [8].

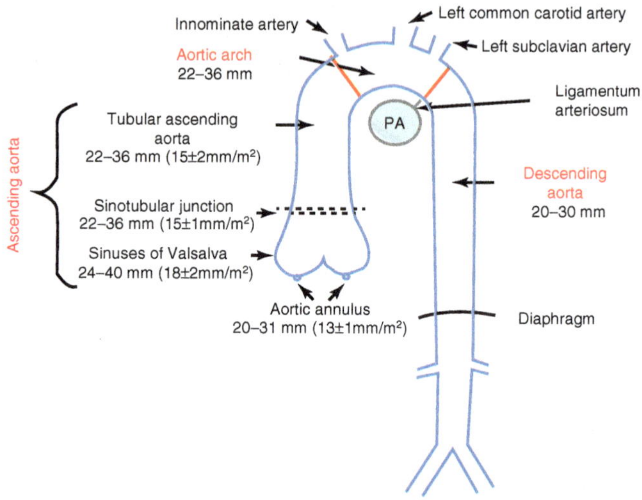

Fig. 6.2 Diagram of ascending and descending aorta with expected diameters in healthy adults [8]. Shows normal range of diameter of each section of aorta. The aorta is divided into thoracic aorta and abdominal aorta. Thoracic aorta is ascending aorta, aortic arch and thoracic descending aorta. Ascending aorta includes aortic annulus, sinuses of Valsalva, sinotubular junction, and proximal ascending aorta. Aortic arch is from brachiocephalic (innominate) artery to arterial ligament. Descending aorta is from arterial ligament to the level of diaphragm. Abdominal aorta is below the level of diaphragm

The location of pain is due to location of dissection; ascending aorta causes anterior chest pain, descending aorta causes back pain, and abdominal aorta causes abdominal pain.

In MFS patients, dissection of most patients is Stanford type A.

From the end of growth phase to 40 years, up to 50 % of undiagnosed or untreated patients die from aortic dissection or rupture, whereas aortic dissection or rupture rarely occur in children or adolescent patients with MFS [12]. Aortic root dilatation is the most common manifestation, and aortic sinus enlargement which causes aortic aneurysm occurs in 50–60 % of adult patients and 50 % of paediatric patients [12].

Januzzi J. et al. [13] have reported about patients with aortic dissection. Five percent of patients developing aortic dissection were patients with MFS. Comparing those with MFS and without MFS, type A was 76 % vs 62 % ($p=0.04$), intramural hematoma was 2 % vs 11 % ($p=0.03$), age was 35 ± 12 vs 64 ± 13 ($p<0.001$), with a history of hypertension was 27 % vs 74 % ($p<0.001$), and with a history of atherosclerosis was 0 % vs 32 % ($p<0.001$) [13].

From another of his reports, 7 % of patients with dissections were under 40 years old. Fifty percent of patients under age 40 years with aortic dissection have MFS, and only 2 % of older (40 and older) patients with aortic dissection have MFS [14].

Risk factors for aortic dissection in Marfan syndrome are as follows: aortic diameter more than 5 cm, progressive aortic dilatation extending beyond sinus of

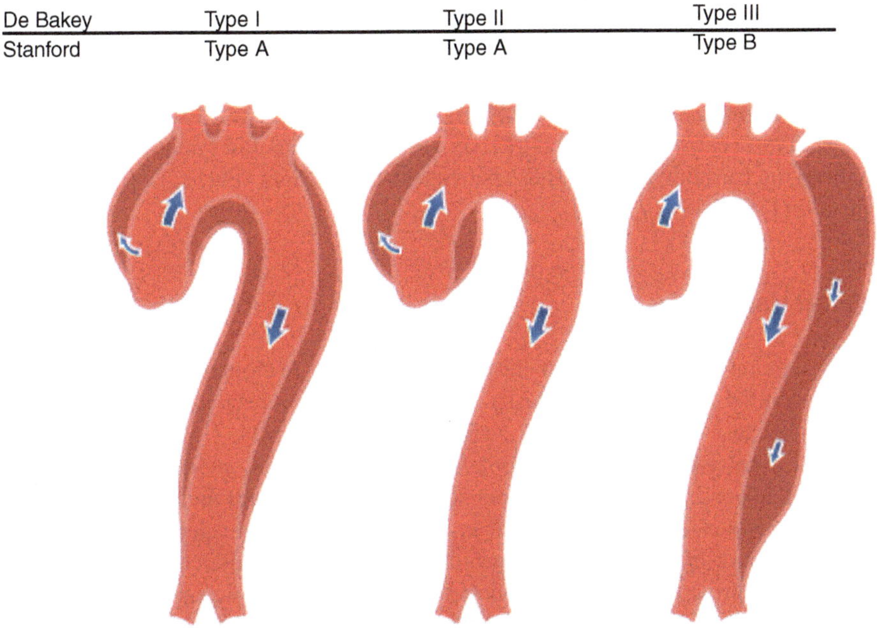

Fig. 6.3 Shows the classification of aortic dissection. De Bakey classification is according to entry level and dissection. De Bakey 1 involves entry in ascending aorta and dissection extends to abdominal aorta. De Bakey 2 involves dissection only of ascending aorta. De Bakey 3 involves entry in descending aorta. De Bakey 3 has subtypes 3A and 3B. Type 3A dissection does not extend to abdominal aorta and 3B extends to abdominal aorta. Stanford classification is according to level of dissection. Stanford type A dissection exists in ascending aorta. Stanford type B dissection does not exist in ascending aorta [5, 6]

Valsalva, rapid aortic growth rate (more than 5 % per year or more than 2 mm per year in adults), and family history of aortic dissection [12] (Fig. 6.3).

Aortic Regurgitation (AR)

Aortic valve regurgitation is caused by aortic annular dilatation or myxomatous degeneration. The associated murmur is heard as high pitched at left sternal border intercostal spaces 3–4 in diastolic phase. Patients have no symptoms during early stage. To evaluate aortic regurgitation severity, colour flow Doppler is essential.

AR severity is evaluated by morphological feature, Doppler index, and quantitative assessment. Ejection volume in each left ventricular contraction increases since the regurgitant volume increases. Thus left ventricular volume in the end-diastolic period becomes larger to maintain cardiac output, and the left atrium enlarges, reflecting the increase of end-diastolic left ventricular pressure and left atrial pressure. The left ventricular ejection fraction is not decreased due to normal or hyperkinetic wall motion in compensation phase. If myocardial damage occurs due to chronic overload, the compensation mechanism collapses and cardiac output cannot be maintained. Myocardial damage spreads to the whole left ventricle and it is important to differentiate this diagnosis from other diseases causing diffuse hypokinesis. Aortic regurgitation is not seen in normal subjects under 40. If mechanical valve lesion or aortic dilatation are seen, pathological aortic regurgitation will be found.

Approximately 25 % of MFS patients have mild (less than 10 %), asymptomatic reduced left ventricular ejection fraction, suggesting impaired systolic function and underlying cardiomyopathy. These patients also have right ventricular systolic dysfunction [15].

Mitral Valve

MFS patients have degenerative mitral valve leaflet with elongation and thickening (myxomatous degeneration). This is due to defective connective tissue and degeneration because of increased TGF-β signaling [16] (Fig. 6.1).

Mitral valve prolapse (MVP) is defined as closing position displacement of one or both leaflets cephalad (or superior) into the left atrium past the annular plane.

The prevalence of isolated MVP is 2–3 % in the general population with the significant risk of severe MR, heart failure, and infective endocarditis. 0.25 % of mitral valve prolapse patients are reported to have MFS. During ventricular contraction, the mitral valve has to withstand its force, and prolapse of posterior leaflet is more common [17]. In 2011, Rybczynski and Treede, reported the prevalence of MVP in MFS is 40 %, severe MR is 12 %, and infective endocarditis is 2.5 % [18]. The prevalence of more severe myxomatous mitral valve thickening with prolapse is 25 % in MFS patients.

They reported the outcome of MVP and MVP related events in 112 patients with MFS. They found that bileaflet MVP affected 62 %, anterior MVP occurring more often than posterior MVP. Mitral Regurgitation (MR) progression was seen in 37 % and it was related to floppy mitral valve and increased indexed end-systolic left ventricle diameters. Mitral valve (MV) infective endocarditis, heart failure, MV replacement and repair were seen in 28 %, predicted by floppy mitral valve and mild or moderate MR. Aortic dilatation, dural ectasia, and new mutation cause were not related to outcome. Neither blood pressure nor medication (Beta-blocker (BB) and Angiotensin Receptor Blocker (ARB)) had any effect on MV related outcome [18].

Habashi et al. studied mice with FBN-1 mutation. They hypothesised that elongation and thickening of the mitral valve leaflet could be caused by increased activation and signaling of TGF-β. When they treated mice with a TGF-β neutralizing antibody, elongation and thickening of leaflet recovered to normal [19].

Mitral valve prolapse is associated with mid-systolic click at apex, especially with the patient lying on the left side. And if it is accompanied by mitral regurgitation, a high-pitched holosystolic murmur is heard. Due to mitral regurgitation, left ventricle and left atrium have volume overload, and heart failure may occur in decompensated phase. Calcification of the valve annulus has also been reported to occur at a greater rate than in normal individuals [5].

Severity of regurgitation is variable. Some paediatric MFS patients have early onset and severe symptoms. In infancy, mitral regurgitation may cause congestive heart failure, pulmonary hypertension, and death. More than 25 % of Marfan syndrome patients have progression of mitral valve prolapse to mitral regurgitation by adulthood, and twice as many women as men demonstrate progressive mitral dysfunction [1].

Tricuspid Valve, Pulmonary Artery

Tricuspid valve prolapse may also occur due to degeneration of tricuspid valve. In a Norwegian study of adult MFS patients, CT or MRI were performed to evaluate the pulmonary artery. In normal subjects, published mean pulmonary diameter was from 24.0 ± 2.0 to 27.2 ± 3.0 mm. More than half of adult patients with MFS had pulmonary artery trunk more than 30 mm, though some (15 %) did not have ascending aortic dilatation [20]. Pulmonary artery dilatation usually occurs at the level of the root [5].

Left Ventricular Dilatation and Dysfunction

If the patient has significant mitral, aortic, or tricuspid regurgitation, left ventricular dilatation and dysfunction may occur due to volume overload. However, De Backer et al. reported some Marfan syndrome patients without significant valve regurgitation showed systolic and diastolic dysfunction independently. Their left ventricular volume in both systolic and diastolic phase was larger than in controls, and ejection fraction was reduced [21]. This was thought to be due to increased left ventricular afterload caused by aortic root stiffness [22]. Extracellular matrix remodelling and abnormal TGF-β due to fibrillin deficiency also contribute to impaired left ventricular function [22].

LV dimension and construction was normal in most of Marfan patients. The LV of 7 % of these patients was dilated but none of them fulfilled criteria for idiopathic Dilated Cardiomyopathy (DCM) [23].

Heart Failure

Heart failure may occur if valve regurgitation becomes severe. Little is written specifically about treatment for heart failure in patients with Marfan syndrome.

Arrhythmia and Sudden Cardiac Death

General

In 1997, A. Savolainen et al. investigated 45 adult patients with Marfan syndrome [24]. The prevalence of cardiac arrhythmias, for example prolonged atrioventricular conduction, ST segment depression and ventricular repolarisation abnormality such as QT interval prolongation and U wave, was higher than in the general population [24].

This was not related to aortic root dilatation, left atrial dilatation, left ventricular dilatation or function. Most arrhythmias were premature atrial or ventricular beats. Moreover, asymptomatic ST depression was also seen in more patients with MFS than in the general population. It was supposed that there would be myocardial abnormality. They thought deficiency of fibrillin in patients with MFS producing microfibril abnormality in the matrix of the heart muscle would affect tissue in the impulse conducting system. Most arrhythmia does not lead to life threatening condition in patients with MFS, however, ventricular arrhythmia may occur in patients with repolarisation abnormality [24].

Yetman et al. reported that ventricular arrhythmia was seen in 21 % of MFS patients, and 4 % died from arrhythmia [28].

Ali Aydin et al. [25] reported that ventricular couplets and non-sustained ventricular tachycardia were seen in 40 %, and PVC more than 10 beats/h was seen in 35 %. PVC and couplet, non-sustained VT and ventricular arrhythmia events were related to NT-pro BNP level elevation and left atrial dilatation. PVC, couplet, and non-sustained VT were related to indexed end-systolic dilatation, moderate mitral regurgitation, and prolonged QTc.

The incidence of ventricular arrhythmia events was 12 %, and sudden cardiac death was 4 %. All arrhythmias were related to NT-pro BNP. Left ventricular dysfunction, and fibrillin-1 gene exon 24–32 mutations increased risk of ventricular arrhythmia event. They reported an 8 % prevalence of ventricular arrhythmic events including sudden cardiac death, much higher than in the general population, and lower than in patients with hypertrophic cardiomyopathy who have a 12 % prevalence [25].

Premature ventricular contraction is an independent risk factor for sudden death. Boris A. Hoffmann et al. reported that 2.1 % of their patients died sudden cardiac death and 6.5 % had sustained ventricular tachycardia. They studied patients' NT-pro BNP, echocardiogram, ECG. They set NT-proBNP >–214.3 pg/ml level as cut-off point. Levels higher than this carried a significant risk factor for sudden cardiac death, and these patients had higher NYHA classification, and decreased left ventricular function. Incidence of sudden cardiac death in MFS is thought to be 0.92 per 1000-person-years. Incidence of sudden cardiac death in those aged 18–50 years is thought to be 0.09 per 1000-person-years, and it is impossible to predict by FBN1 mutation [22].

Discussion About Arrhythmia

As Savolainen et al. [24] reported before, patients with MFS more frequently have dysrhythmia, for example, atrial arrhythmias >1 beat/h, ventricular arrhythmias >1 beat/h, ventricular arrhythmias >10 beats/h, ventricular salvos of >3 beats and R on T phenomenon.

We studied patients at St George's Hospital compared with a control group.

Fifty-five patients fulfilled revised Ghent criteria: 33 patients (60 %) were male, and average age was 34.5 years old. 58.2 % of patients were on medication; beta-blocker, ARB or ACE-I.

The control group consisted of unaffected relatives of cardiac sudden death patients, or healthy volunteers. Of 165 subjects, 94 were male (57.0 %) and the average age was 35.7 years old. Only one control subject was taking beta-blocker.

All of them underwent Holter ECG. 92.7 % of patients with MFS had ventricular ectopy (VE), and 9.8 % of them had >10 beats/h. 73.9 % of the control group had ventricular ectopy, and 4.1 % of them had >10 beats/h. Neither group demonstrated atrial fibrillation, ventricular tachycardia, or significant heart block.

On echocardiogram, mitral valve prolapse (MVP) as a common manifestation in Marfan syndrome was seen in 20 % of patients, in contrast to 1.7 % of the control group ($P<0.05$). Although all those with MVP demonstrated VE, only one had VE >10 beats/h (see Table 6.1).

Ali Aydin et al. studied 80 mutation proven MFS patients [25]. Patients underwent 24 h Holter ECG, 12 lead ECG and echocardiography. They reported 28 out of 80 (35 %) had ventricular premature complexes >10 beats/h, and 16 patients (57 %) had mitral valve prolapse. In our study, 55 patients with MFS underwent 24/48 h Holter ECG and echocardiography. Five out of 55 patients (9.1 %) had ventricular premature complexes >10 beats/h and 1 patient out of 5 had mitral valve prolapse. Ali Aydin also reported that location of mutations in exons 24–32 of the FBN1 gene was a risk factor for ventricular tachycardia event.

In our study, 50 out of 55 patients had fibrillin-1 mutation screening, and a mutation was found in 44 patients (88 %). Seven patients had mutations in exons 24–32. Three patients had missense mutations (1 involving cysteine), 2 patients had nonsense mutations resulting in stop codons, and 2 patients had splice site mutations. Of these 7 patients, 1 patient who had missense mutation affecting cysteine residues in exon 31 had frequent VEs. However, the remaining 6 patients did not have ventricular ectopy or mitral valve prolapse. Our findings did not support the data that mutation in the neonatal region predisposes to VEs. Studies are under way to determine if the actual location of the cysteine affected by the mutation may explain why our results differ from those in the Aydin et al. study.

We recognise that this is a small group with an incomplete data set, but our data regarding incidence of arrhythmia agrees with that in previous publications.

Investigations

Echocardiogram

Echocardiogram is widely-used for evaluation of valve and aortic root, as it is convenient and noninvasive, and can be used in case of emergency. Following initial diagnosis, a second echocardiogram should be performed after 6 months in order to assess the growth of aortic diameter and decide the interval for follow up [26]. After that, in adults, echocardiogram should be performed once a year, unless aortic

Table 6.1 Incidence of arrhythmia in 55 adult Marfan syndrome patients

	VE>0/h	VE>1/h	VE>10/h	VE>30/h
MVP (n=11)	11 (100 %)	6 (55 %)	1 (9.1 %)	0 (0 %)

	Marfan	Control unaffected relatives and healthy volunteers	p value p<0.05 sig
No of subjects	55	165	
Male	33 (60.0 %)	94 (57.0 %)	0.694
Average age (median age)	34.5±12.6 (32)	35.7±12.3 (32)	0.535
Medication			
Beta-blocker	21 (38.2 %)	1 (0.%)	0.000
ARB	12 (21.8 %)	0 (0.0 %)	0.000
ACE-I	3 (5.5 %)	0 (0.0 %)	0.003
None	23 (41.8 %)	164 (99.4 %)	0.000
Holter	55 (100 %)	165 (100 %)	N/A
48 h	41 (74.5 %)	28 (17.0 %)	0.000
VE > 0 beat	51 (92.7 %)	122 (73.9 %)	0.003
VE > 1 beat/h	17 (30.9 %)	16 (9.7 %)	0.000
VE > 10 beats/h	5 (9.1 %)	5 (3.0 %)	0.062
VT	0 (0 %)	1 (0.6 %)	0.563
AF	0 (0 %)	0 (0 %)	N/A
Heart block	0 (0 %)	3 (1.8 %)	0.314
Significant heart block	0 (0 %)	0 (0 %)	N/A
12-lead ECG	21 (38.2 %)	132 (80.0 %)	0.000
Sinus rhythm	21 (100 %)	131 (99.2 %)	0.689
HR (bpm)	61.1±8.6	67.1±13.6	0.05
PR interval (ms)	158.2±21.0	156.1±27.0	0.68
QRS duration (ms)	96.3±11.0	91.9±10.0	0.099
QTc (ms)	403.2±22.7	408.5±42.1	0.396
LVH	4 (19.0 %)	10 (7.6 %)	0.09
T wave inversion (in 2 and more leads)	1 (4.8 %)	4 (3.0 %)	0.678
RSR or pRBBB	4 (19.0 %)	3 (2.3 %)	0.001
CRBBB	0 (0 %)	0 (0 %)	N/A
LBBB	0 (0 %)	1 (0.76 %)	0.689
Echocardiogram	55 (100 %)	118 (71.5 %)	0.000
Aortic root dilation	39 (70.9 %)	7 (5.9 %)	0.000
Aortic root diameter (mm)[a]	39.7±5.4	31.3±4.1	0.000
MVP	11 (20 %)	2 (1.7 %)	0.000

$p<0.05$

[a]Dilation definition: >38 mm diameter or technician comment

diameter is 4.5 cm or over, or there is recent major change in the aorta, when echocardiogram should be performed twice a year [12].

When aortic diameter is estimated, the leading-edge convention in the parasternal long axis view at the end diastolic period is best for visualisation. In order to measure the maximum aortic diameter, apical long axis view of aorta is helpful. Also, it should be parallel to the aortic annular plane [2, 27].

As written above, aortic diameter depends on age, height, gender. Devereux et al. studied aortic root diameters with normal subjects. They found that men had larger aortic diameter, and larger body surface area subjects also had larger aortic diameter. Devereux et al. made Z-score calculation using height, as below [2, 27];

predicted aortic root (cm) for length $= 1.519 + (\text{age} \times 0.010) - (\text{sex} \times 0.247)$
(male = 1, female = 2)
Z-score = (measured diameter – predicted aortic root)/SD
(model SD = 0.215 cm) with an SD of 0.125 cm

Aortic diameter should be checked at annulus, sinus of Valsalva, ST junction, ascending aorta, descending aorta, and abdominal aorta. Annulus is measured during mid systole period [2]. The incidence of aortic dissection is increased in patients with rapid rate of aortic diameter growth compared with slow rate of growth.

CT or MRI CT, MRI, and transesophageal echocardiogram all have high sensitivity and specificity at the time of diagnosis of aortic dissection [12]. CT is used for evaluation of aorta and coronary arteries, and diagnosis of aortic dissection. MRI allows detailed assessment of aorta, valve disease and ventricular size. If patients have chest deformities, MRI is a good tool for evaluation. Evaluation of this systemic condition including whole aorta is possible by MRI without radiation. Two types of measurement of aortic root are used - cusp to commissure and cusp to cusp. It is said that aortic root diameter measured from cusp to commissure in diastole by non-contrast MRI is similar to aortic diameter measured inner edge by echocardiogram [2].

For patients who have had surgery to replace aortic root, CT or MRI should be done before discharge to evaluate beyond the aortic root; aortic arch, descending aorta, abdominal aorta. And it should be done every 6 months until aortic diameter is seen to be stable. Some patients who have had aortic surgery will have distal aortic event [26].

ECG and 24 h ECG

Sometimes abnormal findings are seen, including atrioventricular conduction delay, QT interval prolongation, and ST depression. Perhaps these findings are not due to aortic root diameter, but heart structure and function, and valve condition. However, repolarisation has been thought to be related to left ventricular dilatation [28].

As written in arrhythmia section, it is thought that fibrillin deficiency causes microfibrillar abnormality in the myocardium, and leads to conduction impairment. On the other hand, PQ interval duration is thought to be associated with heart structure [24].

ESC guideline suggests patients who have chest symptoms should have 24 h ECG as ventricular arrhythmia, conduction disorder, and sudden cardiac death may occur in this group [29].

Prevention and Treatment

Daily Life

In the 1970s, Marfan syndrome patients' life expectancy was 40–50 years because of aortic dissection or heart failure from aortic or mitral regurgitation. Due to progression of medical and surgical therapy, life expectancy has improved and now lies within the normal range [30].

Marfan syndrome patients require appropriate exercise, isometric and isokinetic exertion at less than maximal effort. However, to avoid severe cardiovascular complications, they should avoid contact sports which may cause chest trauma, and straining which produces Valsalva strain (breath-holding). Contact sports may also cause ocular complication such as ectopia lentis. Thoracoabdominal cavity pressure increases with Valsalva strain, leads to diminished venous return, causes blood pressure decrease and increased sympathetic nervous tone. This is not recommended because of the risk of dissection or aortic rupture from increasing blood pressure. In general, patients with MFS are recommended low to moderate intensity exercise. And they should check their blood pressure routinely and keep blood pressure under 120/80 mmHg [12, 29]

Risk factors that accelerate expansion of aortic wall should be addressed and modified. Smokers have a higher aortic dilatation expansion rate, and higher occurrence of dissection than non-smokers. Smoking should be avoided by patients with MFS as it is related to vascular complications [31].

About 30 % of patients with MFS have obstructive sleep apnea. It is thought to be related to progression of aortic dilatation as it increases pleural pressure during sleep. Patients who have obstructive sleep apnea should be treated [12]. Sleep apnea is also an independent risk factor for reducing left ventricular ejection fraction and increasing NT-pro BNP [22].

According to European guidelines, systolic blood pressure needs to be kept under 120 mmHg, and under 110 mmHg with aortic dissection [29].

Medical Treatment

To Prevent Aortic Dilatation

β-blocker is currently used for cardiovascular management to reduce aortic root dilatation. As frequency of aortic dissection and rupture are high with hypertensive patients, β-blocker is used to prevent these adverse aortic events in Marfan syndrome. Ideal heart rate is under 60–70 beats per minute and up to 100 beats per minute during exercise [26]. β-blocker inhibits adrenaline β activation release into blood from sympathetic nerves and adrenal gland. In the heart, β-receptor stimulation increases heart rate and cardiac contraction, and excitation conduction in atrioventricular node. Thus β-blocker therapy decreases heart rate, cardiac contraction and myocardial oxygen consumption.

Adrenaline type β1 receptor is related to heart function. There are type β2 receptors in smooth muscle of blood vessel and trachea, and these smooth muscles become relaxed when type β2 receptors are stimulated. β-blocker inhibits relaxation of blood vessel and trachea. Therefore, as β-blocker use risks making diseases involved with smooth muscle contraction worse, β-blocker is contraindicated for patients with diseases involving smooth muscle contraction.

Some studies have shown that β-blocker reduces blood pressure and heart rate, and thus reduces progression of aortic root size [2, 32]. Aortic stiffness is also reduced and aortic distensibility increased [12]. However, there are no reports which indicate that aortic dissection or prophylactic surgery can be avoided by β-blocker [26].

β-blocker is more effective in patients with less aortic dilatation, for example less than 4.0 cm [12]. β-blocker is recommended for use in the early stages regardless of aortic dilatation because the aorta dilates most between the ages of 6–14 years old [26] (See also Chap. 5). In children, the main side effects of β-blocker are bronchospasm, hypotension, bradycardia. β-blocker affects sugar and lipid metabolism, and masks hypoglycemia symptoms, for example palpitation, tremor and hunger [33].

Angiotensin Receptor Blocker (ARB)

As explained previously, TGF-β signaling is excessive due to abnormal fibrillin in patients with MFS. TGF-β is produced when AII combines with AT1 receptor. Increasing activation and signaling cause aneurysm and dissections due to ECM degradation, apoptosis and inflammation. As activation and signaling of TGF-β is increased in Marfan syndrome patients, inhibiting these is felt to be effective [4].

When mice with FBN1 mutation were treated with TGF-β antibody, myxomatous degeneration of aortic and mitral valves was prevented [26, 34]. Use of angiotensin 1 receptor antagonists (Losartan) indicated the same effect. Losartan is one of the angiotensin receptor blockers (ARB) used to control blood pressure. ARB acts on renin-angiotensin pathway. The glomerulus in the kidney senses blood pressure. If blood pressure is low, renin is secreted, and if blood pressure is high, the secretion decreases. Renin effect on angiotensinogen, and angiotensinI(AI) is produced. AI is converted to angiotensinII(AII) by angiotensin conversion enzyme(ACE). AII combines with angiotensinII receptor; when it combines with AT1 receptor in vascular smooth muscle, vasocontraction occurs, and when it combines with AT2 receptor in adrenal cortex, secretion of aldosterone is stimulated. ARB inhibits AII from combining with AT2 receptor and acts as an antihypertensive. Also, TGF-β is produced in endothelium from AT1 receptor and is inhibited by AT2 receptor. ARB blocks AT1 receptor and reduces TGF-β, and so ECM degradation, apoptosis and inflammation are inhibited, thus delaying aneurysm formation [4].

According to a prospective, randomised, controlled trial [35], losartan use reduced aortic root dilatation rate in adult patients with MFS. This study also showed that the reduction of aortic root dilatation rate was irrespective of age, sex, blood pressure, aortic root size, presence of FBN1 mutation and concomitant β-blocker use.

In 2014, Dietz et al. compared the effect of Losartan and Atenolol over 3 years in 608 children and young adults with MFS who were 6 months to 25 years old. They found no significant difference in the rate of aortic root dilatation, aortic surgery, aortic dissection and death [36].

New Drug

In 2008, doxycycline, which is an antibiotic member of the tetracycline family, when administered to mice, inhibited the expression of MMP-2 and MMP-9 both type4 collagenases, was shown to delay elastic fibre disruption and aortic rupture. When doxycycline was compared with atenolol in MFS animal model, animals administered doxycycline had no aortic aneurysm [37].

Doxycycline was thought to affect endothelial function, elastic fibres, and the structure of aortic wall. However, as doxycycline has not been tested in patients with MFS, we do not yet have strong evidence to use this drug for inhibiting aortic dilatation [26].

Management of Ventricular Arrhythmias

As arrhythmias are secondary to other cardiac conditions, it is essential to treat the underlying cardiac disorders to prevent arrhythmia. In addition, patients with MFS should be carefully monitored for early detection of arrhythmia with resting and/or stress ECGs and periodic ambulatory rhythm recordings [38]. As left ventricular dilatation is associated with ventricular arrhythmias in MFS patients, this should be routinely measured and monitored through echocardiography. B-blockers, primarily used to prevent aortic dilatation, are thought to have a parallel protection against arrhythmias [39]. Agents like ARBs and ACEi are likely to play a role in the incidence of arrhythmias indirectly by decreasing the primary cardiac disorder, and directly by modulating alterations in ion channels [40].

However, further research is necessary to elucidate the potential role of RAAS inhibitors for the prevention of cardiac arrhythmias in MFS patients. Furthermore, Hoffmann et al. [22] demonstrated NT-pro BNP to be an independent predictor of adverse arrhythmias in patients with MFS and this new finding might help in selecting patients who are at risk of developing life threatening arrhythmias. Patients at high risk of developing malignant arrhythmias are referred for either an implantable cardiac defibrillator (ICD) or pacemaker [41].

Surgical Treatment

Prophylactic aortic replacement is chosen to avoid aortic dissection, and emergency surgery is required in case of aortic dissection type A. European guidelines also suggest that when aortic diameter reaches 5.0 cm, patients should have surgery [29]. At 4.5 cm, patients are recommended to undergo surgery if they have risk factors for dissection; family history of dissection, size increase more than 3 mm per year, severe aortic regurgitation, or desire for pregnancy [6].

However, sometimes it takes time to consult, see their surgeon and decide a schedule, so 4.8 cm is thought to be a better cut-off for referral. In case of Stanford type A dissection, patients should be sent to surgery, because the mortality within 48 h period is 50 %, perioperative mortality is still 25 %, and some complications remain. Surgery reduces 1 month mortality from 90 to 30 % even in the case of patients without MFS [6].

Aortic root surgery is becoming safer. Mortality of elective surgery is 1.5 %, compared to that of emergency surgery (11.7 %), survival rate at 5 years is 84 %, and at 10 years is 75 %. However, patients have a higher recurrence risk of dissection and aneurysm than in other aortic diseases [29]. In case of Stanford type B dissection, which is seen in 10 % of all aortic dissection in patients with MFS, medical treatment is recommended unless they have complication and required surgery. Patients need to have pain and blood pressure controlled.

Endocarditis

To prevent endocarditis, some patients with MVP, surgical prosthetic material, or personal endocarditis history should take prophylactic antibiotic when they need to have dental procedure or minor surgery. Although infective endocarditis may occur from not only minor surgery or dental procedure, also brushing, chewing, flossing, there is no standardisation about prophylaxis of endocarditis [12, 29]. On the other hand, the National Marfan Foundation recommends prophylaxis of endocarditis for MFS patients who have valvular regurgitation, because although guidelines do not recommend prophylaxis of endocarditis for patients with valvular regurgitation without personal endocarditis history, there is no risk stratification of endocarditis in case of patients with systemic connective tissue disorder [26].

Stent Graft

In case of aortic dissection type B with complications for example, ischemia of lower parts of body, or impending aortic rupture, surgery has higher risk. Stent graft is used to prevent false lumen enlargement. Stent graft may be used for patients in whom open surgery is contraindicated [26].

However, systematic review reported that although MFS patients with dissection who have had stent graft had 2.8 % mortality, 21.6 % patients had periprocedural endoleaks. The average time of occurrence of endoleak was 2.5 years, and the final mortality was 12 % [2]. For these reasons, stent graft for patients with MFS is not recommended.

Summary

Treatment strategies for cardiac manifestations including β-blockers, elective aortic root replacement and mitral valve repair surgery have improved life expectancy in patients with MFS. Despite this improvement, cardiac morbidity remains a problem among patients with MFS. Novel approaches, such as ARBs, are believed to partially exert their beneficial effects on cardiac involvement by reducing TGF-β activity, which has been recognised to play a pivotal role in the pathogenesis of cardiac manifestations observed among MFS patients. However, ARBs have important limitations, and therefore further studies need to be performed to develop more therapies that specifically aim to reduce TGF-β activity.

References

1. Judge DP, Dietz HC. Marfan's syndrome. Lancet. 2005;366:1965–76.
2. Radke RM, Baumgartner H. Diagnosis and treatment of Marfan syndrome: an update. Heart. 2014;100:1382–91.
3. Chiu HH, Wu MH, Chen HC, et al. Epidemiological profile of Marfan syndrome in a general population: a national database study. Mayo Clin Proc. 2014;89:34–42.
4. Pannu H, Tran-Fadulu V, Milewicz DM. Genetic basis of thoracic aortic aneurysms and aortic dissections. Am J Med Genet C Semin Med Genet. 2005;139C:10–6.
5. Cañadas V, Vilacosta I, Bruna I, Fuster V. Marfan syndrome. Part 1: pathophysiology and diagnosis. Nat Rev Cardiol. 2010;7:256–65.
6. Erbel R, Aboyans V, Boileau C, et al. 2014 ESC Guidelines on the diagnosis and treatment of aortic diseases. Eur Heart J. 2014;35:2873–926.
7. Loeys BL, Dietz HC, Braverman AC, et al. The revised Ghent nosology for the Marfan syndrome. J Med Genet. 2010;47:476–85.
8. Evangelista A, Flachskampf FA, Erbel R, et al. Echocardiography in aortic diseases: EAE recommendations for clinical practice. Eur J Echocardiogr. 2010;11:645–58.
9. Campens L. Reference values for echocardiographic assessment of the diameter of the aortic root and ascending aorta spanning all age categories. Am J Cardiol. 2014;114:914–20.
10. Mulder BJM. The distal aorta in the Marfan syndrome. Neth Heart J. 2008;16:382–6.
11. Engelfriet PM, Boersma E, Tijssen JGP, et al. Beyond the root: dilatation of the distal aorta in Marfan's syndrome. Heart. 2006;92:1238–43.
12. Ammash NM, Sundt TM, Connolly HM. Marfan syndrome - diagnosis and management. Curr Probl Cardiol. 2008;33(1):7–39.
13. Januzzi JL. Comparison of aortic dissection in patient with and without Marfan's syndrome. Am J Cardiol. 2004;94:400–2.
14. Januzzi JL. Characterizing the young patient with aortic dissection: results from the International Registry of Aortic Dissection (IRAD). J Am Coll Cardiol. 2004;43:665–9.
15. Alpendurada F. Evidence for Marfan cardiomyopathy. Eur J Heart Fail. 2010;12:1085–91.
16. Judge DP. Mitral valve disease in Marfan syndrome. J Cardiovasc Trans Res. 2011;4:741–7.
17. Weyman AE, Scherrer-Crosbie M. Marfan syndrome and mitral valve prolapse. J Clin Invest. 2004;114:1543–6.
18. Rybczynski M, Treede H. Predictors of outcome of mitral valve prolapse in patients with the Marfan syndrome. Am J Cardiol. 2011;107:268–74.
19. Habashi JP, Judge DP, Holm TM, et al. Losartan, an AT1 antagonist, prevents aortic aneurysm in a mouse model of Marfan syndrome. Science. 2006;312:117–21.

20. Lundby R. The pulmonary artery in patients with Marfan syndrome: a cross-sectional study. Genet Med. 2012;14:922–7.
21. De Backer JF, Devos D, Segers P, et al. Primary impairment of left ventricular function in Marfan syndrome. Int J Cardiol. 2006;112:353–8.
22. Hoffmann A, Rybczynski M, Rostock T. Prospective risk stratification of sudden cardiac death in Marfan's syndrome. Int J Cardiol. 2013;167:2539–45.
23. Meijboom LJ, Timmermans J, van Tintelen JP, et al. Evaluation of left ventricular dimensions and function in Marfan's syndrome without significant valvular regurgitation. Am J Cardiol. 2005;95:795–7.
24. Savolainen A, Kupari M, Toivonen L, et al. Abnormal ambulatory electrocardiographic findings in patients with the Marfan syndrome. J Intern Med. 1997;241:221–6.
25. Aydin A, Adsay BA. Observational cohort study of ventricular arrhythmia in adults with Marfan syndrome caused by FBN1 mutations. PLoS One. 2013;8:1–10.
26. Cañadas V, Vilacosta I, Bruna I, Fuster V. Marfan syndrome. Part 2: treatment and management of patients. Nat Rev Cardiol. 2010;7:266–76.
27. Devereux RB. Normal limits in relation to age, body size and gender of two-dimensional echocardiographic aortic root dimensions in persons >15 years of age. Am J Cardiol. 2012;110:1189–94.
28. Yetman AT, Bornemeier RA, McCrindle BW. Long-term outcome in patients with Marfan syndrome: is aortic dissection the only cause of sudden death? J Am Coll Cardiol. 2003;41:329–32.
29. Baumgartner H, Bonhoeffer P, De Groot NM, et al. ESC guidelines for the management of grown-up congenital heart disease (new version 2010). Eur Heart J. 2010;31:2915–57.
30. Pyeritz RE. Marfan syndrome: 30 years of research equals 30 years of additional life expectancy. Heart. 2009;95:173–6.
31. Boodhwani M, Andelfinger G, Leipsic J, et al. Canadian Cardiovascular Society position statement on the management of thoracic aortic disease. Can J Cardiol. 2014;30:577–89.
32. Benedetto U, Melina G. Surgical management of aortic root disease in Marfan syndrome: a systematic review and meta-analysis. Heart. 2011;97:955–8.
33. Gersony DR, McClaughlin MA. The effect of beta-blocker therapy on clinical outcome in patients with Marfan's syndrome: a meta-analysis. Int J Cardiol. 2007;114:303–8.
34. Habashi JP, Judge DP. Losartan, an AT1 antagonist, prevents aortic aneurysm in a mouse model of Marfan syndrome. Science. 2006;312:117–21.
35. Groenink M. Losartan reduces aortic dilatation rate in adults with Marfan syndrome: a randomized controlled trial. Eur Heart J. 2013;34:3491–500.
36. Lacro RV, Dietz HC, Sleeper LA, et al. Atenolol versus losartan in children and young adults with Marfan's syndrome. N Engl J Med. 2014;371:2061–71.
37. Chung AW, Yang HH, Radomski MW, van Breemen C. Long-term doxycycline is more effective than atenolol to prevent thoracic aortic aneurysm in Marfan syndrome through the inhibition of matrix metalloproteinase-2 and –9. Circ Res. 2008;102:e78–385.
38. Silversides CK, Kiess M, Beauchesne L, et al. Canadian Cardiovascular Society 2009 Consensus Conference on the management of adults with congenital heart disease: Outflow tract obstruction, coarctation of the aorta, tetralogy of Fallot, Ebstein anomaly and Marfan's syndrome. Can J Cardiol. 2010;26:e80–97.
39. Williams A, Davies S, Stuart AG, Wilson DG, Fraser AG. Medical treatment of Marfan syndrome: a time for change. Heart. 2008;94:414–21.
40. Iravanian S, Dudley Jr SC. The Renin-Angiotensin-Aldosterone System (RAAS) and cardiac arrhythmias. Heart Rhythm. 2008;5:s12–7.
41. Xu H-Y, Xu Y-Z, Ling F, et al. Application of CRT-D in a Marfan syndrome patient with chronic heart failure accompanied by ventricular tachycardia and ventricular fibrillation. Zhejiang Univ-Sci B (Biomed & Biotechnol). 2013;14:759–62.

7 Echocardiography in Diagnosis and Management of Patients with Marfan Syndrome

Anna Marciniak and Rajan Sharma

The cardiovascular complications of Marfan syndrome require lifelong monitoring, even after surgical intervention. Echocardiography plays a crucial role in the diagnosis and evaluation of cardiovascular features, follow up and further decision regarding management in patients with Marfan syndrome. Echocardiography is used worldwide, the most widely available and cost effective non invasive technique for evaluating cardiac structures and the proximal aorta. The technique uses ultrasound and is therefore completely safe. A full study takes 30 min. Moreover, machines are now available the size of a smart phone, making this technique attractive for scanning patients repeatedly.

The initial evaluation of patients with Marfan syndrome includes detailed echocardiographic assessment of left ventricular (LV) function, cardiac valves and the aorta. Echocardiographic findings include:

1. Dilatation of the aortic annulus, sinus of Valsalva and ascending aorta.
2. Aortic regurgitation due to aortic root dilatation.
3. Prolapse of the mitral and tricuspid valves with regurgitation.
4. LV dilatation and impaired LV systolic function due to mitral/aortic regurgitation or Marfan Cardiomyopathy.
5. Pulmonary artery dilatation.

Echocardiography is the imaging modality of choice for the diagnosis and ongoing surveillance of these abnormalities.

A. Marciniak, PhD, MRCP • R. Sharma, BSc(Hons), MBBS, MRCP(UK), MD (✉)
Department of Cardiology, St George's Hospital, London, UK
e-mail: annamarciniak@hotmail.co.uk; rajan.sharma@stgeorges.nhs.uk

© Springer-Verlag London 2016

A.H. Child (ed.), *Diagnosis and Management of Marfan Syndrome*,
DOI 10.1007/978-1-4471-5442-6_7

Aorta and Aortic Valve Assessments

Echocardiographic Measurements

When performing transthoracic echocardiographic examination in patients with suspected or confirmed Marfan syndrome it is important to accurately assess the aortic valve, aortic root and the proximal ascending aorta which are well seen in the parasternal long and short axis views (Figs. 7.1 and 7.2). In adults, the aortic diameter measurements should be made [1]:

- In two dimensional long axis plane through the centre of the aortic sinus and the ascending aorta.
- At end diastole (as the aortic pressure is the most stable then. End diastole is also easily identified by the onset of QRS complex).
- From the inner edge to the inner edge defining the aortic lumen.
- At the aortic annulus, aortic sinuses, sinotubular junction and the ascending aorta.

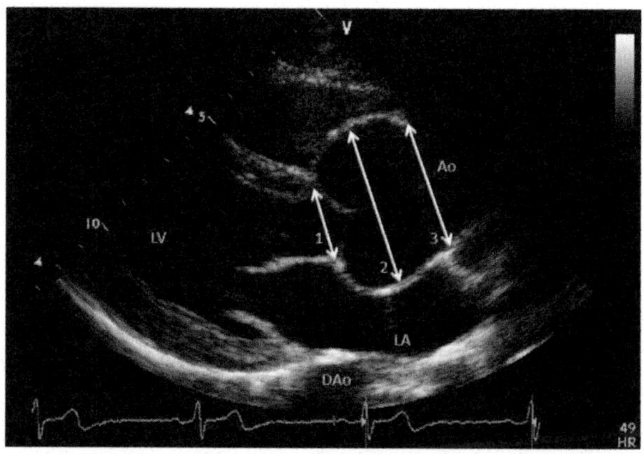

Fig. 7.1 The parasternal long-axis view with dilated aortic sinuses in patient with Marfan syndrome. The regions where aortic diameters are measured for follow up analysis are indicated with *arrows*: *1* aortic valve annulus, *2* aortic sinuses, *3* sinotubular junction, *LA* left atrium, *LV* left ventricle, *Ao* Aorta, *DAo* descending aorta

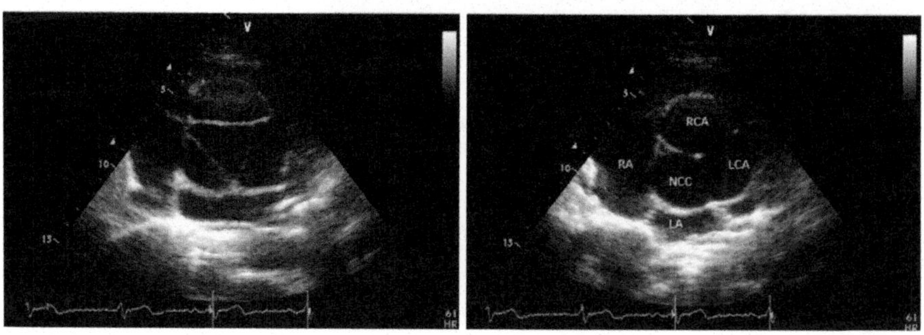

Fig. 7.2 The short-axis view with open aortic valve (*left*). There is a triangular opening of the aortic leaflets, instead of circular, as a result of stretching due to annular dilatation. The short-axis view of the closed aortic valve (*right*). *LA* left atrium, *RA* right atrium, *NCC* non-coronary cusp, *RCA* right coronary cusp, *LCA* left coronary cusp

The key echocardiographic measurement is the aortic diameter at the sinuses of Valsalva (Fig. 7.1) as this is the segment that generally dilates initially and is at the greatest risk for aortic dissection.

Aortic sinus can also be measured with an M-Mode tracing at the level of the valve leaflets when a perpendicular orientation between the ultrasound beam and the aortic sinuses can be obtained. With M-mode tracings a leading edge-to-leading edge measurement convention is used. Depending on the ultrasound penetration, the images of additional segments of the ascending aorta may be obtained by moving the transducer towards the head, one or more intercostal spaces (Fig. 7.3). Image quality is enhanced by positioning the patient in a steep left lateral decubitus position bringing the aorta in contact with the anterior chest wall [1].

To continue assessing the aorta during transthoracic examination, aortic arch is imaged from suprasternal notch or supraclavicular approach with the patient in supine position with the neck extended (Fig. 7.4). Usually only a small segment of

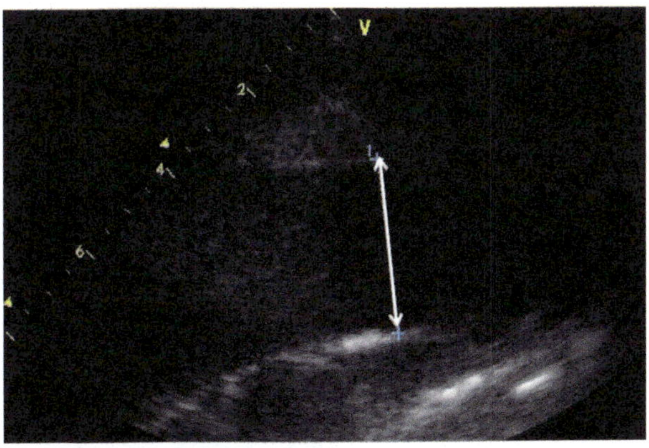

Fig. 7.3 Imaging of the ascending thoracic aorta obtained after moving the transducer one intercostal space toward the head from the standard parasternal long-axis view

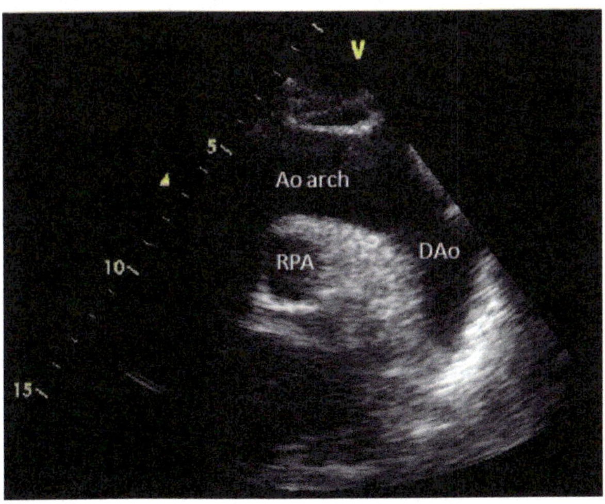

Fig. 7.4 Suprasternal view with aortic arch and descending thoracic aorta. *Ao arch* aortic arch, *DAo*, descending aorta, *RPA* right pulmonary artery

the ascending aorta is visible from the suprasternal notch window but it is variable in different patients [1].

In the assessment of the descending thoracic aorta, it is initially seen in cross section posterior to left atrium in the parasternal long axis (Fig. 7.1). Then from the apical two chamber view a longitudinal section of a segment of the descending aorta is seen by lateral angulation and clockwise rotation of the transducer (Fig. 7.5). Finally from the subcostal approach the distal thoracic and proximal abdominal aorta are seen as it traverses the diaphragm (Fig. 7.6).

The normal values of the aortic diameter are directly proportional to body size throughout normal growth and into adulthood. These normal values were first established by Roman et al. in 1989 and were based on data derived from 135 adult subjects [2]. Given the above average stature and therefore greater body surface

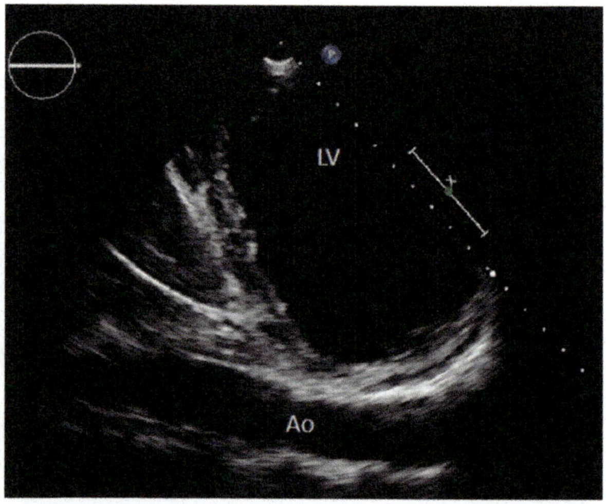

Fig. 7.5 Modified apical 2 chamber view with descending thoracic aorta. *LV* left ventricle, *Ao* aorta

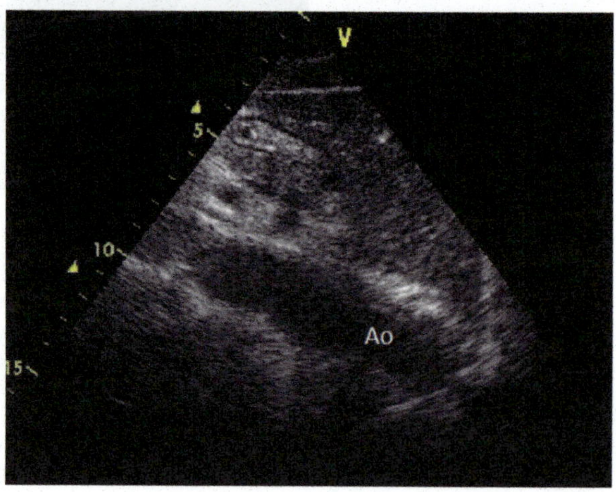

Fig. 7.6 Subcostal view with distal thoracic and proximal abdominal aorta

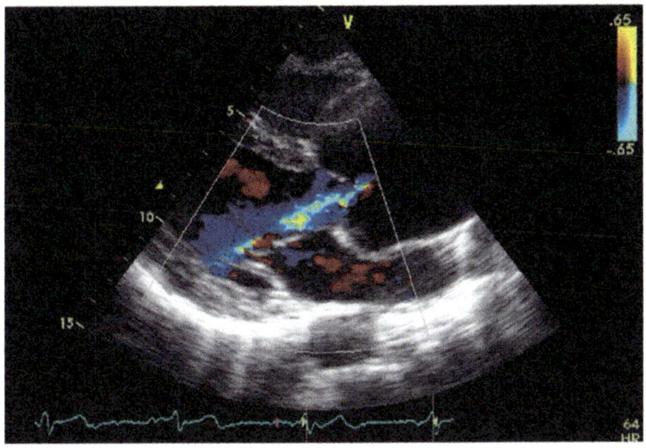

Fig. 7.7 Parasternal long axis view with central jet of aortic regurgitation

area, growing individuals with Marfan syndrome should have their aortic measurements indexed to body surface area [3]. This can be expressed as an aortic size ratio based on gender- and body size-related norms [2, 4] or expressed in relationship to the aortic size in normal population distribution, as a Z score. When considered in these terms, patients with Marfan syndrome with proximal aortic ratios of >1.3 or Z scores >3 are at particular risk [5].

Echocardiography plays an important role in functional evaluation and anatomical inspection of the aortic valve in patients with Marfan syndrome. The aortic annulus dilatation often results in aortic leaflets malcoaptation and a functional aortic regurgitation (Fig. 7.7). The stretching of the leaflets due to dilated aortic annulus causes the triangular shape of the aortic valve, instead of circular, visualised in the parasternal short axis view (Fig. 7.2 left). The detailed assessment of aortic valve morphology i.e., bicuspid vs tricuspid, the presence of calcification and the assessment of the degree of aortic regurgitation are important to guide the planning of surgery. The severity of the aortic regurgitation can be assessed based on quantitative methods like Effective Regurgitant Orifice Area (EROA) and Regurgitant Volume (RVol) and semiquantitative methods like vena contracta and pressure half time.

Monitoring

As recommended in the 2010 ACC/AHA/AATS guidelines for thoracic aortic disease, patients with MFS should have echocardiography performed at the time of diagnosis and 6 months later to determine the aortic root and ascending aortic diameters and their rate of enlargement [6].

According to ESC guidelines from 2010, stable patients need a yearly visit with echocardiography. Cardiac Magnetic Resonance (CMR) should be performed at baseline and repeated at least once in 5 years if the aortic size beyond the root is normal. In the case of aneurysm formation beyond the root, CMR should be repeated at least yearly [7].

Limitations of Echo

The echocardiogram enables us to visualise descending aorta and the blind spot of proximal ascending aorta, therefore computed tomography (CT) or CMR play an important role in imaging of the entire aorta. These studies should be performed every 3–5 years after the initial evaluation, as part of surveillance, as 20 % of Marfan patients may have descending aorta involvement [8].

It is also important to be aware of the differences in aortic measurements between different imaging modalities. The standard echocardiographic conventions established the leading edge to leading edge diameter in end diastole recommended by American Society of Echocardiography [9], however other experts in the literature favor inner edge-to-inner edge diameter [1]. CT or CMR may use either inner edge-to-inner edge or outer edge-to-outer edge, with the external diameter expected to be 2–4 mm larger than the internal one. These measurements also depend upon whether or not contrast agents are utilised.

In CMR/CT the cusp-commissure and cusp-cusp root dimension in sinus planes are assessed, with the latter ones typically being 2–3 mm larger [10]. The cusp-commissure in sinus planes as well as the sinus level in the sagittal LVOT plane correspond to the echocardiographic measurements.

3D echocardiography, CT or CMR also measure the cross sectional area which can be adopted for the acquisition of the views of the different segments. In this situation it is important to avoid oblique imaging of the aorta as this will overestimate the aortic diameter. This usually applies to the measurements of the aortic arch, and the descending thoracic aorta that may take a tortuous course [11].

In the available data, the prevalence and prognostic significance of aortic dilatation in adults have emerged from echocardiography which is a widely available technique. However it is important to complement it with other imaging techniques keeping in mind the difference in the measurements between the imaging modalities.

Management of Aorta Based on Dimensions

In adults, if the aortic diameter is documented as stable over time, then annual imaging is recommended if the aortic dimension is less than 45 mm. If the aortic diameter is ≥45 mm or shows significant growth over time, then more frequent imaging is suggested (e.g., twice yearly) and surgery may be indicated. CMR should be performed at baseline and repeated at least once in 5 years if the aortic size beyond the root is normal. In the case of aneurysm formation beyond the root, CMR should be repeated at least yearly [7].

Transoesophageal Echocardiography

This technique is more invasive and uses a transducer attached to an endoscopy probe. The transducer lies immediately behind the left atrium and therefore allows precise evaluation of the atria, mitral valve and interatrial septum. The shorter distance between the transducer and the aorta allows better evaluation of the severity of aortic regurgitation and higher accuracy for aortic dissection diagnosis. The sensitivity of TOE for aortic dissection diagnosis reaches 99 %, with a specificity of 89 % [12]. Localised aortic dissection of the distal segment of the ascending aorta can be missed – the 'blind spot'.

TOE provides enhanced views of the mitral valve, which now also includes three-dimensional reconstruction to provide detailed information as to the nature of the underlying pathology and helps to visualise the entire mitral valve in the supine position, which the surgical team will find at the time of the surgery. This is very helpful and important when planning mitral valve repair/replacement.

Indications for Surgery

Early identification and establishment of the diagnosis is critical, since prophylactic surgery can prevent aortic dissection and rupture. Indications for surgery are based mainly on aortic diameter and derived from findings based on natural history regarding the risk of complications weighed against the risk of elective surgery. According to ESC guidelines, surgery should be performed in patients with Marfan syndrome, who have a maximal aortic diameter ≥50 mm. A lower threshold of 45 mm can be considered in patients with additional risk factors, including family history of dissection, size increase >3 mm/year (in repeated examinations using the same technique and confirmed by another technique), severe aortic regurgitation, or desire for pregnancy [7]. Patients with marfanoid manifestations due to connective tissue disease, without complete Marfan criteria, should be treated as Marfan patients.

Children

For children with Marfan syndrome, annual imaging is recommended if the aortic dimension is documented as stable over time and not markedly enlarged. There are no validated age-specific absolute aortic diameters that can be used to determine when more frequent imaging should be performed or when prophylactic aortic surgery is indicated. It is recommended that aortic measurements be compared to the body surface area. Sonographic measurement of aortic diameter should be performed annually as long as the increase in aortic size remains proportional to the increase in body surface area. Twice yearly measurements are recommended if aortic size diverges from height when expressed in the same fashion. Individuals under 20 years of age with systemic findings suggestive of Marfan syndrome, but without cardiovascular involvement, should also have annual echocardiograms due to the potential risk of development of aortic disease [13]. Adults with repeatedly normal and stable aortic measurements without a definitive genetic predisposition for aortic enlargement but with a sense of predisposition based upon family history or borderline aortic measurements can be seen at 2–3 year intervals.

Aortic Dissection

The majority of patients with Marfan syndrome present with enlargement of the ascending aorta or a type A dissection. Rarely, a patient presents with a type B dissection involving the descending thoracic aorta, but no data indicate that enlargement of the descending aorta necessarily precedes dissection. Therefore, serial examination of patients with MFS is focused primarily on assessing the ascending aorta.

If aortic dissection is suspected the transthoracic examination includes evaluation of the:

- Ascending aorta from the standard and high parasternal window
- Aortic arch from the suprasternal aortic window
- Descending aorta from the parasternal and apical windows
- Proximal abdominal aorta from a subcostal approach.

The echocardiographic features indicating aortic dissection include the presence of a linear, mobile echogenic structure in the aortic lumen (Fig. 7.8), with pattern of motion different from the aortic wall and the pattern of different colour Doppler flow in true and false lumen which are often associated with the presence of a dilated aortic lumen. In the absence of an identifiable flap there are other signs which may indicate suspected dissection like aortic regurgitation, pericardial effusion and new regional wall motion abnormalities [1]. The sensitivity and specificity of TTE range from 77–80 % to 93–96 %, respectively, for the involvement of the ascending aorta [14–16]. TTE is successful in detecting a distal dissection of the thoracic aorta in only 70 % of patients [16].

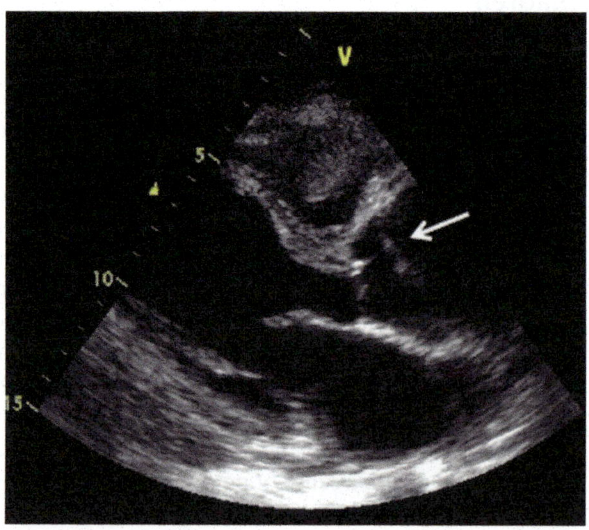

Fig. 7.8 An example of aortic dissection with visible dissection flap (*white arrow*) in patient with Marfan syndrome

Therefore CT, CMR or TOE are often required to confirm the diagnosis and demonstrate the extent of the dissection. These techniques have extremely high (99 %) sensitivity and specificity and the modality used will depend on availability and local expertise. Once diagnosis is made, immediate surgery is required as there is 50 % mortality in first 48 h [17].

Mitral Valve Assessment

Mitral valve prolapse (MVP) is the second most common cardiac manifestation of Marfan syndrome and is thought to be related to myxomatous degeneration of the valvular tissues secondary to underlying extracellular matrix derangements. The biological mechanism for MVP in patients with Marfan syndrome seems to be related, in part, to a genetically induced reduction in the extracellular matrix binding of latent transforming growth factor-β, which leads to a localised increase in TGFβ activity, resulting in elongation and excessive thickening of the mitral valve leaflets [18]. The leaflets' response to repeated mechanical stress may result in the formation of myxomatous valves, even in patients with Marfan syndrome.

In the general population MVP has a prevalence of 3–5 %. In Marfan syndrome, reported prevalence ranges from 28 to 91 % [19, 20]. It has also been shown that valve prolapse becomes more prevalent with increasing age in this group of patients [21]. Kunkala et al. reported that 166 (69 %) of the 239 patients with Marfan syndrome who underwent elective aortic root repair had MVP although only 15 (9 %) of these patients had mitral regurgitation (MR) severity grade >2. This proportion of MR greater than moderate is similar to the reported frequency in MVP patients without connective tissue disorders [18].

Echocardiography is the gold standard for MVP diagnosis and assessment of MR severity and suitability for repair rather than replacement. The mitral leaflets and chordae have an elongated appearance with excessive thickening and a systolic displacement of the leaflets to the left atrium (Fig. 7.9). This displacement in systole is most reliably assessed in parasternal and apical long axis views. The echocardiographic criteria for the diagnosis of mitral valve prolapse are single or bileaflet prolapse ≥2 mm beyond the long-axis annular plane, and leaflet thickening [21]. This is commonly associated with mitral regurgitation which then, as a chronic volume overload condition, may lead to dilatation of the left ventricle and eventually left ventricular impairment, if not operated on in time. These patients often have enlarged atria and develop atrial fibrillation over time, with a high risk of stroke and heart failure [22].

A common complication of mitral valve prolapse is ruptured chordae tendineae which presents as a flail portion of the mitral valve protruding into the left atrium in systole on transthoracic echocardiography. The rupture of mitral chordae may lead to acute mitral regurgitation which may precipitate the acute onset of heart failure or the need for urgent or emergent mitral valve surgery [23–26].

The degree of MR can be assessed using quantitative methods like Effective Regurgitant Orifice Area (EROA), Regurgitant Volume (RVol), and semiquantitative

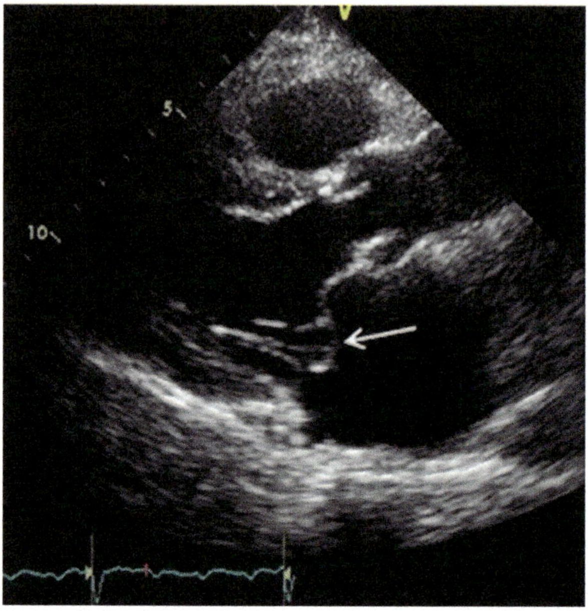

Fig. 7.9 Parasternal long axis view with anterior mitral leaflet prolapse (*white arrow*)

methods like vena contracta, systolic flow reversal in pulmonary vein flow and prominent E wave on mitral inflow.

While performing the transthoracic echo examination there are also numerous clues in the left atrium and ventricle to severe MR [1]:

- The left ventricle is spherically dilated and hyperdynamic
- The left atrium is enlarged at peak systole and has an exaggerated increase in systolic volume
- The mitral valve itself may have one of the lesions consistent with severe MR, such as a flail leaflet.

In situations that impede transthoracic echocardiography (e.g., acoustic shadowing from annular calcium or a mitral prosthesis), TOE provides an unobstructed view. It permits assessment of precisely which of the mitral valve scallops may be affected. The middle scallop of the posterior leaflet (P2) is the most common site of chordal rupture.

It is important to assess the morphology of the mitral valve, the degree of regurgitation and its impact on LV function in patients with Marfan syndrome, as further combined mitral and aortic surgery may be required.

When patients without connective tissue disorders have mitral regurgitation at the time of aortic root replacement, mitral valve intervention is performed if the severity of the MR is at least moderate [27]. Similarly, Marfan patients with mitral valve prolapse and at least moderate mitral regurgitation undergo MV surgery during aortic root replacement.

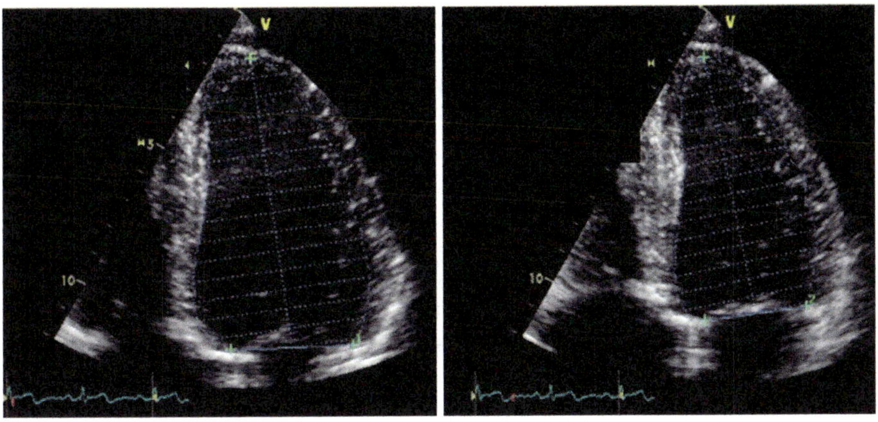

Fig. 7.10 The assessment of left ventricular systolic function using biplane Simpson's technique which involves planimetry of the endocardial border in end diastole (*left*) and end systole (*right*) in apical 4 chamber view. This measurement is then repeated in apical 2 chamber view which then allows automatic calculation of ejection fraction

Marfan Cardiomyopathy

LV abnormalities in patients with Marfan syndrome can occur in the absence of valvular heart disease. These include LV dilatation, LV hypertrophy and impaired LV function. The exact mechanisms are unclear but fibrillin mutation within the myocardium plays a direct role. Up to 25 % Marfan patients may have reduced left ventricular ejection fraction [28].

The echocardiography examination plays an important role in accurately assessing myocardial function and then further monitoring it over time. For reasons of availability, safety and portability, TTE is the gold standard for evaluation of LV size, wall thickness and systolic function. Echocardiography has been the technique of choice for major clinical trials evaluating drug and device treatments in heart failure, revascularization and valve disease. The principle parameter for defining LV systolic function is LV ejection fraction. This is the volume of blood the LV ejects with each heart beat expressed as a percentage of the total volume of blood in the heart at end diastole. The value is determined by modified biplane Simpson technique which involves planimetry of the endocardial border in diastole and end systole (Fig. 7.10). An assumption is then made that ventricular volume is the sum of the volumes of adjacent sets of discs of varying depth and cross sectional area.

Tissue Doppler and deformation imaging with speckle tracking allow evaluation of subclinical cardiac dysfunction but clinical use remains unclear at this stage.

Pregnancy and Marfan Syndrome

Pregnancy and the postpartum period is a high risk time for aortic dissection and rupture in women with Marfan syndrome. The increased risk may be due to increased arterial wall stress associated with the hypervolemic and hyperdynamic circulatory state, or hormonal effects on aortic wall composition [29, 30]. Aortic root dilatation then leads to worsening aortic regurgitation. There is increased risk of aortic dissection with aortic root dilatation in pregnant women with Marfan syndrome, although a normal dimension does not exclude the possibility of dissection [30–32]. The risk of aortic rupture or dissection during pregnancy is difficult to quantify, as limited data are available.

A woman with Marfan syndrome who is contemplating pregnancy should have a screening transthoracic echocardiogram for assessment of aortic root, ascending aorta dimensions, and assessment of possible associated valve or myocardial disease. In addition, imaging of the entire aorta by computed tomography or magnetic resonance imaging, as well as specialist clinical consultation is highly recommended.

Serial clinical assessment should include echocardiographic monitoring in all pregnant women with Marfan syndrome, even among women with baseline aortic root diameter ≤40 mm [33, 34]. The frequency of clinical and imaging follow-up should be individualised depending on patient characteristics. The European Society of Cardiology Guidelines suggest repeat echocardiographic imaging every 4–8 weeks during pregnancy in patients with aortic root or ascending aorta dilatation (diameter >40 mm) [35]. Similarly, the ACC/AHA/AATS guidelines recommend monthly or bimonthly echocardiographic measurement of the aortic root and ascending aortic dimensions in this setting [6].

As noted in the ESC and ACC/AHA/AATS guidelines, magnetic resonance imaging is recommended over computed tomography (CT) for pregnant women with aortic arch, descending or abdominal aortic dilatation, to avoid exposing the mother and fetus to ionizing radiation. The risk of dissection or other serious complications such as heart failure has been estimated to be approximately 1 % in women with Marfan syndrome with an aortic root diameter ≤40 mm. Women with Marfan syndrome with an aortic root diameter >40 mm or rapidly increasing aortic root size are at increased risk of dissection and adverse cardiovascular outcomes [33, 34].

For women with Marfan syndrome with an aortic root diameter ≥45 mm (or >27 mm/m^2), the 2014 ESC guidelines suggest elective repair prior to conception, although limited supporting data are available [33, 34]. This approach differs somewhat from the ACC/AHA/AATS guidelines suggesting that elective repair is reasonable if the aortic diameter exceeds 40 mm in women with Marfan syndrome who are contemplating pregnancy [6]. Although the risk of ascending aortic dissection is reduced with successful surgical correction, there is a risk of aortic dissection in the remaining aorta during subsequent pregnancies [34, 35].

Due to the increased risk of aortic dissection postpartum, the monitoring of patients with Marfan syndrome for complications during the first 4–6 weeks postpartum is very important. Postpartum follow-up may range from one visit for low risk patients to weekly follow-up with imaging during the first few weeks for high risk patients.

The more detailed description of pregnancy management in Marfan patients can be found in Chap. 9.

Echo After Surgery

All patients with Marfan syndrome require lifelong surveillance regardless of the type of surgical procedure they underwent.

After elective surgery and with stable aortic size, a yearly echo and CMR (every 2–3 years) of the thorax are performed to check the condition of the remaining aorta.

After acute dissection or surgical repair of chronic dissection, an initial check-up should be scheduled every 3 months, then every 1–2 years, and include echo and CMR/CT scan of the thorax [17].

In patients who underwent additional aortic or mitral surgery, a complete baseline clinical assessment including echocardiographic examination should be performed 6–12 weeks after surgery [36]. This assessment is of the utmost importance in excluding potential early complications i.e., endocarditis by interpreting clinical changes in symptoms, murmurs and prosthetic sounds. It is important to assess ventricular function, transvalvular gradients to exclude stenosis and paravalvular regurgitation. Transvalvular gradients are best interpreted in comparison with the baseline values, rather than in comparison with theoretical values for a given prosthesis.

Transthoracic echocardiogram should also be performed if any new symptoms occur at any point after valve replacement or if complications are suspected. TOE should be considered in cases of suspected prosthetic dysfunction or endocarditis.

References

1. Otto CM. The textbook of clinical echocardiography. 5th ed. Philadelphia: Elsevier Saunders; 2013. p. 420–2.
2. Roman MJ, Devereux RB, Kramer-Fox R, O'Laughlin JE. Two-dimensional echocardiographic aortic root dimensions in normal children and adults. Am J Cardiol. 1989;64:507–12.
3. Davies RR, Gallo A, Coady MA, Tellides G, Botta DM, Burke B, Coe MP, Kopf GS, Elefteriades JA. Novel measurement of relative aortic size predicts rupture of thoracic aortic aneurysms. Ann Thorac Surg. 2006;81:169–77.
4. Glesby MJ, Pyeritz RE. Association of mitral valve prolapse and systemic abnormalities of connective tissue: a phenotypic continuum. JAMA. 1989;262:523–8.
5. Legget ME, Unger TA, O'Sullivan CK, Zwink TR, Bennett RL, Byers PH, Otto CM. Aortic root complications in Marfan's syndrome: identification of a lower risk group. Heart. 1996;75:389–95.
6. Hiratzka LF, Bakris GL, Beckman JA, et al. ACCF/AHA/AATS/ACR/ASA/SCA/SCAI/SIR/STS/SVM guidelines for the diagnosis and management of patients with thoracic aortic disease. A report of the American College of Cardiology Foundation/American Heart Association Task Force on Practice Guidelines, American Association for Thoracic Surgery, American College of Radiology, American Stroke Association, Society of Cardiovascular Anesthesiologists, Society for Cardiovascular Angiography and Interventions, Society of Interventional Radiology, Society of Thoracic Surgeons, and Society for Vascular Medicine. J Am Coll Cardiol. 2010;55:e27.
7. Baumgartner H, Bonhoeffer P, De Groot NM, de Haan F, Deanfield JE, Galie N, Gatzoulis MA, Gohlke-Baerwolf C, Kaemmerer H, Kilner P, Meijboom F, Mulder BJ, Oechslin E, Oliver JM, Serraf A, Szatmari A, Thaulow E, Vouhe PR, Walma E, Task Force on the Management of

Grown-up Congenital Heart Disease of the European Society of Cardiology (ESC), Association for European Paediatric Cardiology (AEPC), ESC Committee for Practice Guidelines (CPG). ESC Guidelines for the management of grown-up congenital heart disease (new version 2010). Eur Heart J. 2010;31(23):2915–57.
8. Hagan PG, Nienaber CA, Isselbacher EM, et al. The International Registry of Acute Aortic Dissection (IRAD): new insights into an old disease. JAMA. 2000;283:897–903.
9. Lang RM, Badano LP, Mor-Avi V, Afilalo J, Armstrong A, Ernande L, Flachskampf FA, Foster E, Goldstein SA, Kuznetsova T, Lancellotti P, Muraru D, Picard MH, Rietzschel ER, Rudski L, Spencer KT, Tsang W, Voigt JU. Recommendations for cardiac chamber quantification by echocardiography in adults: an update from the American Society of Echocardiography and the European Association of Cardiovascular Imaging. Eur Heart J Cardiovasc Imaging. 2015;16(3):233–70.
10. Burman ED, Keegan J, Kilner PJ. Aortic root measurement by cardiovascular magnetic resonance: specification of planes and lines of measurement and corresponding normal values. Circ Cardiovasc Imaging. 2008;1(2):104–13.
11. Goldstein SA, Evangelista A, Abbara S, Arai A, Asch FM, Badano LP, Bolen MA, Connolly HM, Cuéllar-Calàbria H, Czerny M, Devereux RB, Erbel RA, Fattori R, Isselbacher EM, Lindsay JM, McCulloch M, Michelena HI, Nienaber CA, Oh JK, Pepi M, Taylor AJ, Weinsaft JW, Zamorano JL, Dietz H, Eagle K, Elefteriades J, Jondeau G, Rousseau H, Schepens M. Multimodality imaging of diseases of the thoracic aorta in adults: from the American Society of Echocardiography and the European Association of Cardiovascular Imaging: endorsed by the Society of Cardiovascular Computed Tomography and Society for Cardiovascular Magnetic Resonance. J Am Soc Echocardiogr. 2015;28(2):119–82.
12. Gueret P, Senechal C, Roudaut R. Comparison of trans- esophageal and transthoracic echocardiography in acute aortic dissection. A multicenter prospective study. J Am Coll Cardiol. 1991;17(2s1):A260–A260. doi:10.1016/0735-1097(91)92008-A.
13. Loeys BL, Dietz HC, Braverman AC, et al. The revised Ghent nosology for the Marfan syndrome. J Med Genet. 2010;47(7):476–85. doi:10.1136/jmg.2009.072785.
14. Mintz GS, Kotler MN, Segal BL, Parry WR. Two dimensional echocardiographic recognition of the descending thoracic aorta. Am J Cardiol. 1979;44:232–8.
15. Khandheria BK, Tajik AJ, Taylor CL, Safford RE, Miller Jr FA, Stanson AW, Sinak LJ, Oh JK, Seward JB. Aortic dissection: review of value and limitations of two- dimensional echocardiography in a six-year experience. J Am Soc Echocardiogr. 1989;2:17–24.
16. Iliceto S, Ettorre G, Francioso G, Antonelli G, Biasco G, Rizzon P. Diagnosis of aneurysm of the thoracic aorta. Comparison between two non invasive techniques: two-dimensional echocardiography and computed tomography. Eur Heart J. 1984;5:545–55.
17. Erbel R, Aboyans V, Boileau C, Bossone E, Bartolomeo RD, Eggebrecht H, Evangelista A, Falk V, Frank H, Gaemperli O, Grabenwöger M, Haverich A, Iung B, Manolis AJ, Meijboom F, Nienaber CA, Roffi M, Rousseau H, Sechtem U, Sirnes PA, Allmen RS, Vrints CJ. 2014 ESC guidelines on the diagnosis and treatment of aortic diseases: document covering acute and chronic aortic diseases of the thoracic and abdominal aorta of the adult. The Task Force for the Diagnosis and Treatment of Aortic Diseases of the European Society of Cardiology (ESC). ESC Committee for Practice Guidelines. Eur Heart J. 2014;35(41):2873–2926.
18. Kunkala MR, Schaff HV, Li Z, Volguina I, Dietz HC, LeMaire SA, Coselli JS, Connolly H. Mitral valve disease in patients with Marfan syndrome undergoing aortic root replacement. Circulation. 2013;128:S243–7.
19. Erbel R, Alfonso F, Boileau C, Dirsch O, Eber B, Haverich A, Rakowski H, Struyven J, Radegran K, Sechtem U, Taylor J, Zollikofer CH. Internal reviewers: Klein WW, Mulder B, Providencia LA. Diagnosis and management of aortic dissection. Recommendations of the Task Force on Aortic Dissection, European Society of Cardiology. Eur Heart J. 2001;22:1642–81.
20. Taub CC, Stoler JM, Perez-Sanz T, Chu J, Isselbacher EM, Picard MH, Weyman AE. Mitral valve prolapse in Marfan syndrome: an old topic revisited. Echocardiography. 2009;26:357–64.
21. Hayek E, Gring CN, Griffin BP. Mitral valve prolapse. Lancet. 2005;365:507–18.

22. Détaint D, Faivre L, Collod-Beroud G, Child AH, Loeys BL, Binquet C, Gautier E, Arbustini E, Mayer K, Arslan-Kirchner M, Stheneur C, Halliday D, Beroud C, Bonithon-Kopp C, Claustres M, Plauchu H, Robinson PN, Kiotsekoglou A, De Backer J, Adès L, Francke U, De Paepe A, Boileau C, Jondeau G. Cardiovascular manifestations in men and women carrying a FBN1 mutation. Eur Heart J. 2010;31:2223–9.
23. Freed LA, Levy D, Levine RA, Larson MG, Evans JC, Fuller DL, Lehman B, Benjamin EJ. Prevalence and clinical outcome of mitral-valve prolapse. N Engl J Med. 1999;341:1–7.
24. Kogure K. Pathology of chronic mitral valvular disease in the dog. Nihon Juigaku Zasshi. 1980;42:323–35.
25. Wilcken DE, Hickey AJ. Lifetime risk for patients with mitral valve prolapse of developing severe valve regurgitation requiring surgery. Circulation. 1988;78:10–14.
26. Hickey AJ, Wilcken DE, Wright JS, Warren BA. Primary (spontaneous) chordal rupture: relation to myxomatous valve disease and mitral valve prolapse. J Am Coll Cardiol. 1985;5:1341–6.
27. Barreiro CJ, Patel ND, Fitton TP, Williams JA, Bonde PN, Chan V, Alejo DE, Gott VL, Baumgartner WA. Aortic valve replacement and concomitant mitral valve regurgitation in the elderly: impact on survival and functional outcome. Circulation. 2005;112:I443–7.
28. Kiotsekoglou A, Sutherland GR, Moggridge JC, Nassiri DK, Camm AJ, Child AH. The unravelling of primary myocardial impairment in Marfan syndrome by modern echocardiography. Heart. 2009;95(19):1561–6.
29. Meijboom LJ, Nollen GJ, Merchant N, et al. Frequency of coronary ostial aneurysms after aortic root surgery in patients with the Marfan syndrome. Am J Cardiol. 2002;89:1135–1138.
30. Elkayam U, Ostrzega E, Shotan A, Mehra A. Cardiovascular problems in pregnant women with the Marfan syndrome. Ann Intern Med. 1995;123:117–122.
31. Rossiter JP, Repke JT, Morales AJ, et al. A prospective longitudinal evaluation of pregnancy in the Marfan syndrome. Am J Obstet Gynecol. 1995;173:1599–1606.
32. Lipscomb KJ, Smith JC, Clarke B, et al. Outcome of pregnancy in women with Marfan's syndrome. Br J Obstet Gynaecol. 1997;104:201–206.
33. European Society of Gynecology (ESG), Association for European Paediatric Cardiology (AEPC), German Society for Gender Medicine (DGesGM), et al. ESC guidelines on the management of cardiovascular diseases during pregnancy: the Task Force on the Management of Cardiovascular Diseases during Pregnancy of the European Society of Cardiology (ESC). Eur Heart J. 2011;32(24):3147–3197.
34. Bonow RO, Carabello BA, Chatterjee K, et al. 2008 focused update incorporated into the ACC/AHA 2006 guidelines for the management of patients with valvular heart disease: a report of the American College of Cardiology/American Heart Association Task Force on Practice Guidelines (Writing Committee to revise the 1998 guidelines for the management of patients with valvular heart disease): endorsed by the Society of Cardiovascular Anesthesiologists, Society for Cardiovascular Angiography and Interventions, and Society of Thoracic Surgeons. Circulation. 2008;52(13):e1–142.
35. Meijboom LJ, Vos FE, Timmermans J, et al. Pregnancy and aortic root growth in the Marfan syndrome: a prospective study. Eur Heart J. 2005;26(9):914–920.
36. Vahanian A, Alfieri O, Andreotti F, Antunes MJ, Barón-Esquivias G, Baumgartner H, Borger MA, Carrel TP, De Bonis M, Evangelista A, Falk V, Iung B, Lancellotti P, Pierard L, Price S, Schäfers HJ, Schuler G, Stepinska J, Swedberg K, Takkenberg J, Von Oppell UO, Windecker S, Zamorano JL, Zembala M. Guidelines on the management of valvular heart disease (version 2012). Joint Task Force on the Management of Valvular Heart Disease of the European Society of Cardiology (ESC); European Association for Cardio-Thoracic Surgery (EACTS). Eur Heart J. 2012;33(19):2451–96.

8 Cardiovascular Magnetic Resonance in Marfan Syndrome

Ee Ling Heng and Raad H. Mohiaddin

Introduction

The cardiovascular features and complications of Marfan syndrome (MFS) consist of a spectrum of valvular, myocardial and great vessel pathologies, which require screening and lifelong serial surveillance. Ninety-five percent of deaths in MFS are related to cardiovascular manifestations, with aortic dissection accounting for the most common cause of cardiovascular related mortality [1–3]. Cardiovascular complications are less readily detectable at the early stages compared to ocular and skeletal manifestations, as patients are typically asymptomatic. This brings into focus the relevance of early diagnosis and timely intervention to prevent potentially catastrophic adverse outcomes including death.

Multiple imaging modalities are utilised in the longterm care of MFS patients, but each with their own caveats. Chest radiography is often of limited value in this condition, as the proximal ascending aorta is not well visualised and its temporal sensitivity is poor. Transthoracic echocardiography whilst readily available may pose considerable technical challenges when acoustic windows are limited by the presence of chest wall deformities, thereby preventing comprehensive and reproducible visualisation of the aorta for monitoring dilatation or diagnosing dissection. Computer tomography and cardiac catheterisation are able to supersede the limitations of echocardiography, but suffer the pitfalls of being invasive, involve ionising radiation and contrast media administration. These issues have therefore paved the way for an expanding role for cardiovascular magnetic resonance (CMR) in this patient group.

E.L. Heng, MBBS, BSc, MRCP • R.H. Mohiaddin, FRCR, FRCP, FESC, PhD (✉)
NIHR Cardiovascular Biomedical Research Unit, Royal Brompton and Harefield NHS Foundation Trust and Imperial College London, London, UK
e-mail: e.heng@rbht.nhs.uk; R.Mohiaddin@rbht.nhs.uk

© Springer-Verlag London 2016

A.H. Child (ed.), *Diagnosis and Management of Marfan Syndrome*,
DOI 10.1007/978-1-4471-5442-6_8

CMR is a versatile imaging modality that allows visualisation of the cardiovascular system in any plane with the option for three-dimensional acquisitions and reconstruction; is non-invasive and does not involve x-ray irradiation. CMR is particularly well-suited for the surveillance of individuals with MFS, who invariably require regular imaging from childhood to adolescence and throughout adult life, including child-bearing years in young adult women. CMR eliminates the radiation exposure, which would otherwise be associated with computer tomography surveillance of the aorta. However, the use of CMR is limited in acute clinical settings, due to variable scanner access and longer acquisition times when compared to computer tomography.

Principles of CMR

Understanding the basic principles and details of magnetic resonance imaging (MRI) is invaluable in appreciating the capabilities of the technique and these have been well described many times [4, 5]. Most magnetic resonance studies are of the hydrogen nuclei (protons) in water. Protons spin on their axes and generate a tiny magnetic field and behave as a small magnet, which will align with an applied magnetic field and precess about the field in the same way that a spinning top precesses in a gravitational field (Fig. 8.1). Applying radio waves at the resonance frequency, however, excites some protons to the higher energy antiparallel orientation and these protons initially precess in phase together. The net effect is to rotate the net magnetisation vector at an angle to the applied field, and this initial flip angle is determined by the amount of energy applied. After absorption of energy, the net magnetisation vector precesses and relaxes back to its equilibrium position tracing out a spiral. The rates at which the net magnetisation parallel and perpendicular to the applied field return to equilibrium after a disturbance are called the longitudinal (T_1) and transverse (T_2) relaxation times respectively. They depend upon the fluctuating magnetic fields experienced by the nuclei, and hence upon their biochemical and biophysical environment.

The image is also influenced by the type of imaging sequence used and blood flow in the area of interest. Blood flow effects partly result in the black blood appearance with spin echo imaging, in contrast to gradient echo imaging that produces images in which blood appears white. Spin echo imaging is static and therefore used to delineate cardiovascular anatomy, whilst cine gradient echo images generally relate to cardiac function and blood flow [6].

CMR Sequences

Scanning sequences are necessary to produce images, with components comprising preparation and excitation pulses (to generate contrast between tissues and localise excitation areas), gradient and magnetic field pulses (to form images) followed by

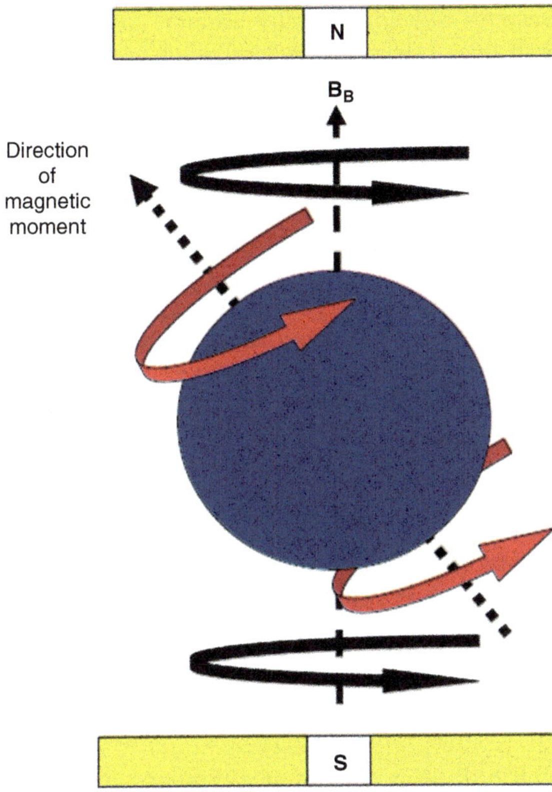

Fig. 8.1 A proton with magnetic moment due to its spin (*red arrows*) approximately aligns with and precesses around the direction of an external magnetic field (B_B)

signal read-outs for data collection. Multiple sequences are acquired in MFS patients to ensure thorough evaluation of the aorta, ventricular function and concomitant valvular pathology. Common sequences applied include:
Spin-echo black blood imaging: delineates aortic anatomy and morphology, in addition to assessing the aortic wall for haematoma or thickening. This sequence is acquired with ECG-gating at end-diastole, sometimes with double-inversion recovery techniques that null the blood signal. Black blood imaging can be repeated after gadolinium administration to identify vessel wall enhancement.

White blood imaging: performed with gradient echo sequences or balanced steady-state free precession (SSFP) techniques. The cine images generated enable measurements to determine ventricular volumes and function, change in aortic diameters between scans and assessment of valvular function by demonstrating turbulent blood flow. Multi-slice static gradient echo sequences may also be acquired in place of black blood images to display cardiovascular anatomy.

Phase contrast velocity mapping: usually acquired to evaluate gradients and blood flow across an area of stenosis or regurgitation. Image contrast is produced by differences in blood flow velocities, which generates two-dimensional images from which peak flow and velocity measurements can be calculated, in addition to plotting time-flow and time-velocity curves. To improve the accuracy of measurements made through a plane transecting a large vessel, correction of background phase offset errors by phase contrast imaging of a static phantom may be required [7].

Contrast-enhanced MR angiography (CE-MRA): T1-weighted spoiled gradient echo imaging performed with intravenous administration of gadolinium contrast to produce a 3D angiogram of the aorta and arch vessels. The contrast administered causes T1 shortening and provides greater signal in the arterial or venous system, thereby enhancing the vessel-to-background contrast-to-noise ratio. Careful timing of image acquisition is necessary to optimise peak enhancement in the vascular system of interest. Maximum intensity projection (MIP) images can then be reconstructed to provide detailed vascular delineation. Although CE-MRA is regarded as the standard technique for imaging the thoracic aorta [8], its application is limited by the need for contrast agents, which restricts its use in patients with renal failure. The acquired images are non ECG gated and image quality may be compromised by suboptimal patient compliance with breath-holds and pulsation artefacts of the aortic root and proximal ascending aorta due to cardiac motion.

Three-dimensional bSSFP: Non-contrast, free-breathing, diaphragmatic navigator and ECG-gated technique [9] which overcomes the limitations of CE-MRA as outlined in the previous section. Numerous respiratory tracking algorithms [10, 11] have been developed, which have resulted in superior image quality of the aortic root [12, 13] compared to CE-MRA, albeit with comparatively slower acquisition times. There is ongoing work seeking to improve scan efficiency for 3D-bSSFP methods.

Gadolinium-enhanced imaging: inversion recovery sequences that are usually taken early after gadolinium contrast administration (~2 min) enable differentiation of slow flow phenomena from thrombus within the cardiac chambers or within the false lumen if a dissection flap is present.

Late gadolinium enhancement with image acquisition from ~10 min post contrast also allows the detection of infarcted myocardium and/or myocardial fibrosis, by exploiting the properties of gadolinium contrast. Kinetic and partition properties of gadolinium cause it to linger in the extracellular space, concentrating in areas of cell necrosis or fibrosis as a result of local extracellular expansion. The signal intensity of normal myocardium can be set to zero with varied inversion times, which leads to high signal intensities in infarcted and fibrotic areas [14].

A proposed CMR protocol for MFS is outlined in Table 8.1. This can be used in part or in its entirety on a case by case scenario [15, 16]:

Table 8.1 CMR protocol with recommended sequences, and optional sequences to be considered for inclusion in *italics*

Localisers and multislice scouts	Half-fourier single shot turbo spin echo or multislice SSFP stacks in transaxial/coronal/sagittal views
SSFP cines	Two and four chamber views
	Short-axis stack encompassing LV and RV
	LVOT views and aortic valve
	Aortic arch (in 'candy/hockey stick' view)
	Mitral valve stack
	Aortic sinus stack
Velocity mapping	Aortic flow (assessment of AR)
	Flow through true vs false lumen if dissection present *(optional)*
Turbo spin echo (T1/T2)	Vessel wall assessment in transaxial/sagittal oblique slices *(optional)*
3D SSFP CE-MRA	Aortic arch and branch vessels assessment
Late Gadolinium Enhancement	LV scar assessment in long axis and short axis stack views *(optional)*

AR aortic regurgitation, *CE-MRA* Contrast-enhanced magnetic resonance angiography, *LV* left ventricle, *LVOT* left ventricular outflow tract, *RV* right ventricle, *SSFP* steady-state free precession, *3D* three-dimensional

Role of CMR in Marfan Syndrome

CMR is central in providing diagnostic and follow-up imaging data in patients with MFS. Current European guidelines recommend dual imaging modalities for diagnosis and surveillance in MFS, with the second modality being either CMR or computer tomography, during which the entire aorta should be imaged at baseline [17]. Thereafter, CMR should be repeated at least once every 5 years if the aortic dimensions beyond the root are normal. When there is known aneurysm formation, CMR should be undertaken at least annually. European and American guidelines advocate more frequent imaging if the maximal aortic diameter >4.5 cm or if significant growth from baseline is evident [17–19].

The response to medical therapy in MFS can be evaluated with CMR. Pharmacotherapy is targeted at reducing the rate of aortic dilatation and risk of aortic dissection with beta-blockers and angiotensin receptor blockers (via angiotension converting enzyme (ACE) inhibitors or angiotensin II receptor antagonists). An early randomised controlled trial investigated the effects of beta-blockade on aortic root diameters as determined by echocardiography, with propanolol appearing to retard the rate of aortic dilatation [20]. The study findings prompted numerous further studies, and propelled beta-blocker into the mainstay of medical treatment in MFS. However, subsequent meta-analyses have reported inconsistencies in the beneficial effects of beta-blockers [21–23]. Angiotensin II and Type 2 receptor expression are known to be increased in MFS aortas and associated with cystic medial degeneration [24]. ACE inhibitors and angiotensin II receptor antagonists have therefore been trialled in MFS, with evidence of reduction in aortic stiffness and aortic root diameters when prescribed in isolation or combined with beta-blockade [25, 26]. There was no clear benefit of an angiotensin II receptor over beta-blockade in a recent head-to-head analysis [27]. Current drug therapy trials in MFS examining the impact of losartan and combination therapy have either incorporated CMR into the study protocol or chosen CMR as the primary imaging technique for assessing aortic dilatation rates as outcome measures of therapeutic effectiveness [28–30].

CMR is the technique of choice for longterm follow-up after surgical intervention in MFS for the surveillance of new aneurysm formation or further dissection. Whilst computer tomography provides similar accuracy to CMR, the need for potentially nephrotoxic contrast media and ionising radiation exposure limits its repeated application. Furthermore, CMR is recognised to have an equivalent sensitivity and specificity to computer tomography for the diagnosis of suspected aortic dissection, but is more accurate when the pre-test probability is high [31]. When transoesophageal echocardiography was compared directly with CMR, a better specificity of CMR was demonstrated due to lower false positive rates. If aortic dissection is present, CMR allows concurrent evaluation of the aortic valve for cusp involvement and quantification of aortic regurgitation (if present). The entry and exit points of a dissected aorta can usually be identified by gradient echo images with velocity measurements. Velocity mapping seals the diagnosis by demonstrating differences in flow velocities in the true and false lumina.

Advantages and Limitations of CMR in Marfan Syndrome

The main strengths of CMR arise from its multi-planar image acquisition approach without the use of ionising radiation, thereby allowing biventricular volume and functional measurement regardless of cardiac chamber anatomy which may be distorted by associated skeletal malformations. Specific to MFS, CMR is able to identify anatomical variants of aortic dissection, as well as assess involvement of vascular branches and the aortic valve. It is also unrivalled as a non-invasive technique for tissue characterisation, particularly for the detection and quantification of myocardial fibrosis.

In spite of its numerous advantages, the use of CMR is not ubiquitous as it is contraindicated in patients with claustrophobia, metallic implants (such as some types of cerebral aneurysm clips) and non MR-conditional pacemakers. A comprehensive resource for magnetic resonance safety can be obtained at mrisafety.com. The need for patient co-operation and longer scan times in contrast to computer tomography restricts its use in unstable patients when they present as emergencies. When focussed on aortic assessment, CMR is not always able to evaluate aortic valve calcification of anchoring zones. Image quality in CMR is dependent upon optimisation of multiple sequence parameters, and an operator learning curve is therefore inevitable and should be taken into consideration [15]. Lastly, the administration of gadolinium based contrast in patients with severe renal impairment (estimated glomerular filtration rate <30 ml/min) is recognised as a potential risk for nephrogenic systemic fibrosis [32]. However, the risk is very small particularly when using more stable cyclic compounds.

Specific Applications of CMR in Marfan Syndrome

Anatomy and Function

Cardiac and vascular anatomical details can be demonstrated by CMR in any plane in patients with MFS. Images in standardised views can be planned from transaxial, coronal and sagittal multislice series. Extra-cardiac features of MFS can sometimes be visualised within the field of view of CMR, providing additional anatomical information. For example, skeletal abnormalities (such as scoliosis and pectus excavatum) can result in thoracic cavity distortion and displacement of the heart in this patient cohort, which then adversely impacts upon ventricular function (Fig. 8.2). Features of dural ectasia may also be visible on sagittal and coronal acquisitions in which the lumbosacral spine is imaged alongside the heart [33, 34].

CMR is considered the gold standard for biventricular volumetric and functional measurement. Ventricular volumes can be derived from the summation of disks

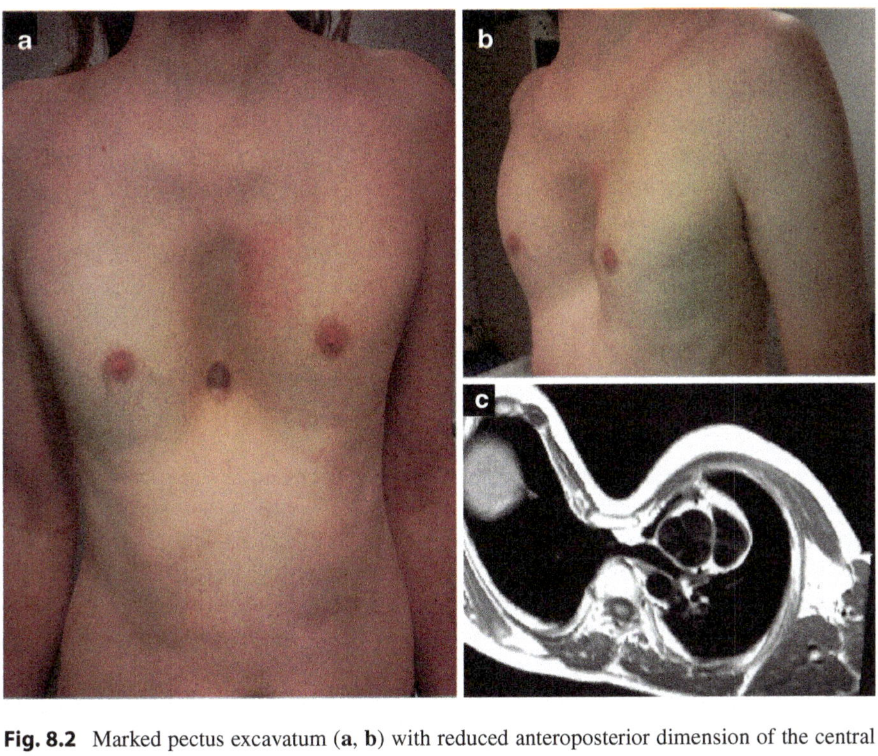

Fig. 8.2 Marked pectus excavatum (**a**, **b**) with reduced anteroposterior dimension of the central thorax seen on transaxial turbo spin-echo imaging (**c**)

method, either by manual planimetry or semi-automated segmentation software (Fig. 8.3). Volumetric analysis by manual planimetry involves delineating the epicardial and endocardial borders at end-diastole, as well as endocardial borders at end-systole. Simpson's rule is then used to derive volumes and mass, with subtraction of systolic volume from diastolic volume to obtain ejection fraction [35]. Manual contouring is time consuming and has been largely replaced by a variety of semi-automated segmentation software in which similar principles are applied. When interpreting ventricular volumes and function, it is worth noting that different imaging sequences produce systematic differences in measurements. SSFP imaging tends to produce slightly larger ventricular volumes and stroke volumes with smaller ventricular mass, possibly related to superior contrast between myocardium and the blood pool compared to gradient echo cine sequences [36]. Normative reference values should therefore be applied specific to the sequence.

Cardiomyopathy

In Marfan patients, there has been growing awareness of a Marfan-associated cardiomyopathy since the first description of myocardial involvement in 1985 [37], with subsequent identification of a dilated cardiomyopathy phenotype [38, 39]. Mild biventricular impairment of ejection fraction and elevated volumes as quantified by CMR has been reported in asymptomatic MFS patients without significant valvular abnormalities [40, 41]. CMR is advantageous over echocardiography in evaluating these often subtle changes in Marfan patients with superior reproducibility and therefore lower sample sizes required to demonstrate clinically relevant changes in LV size and function [42]. This clinical entity has also been recognised in a small subset of patients with MFS who have undergone cardiac surgery [43].

Whilst ventricular impairment seen in patients with MFS may relate directly to myocardial factors, it is worth recognising that pectus excavatum may independently cause ventricular dysfunction through sternal compression which causes cardiac geometric distortion. This then negatively impacts upon cardiopulmonary function, which can be improved or partially reversed by surgical correction with the Nuss procedure [44, 45].

Vascular

CMR vascular assessment in a patient with MFS is focussed on the vulnerable aorta, which is subjected to endothelial shear and intrinsic wall stresses, which over time leads to thinning of the aortic wall that dilates and loses distensibility. This sequence of events directly increases the risk of aneurysm formation throughout the course of the aorta, but particularly at the aortic root (Fig. 8.4) [38]. There is a male preponderance of aortic dilatation and subsequent dissection. The risk of aortic dilatation and dissection increases with age and aortic diameters, with aortic dilatation present in 96 % of MFS patients with a fibrillin 1 (FBN1) mutation by the age of 60 years [46]. Aortic dilatation remains the best predictor for a future aortic event [47], and meticulous measurements and surveillance are therefore paramount.

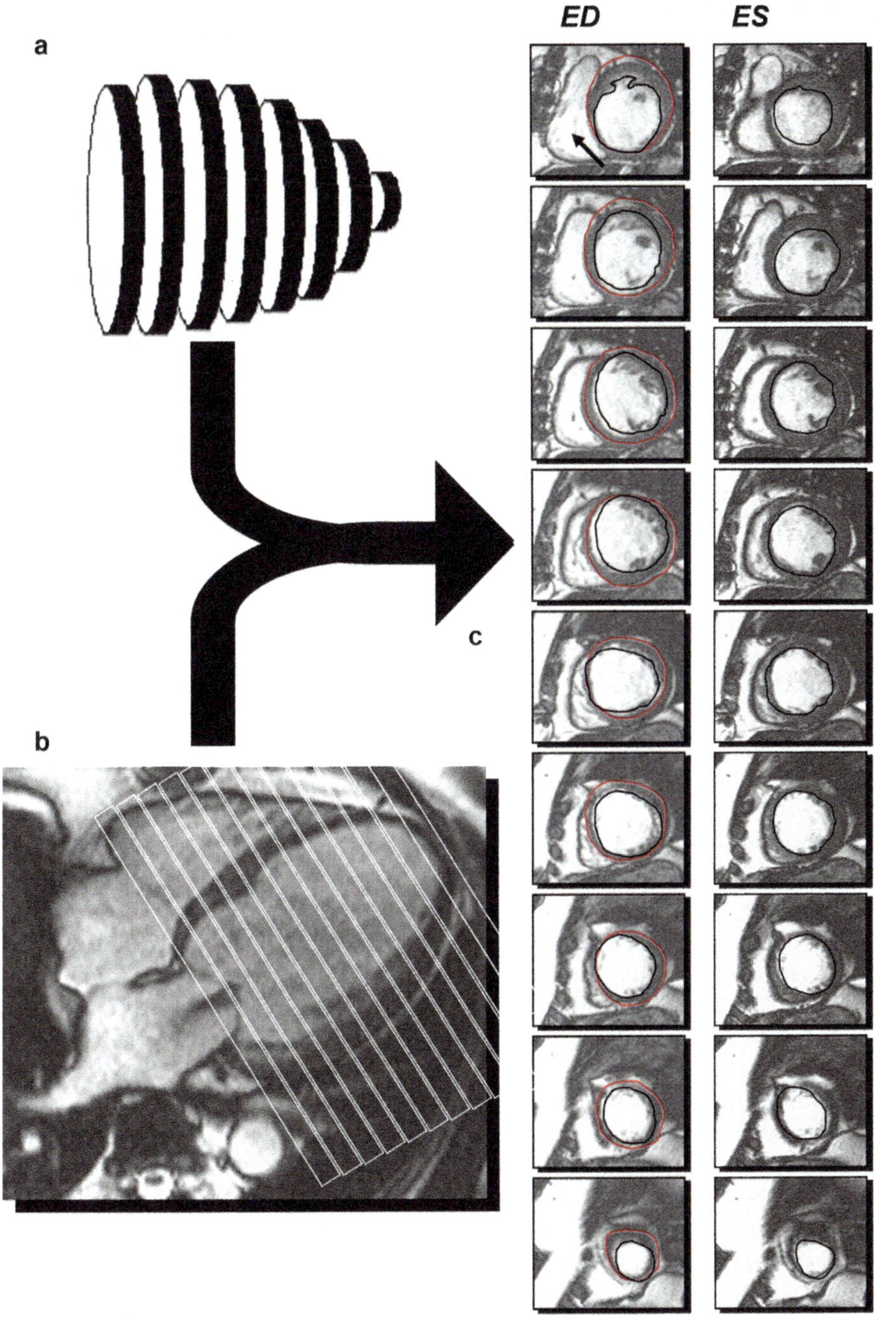

Fig. 8.3 Volumetric analysis with CMR by summation of disks method (for which pre-defined slice thickness are illustrated in panels **a** and **b**, which are then acquired to produce the corresponding short-axis stack shown in panel **c**. Each row in panel c represents a single level acquisition). The epicardial (in *red*) and endocardial (in *black*) borders in diastole and endocardial borders in systole are then delineated. *ED* end diastole, *ES* end systole

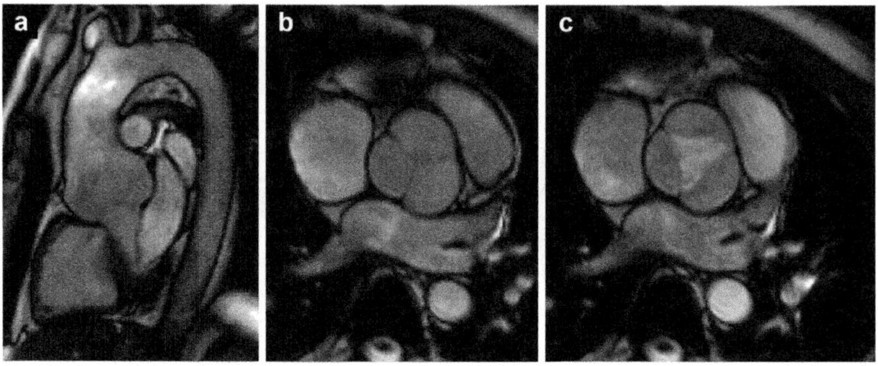

Fig. 8.4 Dilated aortic root at sinus level (**a**) with 'en face' view of aortic valve sinuses in end diastole (**b**) and end systole (**c**)

Decision making for timing of surgical intervention often relies on serial CMR-derived measurements. Measurement of aortic diameters should be made perpendicular to the longitudinal or flow axis of the aorta and at standard anatomic locations to avoid serial measurement error. Guidelines recommend that the external diameter of the aorta should be measured with CMR and the widest aortic root diameter (usually at mid-sinus level) should be quoted [19]. However, internal diameters are still measured for continuity in selected centres [16].

Apart from imaging the aorta, it is also important to visualise the main and branch pulmonary arteries as dilatation of the main pulmonary artery occurs in >10 % of MFS patients, although associated pulmonary trunk aneurysms are rare.

The Aorta: Aortic Aneurysm and Dissection

An aneurysm is a 'permanent localised dilatation of the artery', which increases by ≥50 % of the expected normal diameter as defined by the American guidelines [19]. Aortic dilatation in MFS typically affects the aortic root and proximal ascending aorta with effacement of the sinotubular junction. Asymmetrical aortic root dilatation which is often seen in MFS may be implicated in aortic root dissection [48].

The aorta is particularly well visualised with CMR due to its size, relative immobility and natural contrast between the vessel wall and moving blood within it. When an aortic aneurysm is known of or suspected, CMR enables accurate localisation, delineation of the extent of the aneurysm(s) and its relation to neighbouring branch vessels (Fig. 8.5). Luminal dimensions of aneurysms can be measured and compared between carefully aligned serial scans in similar planes to establish progression (that is, rate of change). When comparisons of successive aortic dimensions are to be taken, it is vital not only to consider equivalent image planes, but to ensure that these are acquired in similar phases of the cardiac cycle with ideally the same sequence type (be it black-blood imaging, SSFP cine images, contrast-enhanced MRA or 3D SSFP). Reference values are available for CMR-derived aortic root and aortic dimensions with sinus-sinus and sinus-commissure measurements shown to be comparable with echocardiographic data [49–51]. In addition,

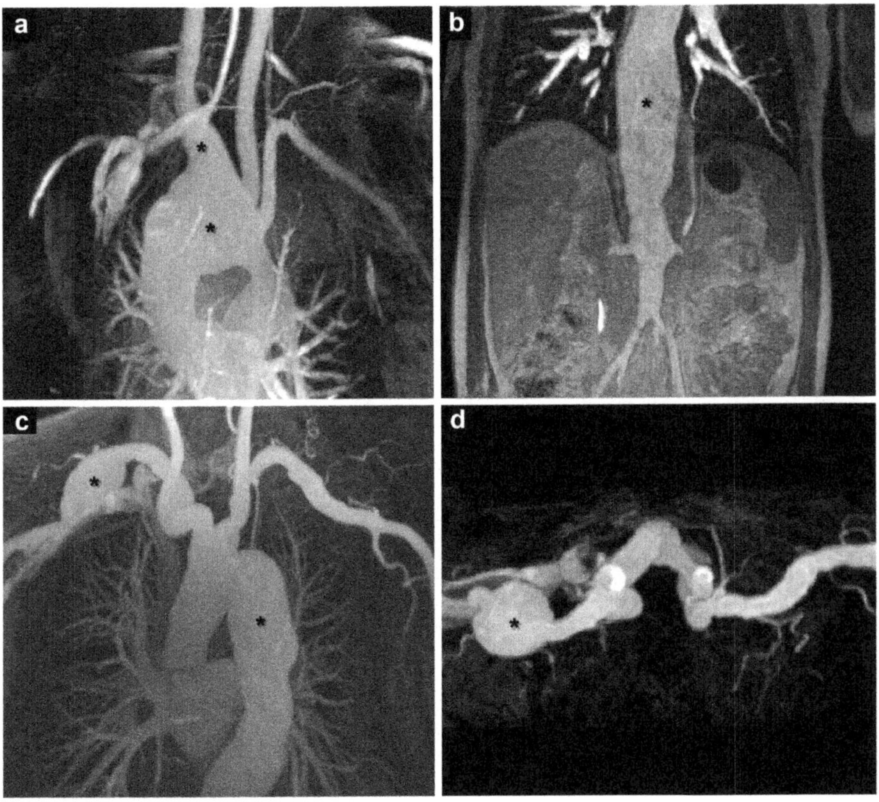

Fig. 8.5 Coronal orientation maximal intensity projection (MIP) images from contrast-enhanced MR angiography illustrating aneurysms of the ascending, descending and abdominal aorta, with involvement of the brachiocephalic artery in the same patient with Marfan syndrome (aneurysms marked *) in panels **a** and **b**. Right subclavian artery and descending aortic aneurysms in second patient with Marfan syndrome in coronal (panel **c**) and transaxial (panel **d**) reconstructions

non-contrast 3D-navigated balanced SSFP sequences can be acquired as a promising alternative method for accurate and reproducible aortic measurements [9, 52].

CMR examination of a suspected aortic dissection should provide diagnostic information that includes anatomical delineation of the origin and extension of the intimal flap, associated valvular abnormalities and flow in affected aortic branches. Spin echo and cine imaging should be undertaken early during the scan in multiple planes (e.g. transaxial and sagittal) to detect the presence of an intraluminal intimal flap. In haemodynamically stable patients, gradient echo imaging and phase contrast flow images can be acquired to quantify aortic regurgitation in Type A dissections (Fig. 8.6), as well as differentiate between the true and false lumens. The false lumen can be identified from remnants of dissected aortic media attaching as 'webs' to the outer luminal wall. High signal intensities may also be visible in the periaortic space adjacent to the descending aorta or pericardium, reflecting blood leakage through the rupture site. A bloody pericardial effusion heralds impending rupture of

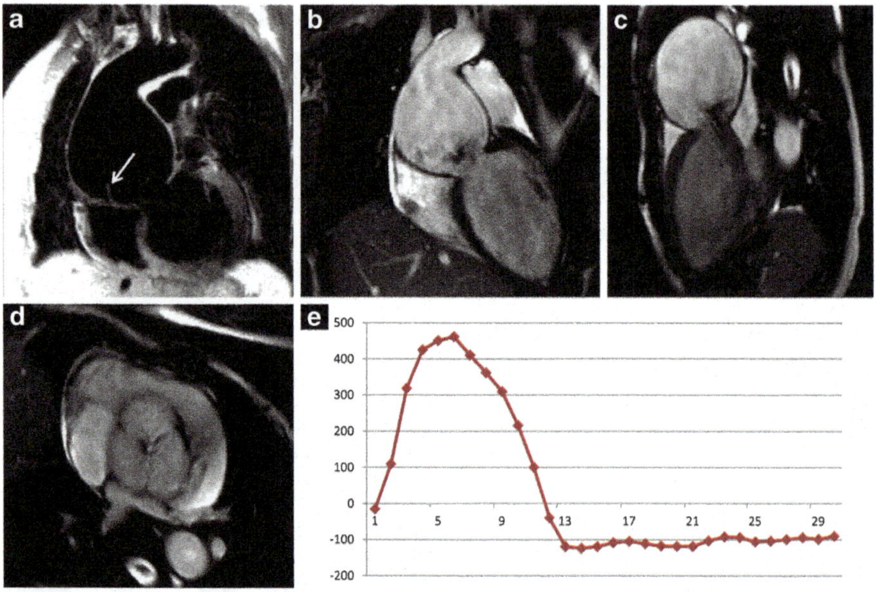

Fig. 8.6 Spin-echo image (**a**) and balanced SSFP image (**b**) of significantly dilated aortic root and proximal ascending aorta with type A dissection flap (*arrowed*). There is associated functional severe eccentric aortic regurgitation (**c**) with central coaptation defect seen at sinus level (**d**). The flow-time curve across the aortic valve (**e**) allows derivation of forward and regurgitant flows, with systolic forward and diastolic reversed flow

the ascending aorta into the pericardial space [53]. Thereafter, 3D CE-MRA should be undertaken as to seal the diagnosis and complete anatomical definition of the dissection particularly when involvement of the arch vessels and branch arteries are suspected. CMR has been shown to be the superior imaging technique for the prompt diagnosis of aortic dissection in stable patients, and current guidelines recommend whole aorta imaging with CMR or computer tomography in every Marfan patient [17, 54, 55].

The aortic wall can also be assessed for aortic dissection, intramural haematoma, mural thrombus, aortitis and para-aortic haematomas (Fig. 8.7) [56]. The descending aorta should not be neglected during aortic surveillance in MFS patients, as 20 % of dissections originate in the descending aorta and occur independently of ascending aorta dilatation. Furthermore, in patients with a history of aortic dissection, secondary dissections appear to disproportionately affect the descending aorta [57].

Valvular Pathology and Flow Assessment

Aortic, mitral and tricuspid valve involvement is recognised in MFS, and can be detected and quantified by cine MR imaging, volumetric analysis and great vessel

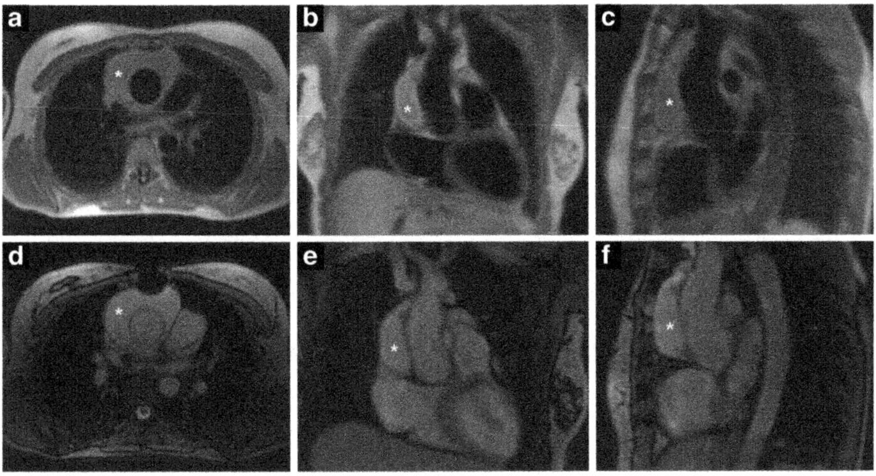

Fig. 8.7 Para-aortic haematoma (*) in Marfan patient 1 year after aortic root replacement surgery. Transaxial (**a**, **d**), coronal (**b**, **e**) and sagittal (**c**, **f**) views with turbo spin-echo imaging (**a**–**c**) and balanced SSFP imaging (**d**–**f**)

phase contrast velocity mapping. CMR not only provides a visual estimate of the severity of valvar regurgitation analogous to echocardiography, but also provides the added advantage of valvular regurgitant fraction quantification. This measurement can be serially charted to detect asymptomatic progression of valvular regurgitation.

Mitral Valve Prolapse and Regurgitation

The incidence of mitral valve prolapse and regurgitation increases with age in MFS. Mitral valve pathology is present in up to 80 % of adult MFS patients, with an increased prevalence of bileaflet and anterior leaflet prolapse when compared to myxomatous mitral valve disease [46, 58, 59]. Progression of mitral regurgitation may require surgical intervention with mitral valve repair or replacement [60, 61].

Mitral valve prolapse is defined as systolic displacement of one or both leaflets >2 mm from the mitral annulus plane in the LVOT view [62]. Mitral valve anatomy and regurgitation can be visualised in left ventricular long axis views and in short-axis planes transecting the mitral valve. Balanced SSFP cine imaging in the LVOT view is often optimal for detecting mitral valve prolapse [63]. When mitral regurgitation is present, a mitral valve stack should be acquired, consisting of a contiguous stack of 5 mm slices aligned to the mitral valve inflow across the coaptation line to determine the anatomical basis for regurgitation. This will identify the scallops of both leaflets implicated.

The degree of mitral regurgitation can be calculated from ventricular volumes and phase-contrast velocity mapping of the aortic valve. The aortic forward flow is measured from through-plane velocity mapping in a transaxial plane, transecting the aorta at the level of the sinotubular junction. The stroke volume of each ventricle is derived from a summation of the area of contiguous short-axis slices through the heart at end-diastole and end-systole. As the stroke volume ratio between the right and left ventricles approximate to unity over an imaging period of minutes, any differences seen would therefore reflect the severity of valvular regurgitation when there is an isolated valve lesion present [64]. The severity of mitral regurgitation can then be worked out:

$$\text{Mitral regurgitant volume}(\text{ml}) = \text{LV stroke volume} - \text{aortic forward flow}$$

$$\text{Mitral regurgitant fraction} = \text{mitral regurgitant volume} / \text{LV stroke volume} \times 100\ \%$$

The Aortic Valve

Aortic valve dysfunction in MFS is usually secondary to annular dilatation with aortic regurgitation present in up to 50 % in reported series [65]. Aortic valve anatomy and regurgitation can be imaged (similar to the mitral valve) with balanced SSFP cine imaging in left ventricular long axis and valvular 'en face' views. If and when relevant, the degree of aortic regurgitation can be derived from phase-contrast through-plane velocity mapping transecting the aorta at the level of the sinotubular junction or from stroke volume calculations (if aortic regurgitation is present as an isolated valvular lesion).

The aortic regurgitant fraction from velocity mapping is derived from the regurgitant volume/aortic forward flow in systole × 100 %; whilst by stroke volume measurements, it is calculated from the stroke volume difference between left and right ventricles/LV stroke volume × 100 %. Holodiastolic flow reversal may be present in the descending thoracic aorta or abdominal aorta, and can be ascertained from through-plane phase-contrast velocity mapping and velocity-time plots at the relevant aortic levels.

Late Gadolinium Enhancement (LGE)

LGE CMR facilitates the detection and diagnosis of concurrent myocardial pathology in Marfan patients, including myocarditis, myocardial infarction (Fig. 8.8),

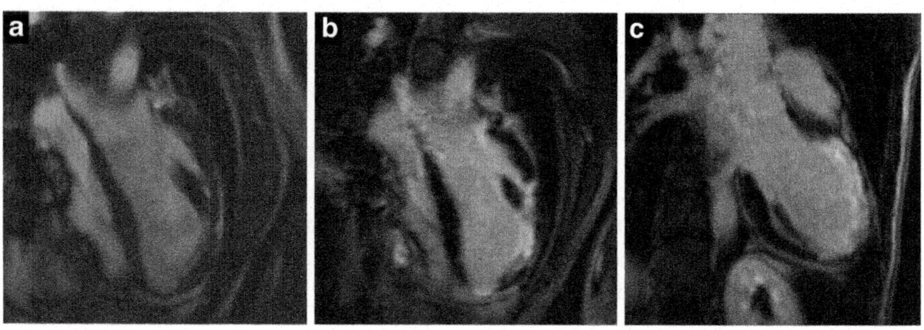

Fig. 8.8 Transmural late gadolinium enhancement reflecting anterolateral myocardial infarction during peri-operative period of aortic root replacement. Balanced SSFP imaging shows thinned mid to apical anterolateral wall and apex (**a**) with LGE in corresponding regions in four chamber view (**b**) and two chamber view (**c**)

fibrosis or infiltration. Papillary muscle enhancement may be seen in patients with mitral valve prolapse, in whom evidence of papillary muscle dysfunction is evident. Subendocardial or transmural LGE may be seen in Marfan patients with aortic dissections that cause coronary ostial occlusion.

Biophysical Properties of the Aortic Wall

The histological hallmark of MFS is that of 'cystic medial necrosis', with degradation of the extracellular matrix. At a microscopic level, elastic lamella and smooth muscle fibre disruption, and hypertrophy with increased vascular channels from the media to adventitia are evident. MFS is not only a consequence of structural connective tissue pathology, but also implicates binding protein dysregulation via transforming growth factor–β (TGFβ) [66].

These molecular pathological changes translate to reduced aortic distensibility and compliance at the macroscopic level. Aortic distensibility is defined as the percentage luminal increase per pressure increase during a cardiac cycle (in mmHg) or the propagation velocity of the pulse wave through the aorta (known as pulse wave velocity or flow wave velocity). Arterial compliance is the reciprocal of the resistance to deformation and defined by the change in volume per unit change in pressure (micro millilitre/mmHg). Compliance is typically greatest in the ascending aorta compared to the arch and lowest in the descending aorta in healthy individuals, and decreases with age [67].

Regional aortic distensibility can be measured from high-resolution cine imaging in a plane perpendicular to the aortic region of interest (ascending or descending aorta), together with the aortic pulse pressure derived from a sphygmomanometer at the level of the brachial artery (Fig. 8.9) in accordance to the formula:

$$\text{Aortic distensibility} = \left(A_{\text{max}} - A_{\text{min}}\right) / A_{\text{min}} \times \text{pulse pressure}$$

In which A_{max} = maximal aortic area (mm^2), A_{min} = minimal aortic area (mm^2) and pulse pressure is the difference between systolic and diastolic blood pressure (mmHg). The aortic luminal area in systole (A_{max}) and diastole (A_{min}) are either manually contoured from the relevant cine frames or derived from an automated algorithm [67, 68].

Regional arterial compliance is derived by calculating the change in volume of the aortic segment of interest:

$$\text{Aortic compliance} = \left(A_{\text{max}} - A_{\text{min}}\right) \times \text{slice thickness} / \text{pulse pressure}$$

Aortic pulse wave velocity is expressed as the ratio between the distance separating two points of interest within the vessel and the time taken for pressure/velocity waveform to traverse this distance, and typically increases as distensibility decreases [69]. Phase contrast through-plane velocity mapping is acquired perpendicular to the aortic lumen at two different levels (typically ascending and descending thoracic aorta at the level of the pulmonary artery bifurcation), generating a phase velocity map. The mean flow velocity across the cross-sectional area of the vessel can then

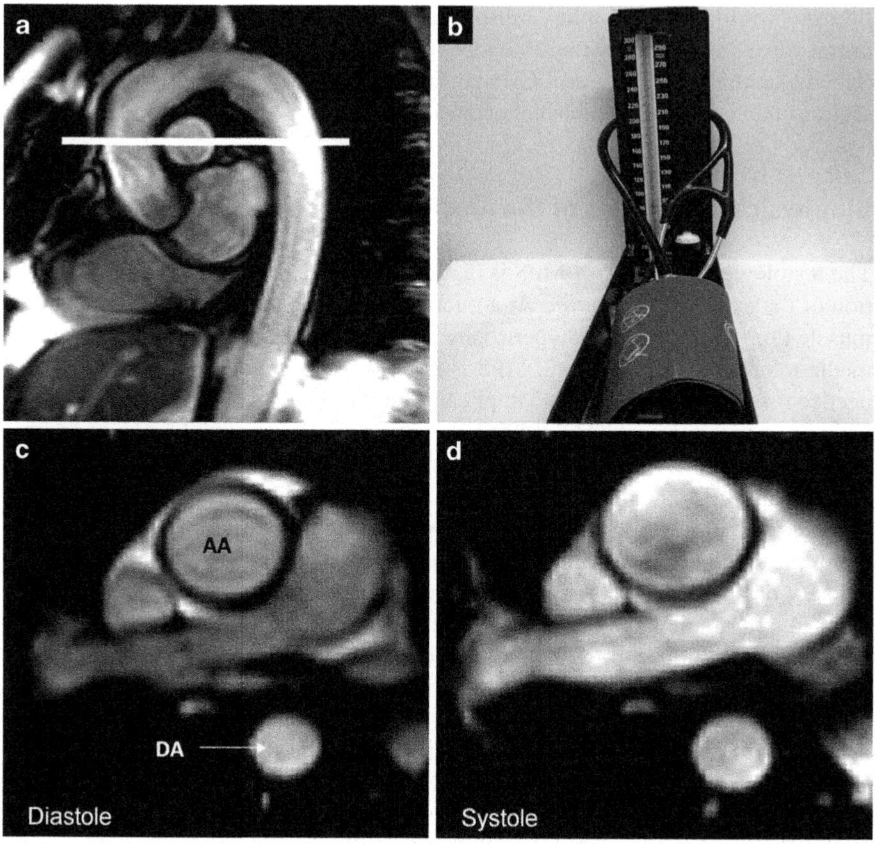

Fig. 8.9 Regional aortic distensibility obtained at level demarcated in sagittal oblique orientation (**a**) with corresponding oblique transaxial planes in diastole (**c**) and systole (**d**). The brachial blood pressure should be measured concurrently (**b**). *AA* ascending aorta, *DA* descending aorta

be plotted as a function of time across both levels to obtain the transit time of the foot of the flow wave (Fig. 8.10). There are multiple methods for obtaining transit time estimations with high reproducibility of calculated pulse wave velocities [70].

Aortic distensibility has been shown to be a predictor of progressive aortic dilatation and aortic events in MFS when measured by CMR [71, 72]. Decreased aortic distensibility and increased flow wave velocity has been detected in non-dilated aortas in patients with MFS, with variations in distensibility seen at different regions of the aorta. Distensibility has therefore been proposed as a potential biomarker of early aortic involvement in MFS before overt dilatation occurs [73–75], and may play a role in family screening or risk stratification. It has also been applied to assess the response to beta-blocker therapy prescribed to mediate aortic root dilatation in patients with MFS. Beta-blockade produced a significant increase in aortic distensibility at multiple levels in tandem with a reduction in pulse wave velocity in patients with MFS when compared to control subjects [76].

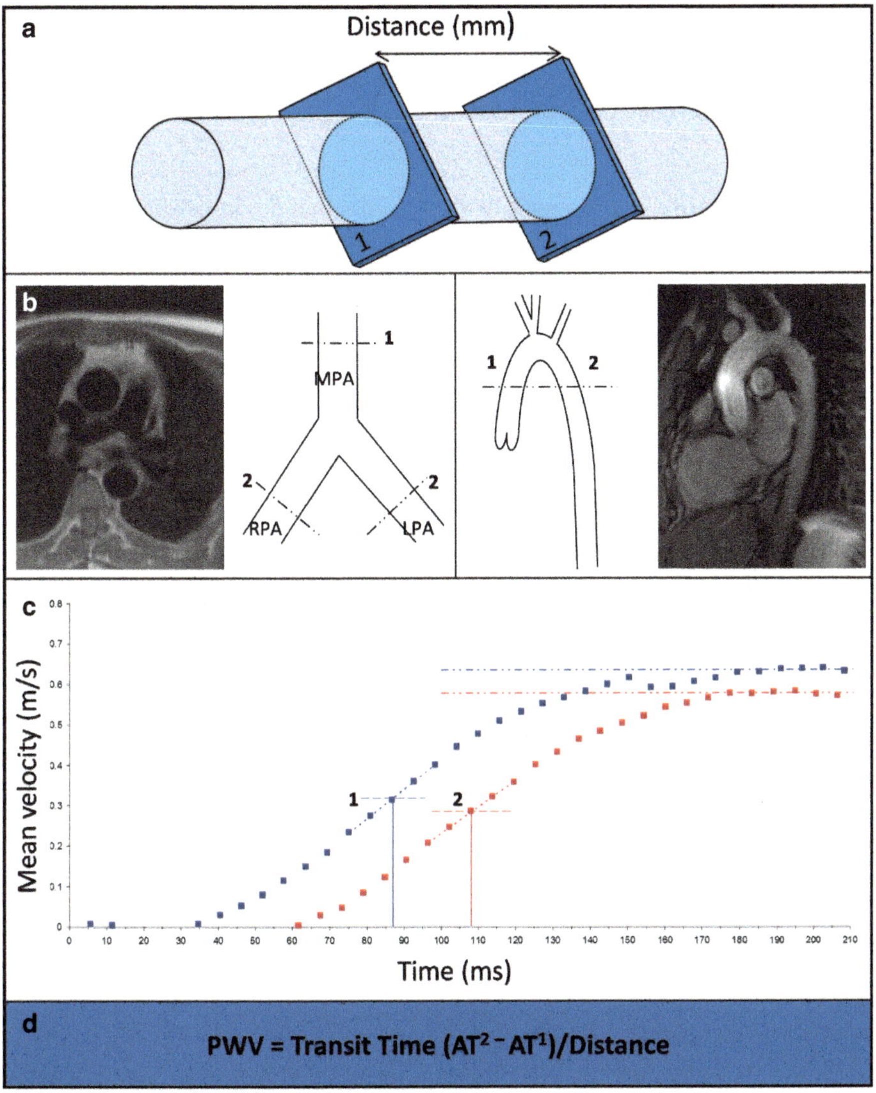

Fig. 8.10 Pulse wave velocity assessment with phase velocity acquisition at points 1 and 2 (planes for pulmonary arteries and aorta illustrated) in (**b**). The distance between the 2 points is measured as in (**a**). The pulse wave velocity is calculated from the transit time (defined as the difference in arrival time of the flow wave and points 1–2) divided by the distance in (**c**) and (**d**) [53]

Post Surgical Surveillance

Aortic surgical intervention may be indicated electively or acutely with emergency presentations in Marfan patients. Surgery for aortic dilatation is indicated when the external diameter of the dilated aortic segment exceeds 5 cm, or if any concomitant factors are present:

- Progressive aortic dilatation >0.2–0.5 cm/year
- Family history of aortic dissection
- Presence of significant aortic or mitral regurgitation, or
- If pregnancy is contemplated in women with maximal aortic dimension >4 cm [17–19]

Surgery is performed to repair or replace diseased aortic tissue, with various surgical procedures available targeted towards aortic valve, root and/or arch replacement. More recent surgical approaches have enabled valve-sparing procedures (such as the Yacoub and David techniques) to preserve anatomically normal aortic valves when aortic root or arch surgery is required [77–79]. The Bentall composite graft can be implanted in patients in whom complete replacement of the aortic valve and ascending aorta is desired, with reimplantation of the coronary artery ostia into the aortic prosthesis [80]. A surgical technique involving an 'aortic wrap' has also been developed in the last decade to proactively mitigate ongoing aortic root dilatation (see section below on PEARS).

Whilst the life expectancy of patients with MFS has improved with timely aortic surgery for aneurysms and dissection at first presentation, the majority remain susceptible to further events, with 70 % of a series of 192 MFS patients developing subsequent vascular system aneurysms or dissections [81]. Regular CMRs post surgical intervention has been shown to effectively detect and monitor complications such as peri-prosthetic haematomas, false aneurysms, residual chronic dissection and aneurysm formation in sections of native aorta [82]. CMR imaging of the aorta should be considered during the same admission after surgical intervention for aortic dissection, and then at 1, 3, 6 and 12 months post-intervention. If post-operative findings are stable, annual imaging should then be carried out. In patients who have undergone aortic root repair or aortic valve replacement, CMR should be contemplated pre-discharge and annually thereafter [19].

Other post surgical complications that can be assessed by CMR include peri-prosthetic leaks, haemopericardium, intra-cardiac thrombus, peri-operative myocardial infarction and infection (Fig. 8.11).

Prosthetic Valves

CMR can be performed after prosthetic valve replacement surgery for longterm monitoring of valve function and late complications. Prosthetic valves and almost all metallic surgical and interventional implants within the chest are non-ferromagnetic and safe within 1.5 or 3 T magnetic fields, including sternal wires, clips, stents and occlusion devices. The guidelines recommend doing the CMR scan at least 6 weeks after surgery to allow fibrosis to settle in. Localised artefact around the prosthetic valve should be anticipated, although modern implants may cause less localised artefact within the magnetic field, and valve function is not usually adversely affected [83–85]. Localised artefact arises around prosthetic valves as they do not contain mobile hydrogen ions, resulting in distortion of the local magnetic field with signal loss for a variable distance around the prosthesis. The distortion is less pronounced in spin echo images as compared to gradient echo images,

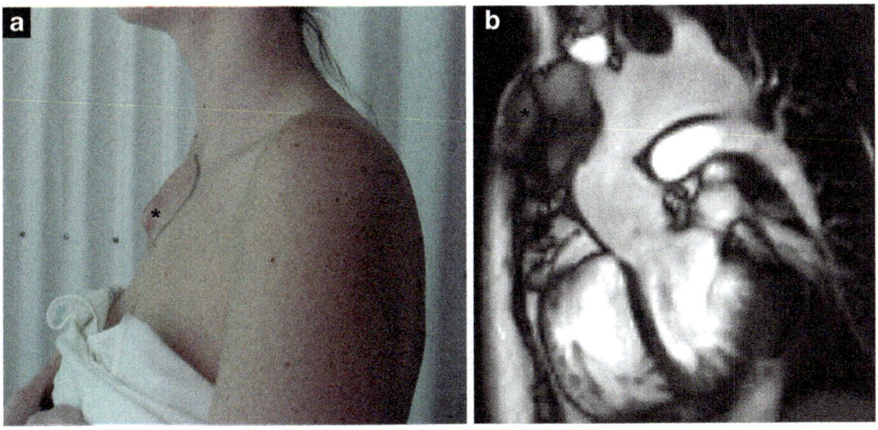

Fig. 8.11 Subcutaneous infected collection (marked *) post aortic root and ascending aorta replacement with infected Dacron graft seen superficially (**a**) and on balanced SSFP imaging (**b**) (Reproduced from Dormand and Mohiaddin [16])

and can introduce inaccuracies in establishing the assessment of turbulent jets in the region of the prosthetic valve.

Aortic Surveillance After Personalised External Aortic Root Support (PEARS)

The personalised external aortic root support (PEARS) system was developed in 2004 as a conservative approach to halt aortic root dilatation and circumvent aortic dissection in Marfan patients (Fig. 8.12) [87]. CMR is the main imaging modality utilised in surgical planning and subsequent post-operative surveillance at 6 months, 1 year and annually thereafter. Pre-procedural CMR spatial data is utilised to replicate the patient's aorta to guide production of a customised external mesh support, designed to accommodate the aortic sinuses and coronary artery origins without impingement [88, 89]. The operation is typically performed without cardiopulmonary bypass on a beating heart. During the course of mean 4.4 years (range 1.4–8.8 years) follow-up in 30 patients, there is conservation of the aortic valve and root architecture. There has been one perioperative death in the first 50 patients. No aortic, cerebral or aortic valve related events have occurred after 133 patient-years of follow-up. PEARS stabilises aortic root dimensions with outcomes comparable to valve-sparing aortic root replacement surgery [90].

Emerging CMR Applications in Marfan Syndrome: Flow-Sensitive 4D MRI

Time resolved three-dimensional phase contrast MRI with three-directional velocity encoding (also known as flow-sensitive 4D MRI) appears to be relevant for illustrating the morphology and abnormal flow dynamics in MFS that contribute to

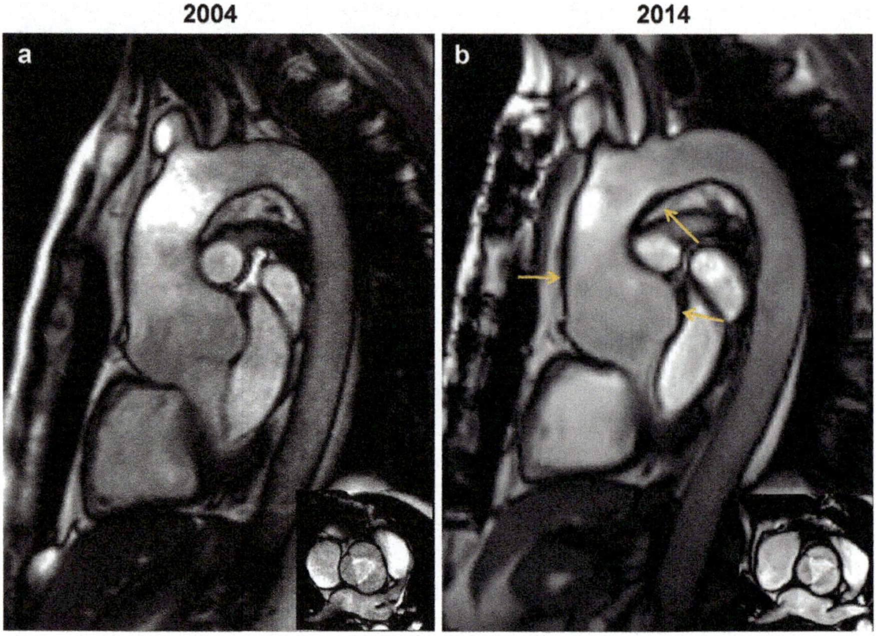

Fig. 8.12 Patient with Marfan syndrome before (**a**) and after (**b**) Personalised External Aortic Root Support (PEARS) with stable aortic root dimensions. Balanced SSFP imaging of aorta in sagittal oblique view and transaxial plane at aortic valve level (*inset*). Thickening of the ascending aortic walls can be seen (**b**) as a result of mesh incorporation, forming a mesh-aortic composite wall (*arrowed*) (From Treasure et al. [86]. Copyright © 2015 Massachusetts Medical Society. Reprinted with permission)

aortic pathology, which may in turn impact upon post-surgical outcomes. Flow-sensitive 4D MRI is acquired with cardiac ECG and respiratory navigator gating with a 3D phase-contrast pulse sequence. The data acquired is then corrected for eddy currents, gradient (Maxwell) terms and velocity aliasing [91, 92], before software facilitated post-processing to generate flow visualisations (Fig. 8.13). Various parameters can be derived from the analysis of flow-sensitive 4D MRI data including alterations in wall shear stress, normalised flow displacement, in addition to the presence of helix and vortex flow [94–97]. The technique has also been extended to derive transient pressure indexes that reflect spatiotemporal distributions of relative pressure and its components in the aorta [98, 99].

As MFS patients remain susceptible to further aortic complications of aneurysms and dissections most commonly distal to their index dissection, flow-sensitive 4D MRI has shown early promise in small patient series in identifying abnormal aortic wall shear stresses that may predispose to the development of these complications [100, 101]. Alterations in wall shear stress in MFS patients without significant aortic dilatation have been elucidated. It has also been postulated that the loss of aortic sinus integrity after root replacement surgery in MFS may negatively affect aortic

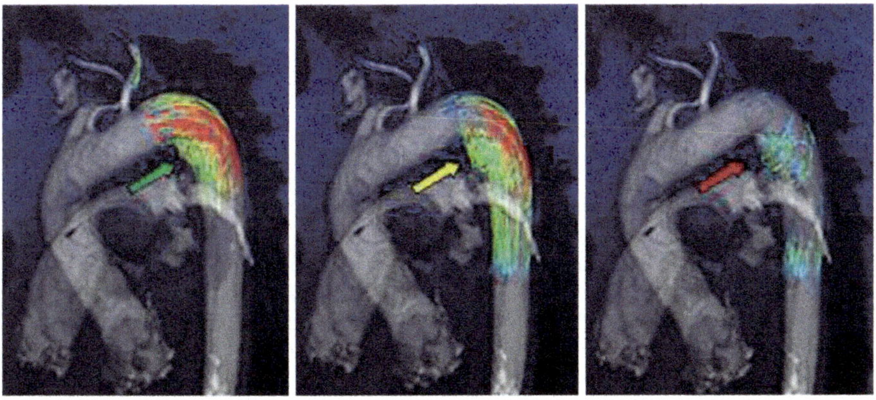

Fig. 8.13 4D flow images of the aorta of a patient with Marfan syndrome with arrows indicating regions of turbulent vortex formation (Reproduced from Pitcher et al. [93])

valve function through loss of supravalvular flow vortices, which would otherwise allow sharing of shear stress and load [102].

Disturbances to helical and vortical flows have been described in MFS. Helical flow is defined as a circular or 'corkscrew-like' motion where the predominant flow occurs along the axis of rotation, whereas vortex flow consists of particles revolving around a point within a vessel, in which the rotational direction deviates >90° from the physiological flow direction. Helix flow can be subdivided into global helix formation of the whole vessel or local helix flow which only affects a circumscribed section of the vessel. Increased local helical flow has been demonstrated in the ascending aortas of MFS patients in association with aortic sinus dilatation. Increased global helical and vortex flows have also been found in the descending aorta, together with evidence of local helix flow in the left subclavian artery. These factors in combination may be implicated in the formation of Type B dissections, due to flow alterations in the proximal descending aorta, which induces pathological shear forces of the vessel wall [96]. Flow-sensitive 4D MRI is currently restricted to the research domain in MFS patients, but may have important contributions to make towards clinical decision making in this patient cohort.

Conclusion

The diagnosis and management of cardiovascular manifestations of MFS remain pivotal to the lifelong care of these patients, with surveillance by CMR forming an integral component of the available imaging armamentarium. CMR is not only able to non-invasively provide accurate and reproducible myocardial and vascular assessment, but may increasingly provide mechanistic insight into the disease pathophysiology and aid in timing of interventions to optimise clinical outcomes.

Acknowledgements This work is supported by the NIHR Cardiovascular Biomedical Research Unit of the Royal Brompton and Harefield NHS Foundation Trust and Imperial College London.

References

1. Murdoch JL, Walker BA, Halpern BL, Kuzma JW, McKusick VA. Life expectancy and causes of death in the Marfan syndrome. N Engl J Med. 1972;286:804–8.
2. Krause KJ. Marfan syndrome: literature review of mortality studies. J Insur Med (New York, NY). 2000;32:79–88.
3. Silverman DI, Burton KJ, Gray J, Bosner MS, Kouchoukos NT, Roman MJ, Boxer M, Devereux RB, Tsipouras P. Life expectancy in the Marfan syndrome. Am J Cardiol. 1995;75:157–60.
4. Ridgway JP. Cardiovascular magnetic resonance physics for clinicians: part I. J Cardiovasc Magn Reson Off J Soc Cardiovasc Magn Reson. 2010;12:71.
5. Biglands JD, Radjenovic A, Ridgway JP. Cardiovascular magnetic resonance physics for clinicians: part II. J Cardiovasc Magn Reson Off J Soc Cardiovasc Magn Reson. 2012;14:66.
6. Mohiaddin RH, Longmore DB. Functional aspects of cardiovascular nuclear magnetic resonance imaging. Techniques and application. Circulation. 1993;88:264–81.
7. Chernobelsky A, Shubayev O, Comeau CR, Wolff SD. Baseline correction of phase contrast images improves quantification of blood flow in the great vessels. J Cardiovasc Magn Reson Off J Soc Cardiovasc Magn Reson. 2007;9:681–5.
8. Krinsky GA, Rofsky NM, DeCorato DR, Weinreb JC, Earls JP, Flyer MA, Galloway AC, Colvin SB. Thoracic aorta: comparison of gadolinium-enhanced three-dimensional MR angiography with conventional MR imaging. Radiology. 1997;202:183–93.
9. Amano Y, Takahama K, Kumita S. Non-contrast-enhanced MR angiography of the thoracic aorta using cardiac and navigator-gated magnetization-prepared three-dimensional steady-state free precession. J Magn Reson Imaging JMRI. 2008;27:504–9.
10. Jhooti P, Keegan J, Firmin DN. A fully automatic and highly efficient navigator gating technique for high-resolution free-breathing acquisitions: continuously adaptive windowing strategy. Magn Reson Med Off J Soc Magn Reson Med/Soc Magn Reson Med. 2010;64:1015–26.
11. Jhooti P, Haas T, Kawel N, Bremerich J, Keegan J, Scheffler K. Use of respiratory biofeedback and CLAWS for increased navigator efficiency for imaging the thoracic aorta. Magn Reson Med Off J Soc Magn Reson Med/Soc Magn Reson Med. 2011;66:1666–73.
12. Francois CJ, Tuite D, Deshpande V, Jerecic R, Weale P, Carr JC. Unenhanced MR angiography of the thoracic aorta: initial clinical evaluation. AJR Am J Roentgenol. 2008;190:902–6.
13. Kawel N, Jhooti P, Dashti D, Haas T, Winter L, Zellweger MJ, Buser PT, Keegan J, Scheffler K, Bremerich J. MR-imaging of the thoracic aorta: 3D-ECG- and respiratory-gated bSSFP imaging using the CLAWS algorithm versus contrast-enhanced 3d-MRA. Eur J Radiol. 2012;81:239–43.
14. Camm JA, Luscher TA, Serruys PW. The ESC textbook of cardiovascular medicine. Oxford/New York: Oxford University Press; 2009.
15. Kilner PJ, Geva T, Kaemmerer H, Trindade PT, Schwitter J, Webb GD. Recommendations for cardiovascular magnetic resonance in adults with congenital heart disease from the respective working groups of the European Society of Cardiology. Eur Heart J. 2010;31:794–805.
16. Dormand H, Mohiaddin RH. Cardiovascular magnetic resonance in Marfan syndrome. J Cardiovasc Magn Reson Off J Soc Cardiovasc Magn Reson. 2013;15:33.
17. Baumgartner H, Bonhoeffer P, De Groot NM, de Haan F, Deanfield JE, Galie N, Gatzoulis MA, Gohlke-Baerwolf C, Kaemmerer H, Kilner P, Meijboom F, Mulder BJ, Oechslin E, Oliver JM, Serraf A, Szatmari A, Thaulow E, Vouhe PR, Walma E, Task Force on the Management of Grown-up Congenital Heart Disease of the European Society of Cardiology, Association for European Paediatric Cardiology, ESC Committee for Practice Guidelines (CPG). ESC guidelines for the management of grown-up congenital heart disease (new version 2010). Eur Heart J. 2010;31:2915–57.
18. Erbel R, Aboyans V, Boileau C, Bossone E, Bartolomeo RD, Eggebrecht H, Evangelista A, Falk V, Frank H, Gaemperli O, Grabenwoger M, Haverich A, Iung B, Manolis AJ, Meijboom

F, Nienaber CA, Roffi M, Rousseau H, Sechtem U, Sirnes PA, Allmen RS, Vrints CJ. 2014 ESC guidelines on the diagnosis and treatment of aortic diseases: document covering acute and chronic aortic diseases of the thoracic and abdominal aorta of the adult. The task force for the diagnosis and treatment of aortic diseases of the European Society of Cardiology (ESC). Eur Heart J. 2014;35:2873–926.

19. Hiratzka LF, Bakris GL, Beckman JA, Bersin RM, Carr VF, Casey Jr DE, Eagle KA, Hermann LK, Isselbacher EM, Kazerooni EA, Kouchoukos NT, Lytle BW, Milewicz DM, Reich DL, Sen S, Shinn JA, Svensson LG, Williams DM. 2010 ACCF/AHA/AATS/ACR/ASA/SCA/SCAI/SIR/STS/SVM guidelines for the diagnosis and management of patients with thoracic aortic disease. A report of the American College of Cardiology Foundation/American Heart Association task force on practice guidelines, American Association for Thoracic Surgery, American College of Radiology, American Stroke Association, Society of Cardiovascular Anesthesiologists, Society for Cardiovascular Angiography and Interventions, Society of Interventional Radiology, Society of Thoracic Surgeons, and Society for Vascular Medicine. J Am Coll Cardiol. 2010;55:e27–129.
20. Shores J, Berger KR, Murphy EA, Pyeritz RE. Progression of aortic dilatation and the benefit of long-term beta-adrenergic blockade in Marfan's syndrome. N Engl J Med. 1994;330:1335–41.
21. Gersony DR, McClaughlin MA, Jin Z, Gersony WM. The effect of beta-blocker therapy on clinical outcome in patients with Marfan's syndrome: a meta-analysis. Int J Cardiol. 2007;114:303–8.
22. Engelfriet P, Mulder B. Is there benefit of beta-blocking agents in the treatment of patients with the Marfan syndrome? Int J Cardiol. 2007;114:300–2.
23. Gao L, Mao Q, Wen D, Zhang L, Zhou X, Hui R. The effect of beta-blocker therapy on progressive aortic dilatation in children and adolescents with Marfan's syndrome: a meta-analysis. Acta Paediatrica (Oslo, Norway: 1992). 2011;100:e101–5.
24. Nagashima H, Sakomura Y, Aoka Y, Uto K, Kameyama K, Ogawa M, Aomi S, Koyanagi H, Ishizuka N, Naruse M, Kawana M, Kasanuki H. Angiotensin II type 2 receptor mediates vascular smooth muscle cell apoptosis in cystic medial degeneration associated with Marfan's syndrome. Circulation. 2001;104:I282–7.
25. Ahimastos AA, Aggarwal A, D'Orsa KM, Formosa MF, White AJ, Savarirayan R, Dart AM, Kingwell BA. Effect of perindopril on large artery stiffness and aortic root diameter in patients with Marfan syndrome: a randomized controlled trial. JAMA. 2007;298:1539–47.
26. Brooke BS, Habashi JP, Judge DP, Patel N, Loeys B, Dietz 3rd HC. Angiotensin II blockade and aortic-root dilation in Marfan's syndrome. N Engl J Med. 2008;358:2787–95.
27. Lacro RV, Dietz HC, Sleeper LA, Yetman AT, Bradley TJ, Colan SD, Pearson GD, Selamet Tierney ES, Levine JC, Atz AM, Benson DW, Braverman AC, Chen S, De Backer J, Gelb BD, Grossfeld PD, Klein GL, Lai WW, Liou A, Loeys BL, Markham LW, Olson AK, Paridon SM, Pemberton VL, Pierpont ME, Pyeritz RE, Radojewski E, Roman MJ, Sharkey AM, Stylianou MP, Wechsler SB, Young LT, Mahony L. Atenolol versus losartan in children and young adults with Marfan's syndrome. N Engl J Med. 2014;371:2061–71.
28. Radonic T, de Witte P, Baars MJ, Zwinderman AH, Mulder BJ, Groenink M. Losartan therapy in adults with Marfan syndrome: study protocol of the multi-center randomized controlled compare trial. Trials. 2010;11:3.
29. Groenink M, den Hartog AW, Franken R, Radonic T, de Waard V, Timmermans J, Scholte AJ, van den Berg MP, Spijkerboer AM, Marquering HA, Zwinderman AH, Mulder BJ. Losartan reduces aortic dilatation rate in adults with Marfan syndrome: a randomized controlled trial. Eur Heart J. 2013;34:3491–500.
30. Moberg K, De Nobele S, Devos D, Goetghebeur E, Segers P, Trachet B, Vervaet C, Renard M, Coucke P, Loeys B, De Paepe A, De Backer J. The Ghent Marfan trial – a randomized, double-blind placebo controlled trial with losartan in Marfan patients treated with beta-blockers. Int J Cardiol. 2012;157:354–8.
31. Shiga T, Wajima Z, Apfel CC, Inoue T, Ohe Y. Diagnostic accuracy of transesophageal echocardiography, helical computed tomography, and magnetic resonance imaging for suspected

thoracic aortic dissection: systematic review and meta-analysis. Arch Intern Med. 2006;166:1350–6.
32. Reiter T, Ritter O, Prince MR, Nordbeck P, Wanner C, Nagel E, Bauer WR. Minimizing risk of nephrogenic systemic fibrosis in cardiovascular magnetic resonance. J Cardiovasc Magn Reson Off J Soc Cardiovasc Magn Reson. 2012;14:31.
33. Oosterhof T, Groenink M, Hulsmans FJ, Mulder BJ, van der Wall EE, Smit R, Hennekam RC. Quantitative assessment of dural ectasia as a marker for Marfan syndrome. Radiology. 2001;220:514–8.
34. Knirsch W, Kurtz C, Haffner N, Binz G, Heim P, Winkler P, Baumgartner D, Freund-Unsinn K, Stern H, Kaemmerer H, Molinari L, Kececioglu D, Uhlemann F. Dural ectasia in children with Marfan syndrome: a prospective, multicenter, patient-control study. Am J Med Genet A. 2006;140:775–81.
35. Lorenz CH, Walker ES, Morgan VL, Klein SS, Graham Jr TP. Normal human right and left ventricular mass, systolic function, and gender differences by cine magnetic resonance imaging. J Cardiovasc Magn Reson Off J Soc Cardiovasc Magn Reson. 1999;1:7–21.
36. Moon JC, Lorenz CH, Francis JM, Smith GC, Pennell DJ. Breath-hold flash and FISP cardiovascular MR imaging: left ventricular volume differences and reproducibility. Radiology. 2002;223:789–97.
37. Fujiseki Y, Okuno K, Tanaka M, Shimada M, Takahashi M, Kawanishi K. Myocardial involvement in the Marfan syndrome. Jpn Heart J. 1985;26:1043–50.
38. Keane MG, Pyeritz RE. Medical management of Marfan syndrome. Circulation. 2008;117:2802–13.
39. Kahveci G, Erkol A, Yilmaz F. Dilated cardiomyopathy in a patient with Marfan syndrome accompanied by chronic type A aortic dissection and right atrial thrombus. Intern Med (Tokyo, Japan). 2010;49:2583–6.
40. Alpendurada F, Wong J, Kiotsekoglou A, Banya W, Child A, Prasad SK, Pennell DJ, Mohiaddin RH. Evidence for Marfan cardiomyopathy. Eur J Heart Fail. 2010;12:1085–91.
41. De Backer JF, Devos D, Segers P, Matthys D, Francois K, Gillebert TC, De Paepe AM, De Sutter J. Primary impairment of left ventricular function in Marfan syndrome. Int J Cardiol. 2006;112:353–8.
42. Grothues F, Smith GC, Moon JC, Bellenger NG, Collins P, Klein HU, Pennell DJ. Comparison of interstudy reproducibility of cardiovascular magnetic resonance with two-dimensional echocardiography in normal subjects and in patients with heart failure or left ventricular hypertrophy. Am J Cardiol. 2002;90:29–34.
43. Hetzer R, Siegel G, Delmo Walter EM. Cardiomyopathy in Marfan syndrome. Eur J Cardiothorac Surg Off J Eur Assoc Cardiothorac Surg. 2015; pii:ezv073 [Epub ahead of print].
44. Saleh RS, Finn JP, Fenchel M, Moghadam AN, Krishnam M, Abrazado M, Ton A, Habibi R, Fonkalsrud EW, Cooper CB. Cardiovascular magnetic resonance in patients with pectus excavatum compared with normal controls. J Cardiovasc Magn Reson Off J Soc Cardiovasc Magn Reson. 2010;12:73.
45. Zagrosek A, von Knobelsdorff-Brenkenhoff F, Polleichtner S, Schaarschmidt K, Schulz-Menger J. Hemodynamic impact of surgical correction of pectus excavatum – a cardiovascular magnetic resonance study. J Cardiovasc Magn Reson Off J Soc Cardiovasc Magn Reson. 2011;13:P190.
46. Detaint D, Faivre L, Collod-Beroud G, Child AH, Loeys BL, Binquet C, Gautier E, Arbustini E, Mayer K, Arslan-Kirchner M, Stheneur C, Halliday D, Beroud C, Bonithon-Kopp C, Claustres M, Plauchu H, Robinson PN, Kiotsekoglou A, De Backer J, Ades L, Francke U, De Paepe A, Boileau C, Jondeau G. Cardiovascular manifestations in men and women carrying a FBN1 mutation. Eur Heart J. 2010;31:2223–9.
47. Silverman DI, Gray J, Roman MJ, Bridges A, Burton K, Boxer M, Devereux RB, Tsipouras P. Family history of severe cardiovascular disease in Marfan syndrome is associated with increased aortic diameter and decreased survival. J Am Coll Cardiol. 1995;26:1062–7.
48. Meijboom LJ, Groenink M, van der Wall EE, Romkes H, Stoker J, Mulder BJ. Aortic root asymmetry in Marfan patients; evaluation by magnetic resonance imaging and comparison with standard echocardiography. Int J Card Imaging. 2000;16:161–8.

49. Burman ED, Keegan J, Kilner PJ. Aortic root measurement by cardiovascular magnetic resonance: specification of planes and lines of measurement and corresponding normal values. Circ Cardiovasc Imaging. 2008;1:104–13.
50. Davis AE, Lewandowski AJ, Holloway CJ, Ntusi NA, Banerjee R, Nethononda R, Pitcher A, Francis JM, Myerson SG, Leeson P, Donovan T, Neubauer S, Rider OJ. Observational study of regional aortic size referenced to body size: production of a cardiovascular magnetic resonance nomogram. J Cardiovasc Magn Reson Off J Soc Cardiovasc Magn Reson. 2014;16:9.
51. Kaiser T, Kellenberger CJ, Albisetti M, Bergstrasser E, Valsangiacomo Buechel ER. Normal values for aortic diameters in children and adolescents – assessment in vivo by contrast-enhanced CMR-angiography. J Cardiovasc Magn Reson Off J Soc Cardiovasc Magn Reson. 2008;10:56.
52. Bhatla P, Nielsen JC. Cardiovascular magnetic resonance as an alternate method for serial evaluation of proximal aorta: comparison with echocardiography. Echocardiography (Mount Kisco, NY). 2013;30:713–8.
53. Manning WJ, Pennell DJ. Cardiovascular magnetic resonance. Philadelphia: Saunders Elsevier; 2010.
54. Nienaber CA, von Kodolitsch Y, Nicolas V, Siglow V, Piepho A, Brockhoff C, Koschyk DH, Spielmann RP. The diagnosis of thoracic aortic dissection by noninvasive imaging procedures. N Engl J Med. 1993;328:1–9.
55. Nienaber CA, Spielmann RP, von Kodolitsch Y, Siglow V, Piepho A, Jaup T, Nicolas V, Weber P, Triebel HJ, Bleifeld W. Diagnosis of thoracic aortic dissection. Magnetic resonance imaging versus transesophageal echocardiography. Circulation. 1992;85:434–47.
56. Nienaber CA, von Kodolitsch Y, Petersen B, Loose R, Helmchen U, Haverich A, Spielmann RP. Intramural hemorrhage of the thoracic aorta. Diagnostic and therapeutic implications. Circulation. 1995;92:1465–72.
57. Mimoun L, Detaint D, Hamroun D, Arnoult F, Delorme G, Gautier M, Milleron O, Meuleman C, Raoux F, Boileau C, Vahanian A, Jondeau G. Dissection in Marfan syndrome: the importance of the descending aorta. Eur Heart J. 2011;32:443–9.
58. Pyeritz RE, Wappel MA. Mitral valve dysfunction in the Marfan syndrome. Clinical and echocardiographic study of prevalence and natural history. Am J Med. 1983;74:797–807.
59. Bhudia SK, Troughton R, Lam BK, Rajeswaran J, Mills WR, Gillinov AM, Griffin BP, Blackstone EH, Lytle BW, Svensson LG. Mitral valve surgery in the adult Marfan syndrome patient. Ann Thorac Surg. 2006;81:843–8.
60. Fuzellier JF, Chauvaud SM, Fornes P, Berrebi AJ, Lajos PS, Bruneval P, Carpentier AF. Surgical management of mitral regurgitation associated with Marfan's syndrome. Ann Thorac Surg. 1998;66:68–72.
61. Bernhardt AM, Treede H, Detter C, Rybczynski M, Sheikhzadeh S, Wagner FM, Von Kodolitsch Y, Reichenspurner H. Results of modern mitral valve repair in patients with Marfan syndrome. Thorac Cardiovasc Surg. 2014;62:35–41.
62. Hayek E, Gring CN, Griffin BP. Mitral valve prolapse. Lancet. 2005;365:507–18.
63. Han Y, Peters DC, Salton CJ, Bzymek D, Nezafat R, Goddu B, Kissinger KV, Zimetbaum PJ, Manning WJ, Yeon SB. Cardiovascular magnetic resonance characterization of mitral valve prolapse. JACC Cardiovasc Imaging. 2008;1:294–303.
64. Underwood SR, Klipstein RH, Firmin DN, Fox KM, Poole-Wilson PA, Rees RS, Longmore DB. Magnetic resonance assessment of aortic and mitral regurgitation. Br Heart J. 1986;56:455–62.
65. Alpendurada F, Mohiaddin RH. Prevalence of cardiovascular manifestations in patients with Marfan syndrome: a cardiovascular magnetic resonance study. J Cardiovasc Magn Reson Off J Soc Cardiovasc Magn Reson. 2008;10:A164.
66. Ng CM, Cheng A, Myers LA, Martinez-Murillo F, Jie C, Bedja D, Gabrielson KL, Hausladen JM, Mecham RP, Judge DP, Dietz HC. TGF-beta-dependent pathogenesis of mitral valve prolapse in a mouse model of Marfan syndrome. J Clin Invest. 2004;114:1586–92.
67. Mohiaddin RH, Underwood SR, Bogren HG, Firmin DN, Klipstein RH, Rees RS, Longmore DB. Regional aortic compliance studied by magnetic resonance imaging: the effects of age, training, and coronary artery disease. Br Heart J. 1989;62:90–6.

68. Rueckert D, Burger P, Forbat SM, Mohiaddin RD, Yang GZ. Automatic tracking of the aorta in cardiovascular MR images using deformable models. IEEE Trans Med Imaging. 1997;16:581–90.
69. Mohiaddin RH, Firmin DN, Longmore DB. Age-related changes of human aortic flow wave velocity measured noninvasively by magnetic resonance imaging. J Appl Physiol (Bethesda, Md: 1985). 1993;74:492–7.
70. Dogui A, Redheuil A, Lefort M, DeCesare A, Kachenoura N, Herment A, Mousseaux E. Measurement of aortic arch pulse wave velocity in cardiovascular MR: comparison of transit time estimators and description of a new approach. J Magn Reson Imaging JMRI. 2011;33:1321–9.
71. Nollen GJ, Groenink M, Tijssen JG, Van Der Wall EE, Mulder BJ. Aortic stiffness and diameter predict progressive aortic dilatation in patients with Marfan syndrome. Eur Heart J. 2004;25:1146–52.
72. De Witte P, Radonic T, Laan K, Zwinderman AH, Mulder B, Groenink M. Aortic distensibility is a predictor for aortic events in patients with Marfan syndrome: a 12 year-survival analysis. J Am Coll Cardiol. 2010;55:A40.E378.
73. Groenink M, de Roos A, Mulder BJ, Verbeeten Jr B, Timmermans J, Zwinderman AH, Spaan JA, van der Wall EE. Biophysical properties of the normal-sized aorta in patients with Marfan syndrome: evaluation with MR flow mapping. Radiology. 2001;219:535–40.
74. Hirata K, Triposkiadis F, Sparks E, Bowen J, Wooley CF, Boudoulas H. The Marfan syndrome: abnormal aortic elastic properties. J Am Coll Cardiol. 1991;18:57–63.
75. Fattori R, Bacchi Reggiani L, Pepe G, Napoli G, Bna C, Celletti F, Lovato L, Gavelli G. Magnetic resonance imaging evaluation of aortic elastic properties as early expression of Marfan syndrome. J Cardiovasc Magn Reson Off J Soc Cardiovasc Magn Reson. 2000;2:251–6.
76. Groenink M, de Roos A, Mulder BJ, Spaan JA, van der Wall EE. Changes in aortic distensibility and pulse wave velocity assessed with magnetic resonance imaging following beta-blocker therapy in the Marfan syndrome. Am J Cardiol. 1998;82:203–8.
77. Yacoub MH, Gehle P, Chandrasekaran V, Birks EJ, Child A, Radley-Smith R. Late results of a valve-preserving operation in patients with aneurysms of the ascending aorta and root. J Thorac Cardiovasc Surg. 1998;115:1080–90.
78. Tambeur L, David TE, Unger M, Armstrong S, Ivanov J, Webb G. Results of surgery for aortic root aneurysm in patients with the Marfan syndrome. Eur J Cardiothorac Surg Off J Eur Assoc Cardiothorac Surg. 2000;17:415–9.
79. David TE, Armstrong S, Ivanov J, Feindel CM, Omran A, Webb G. Results of aortic valve-sparing operations. J Thorac Cardiovasc Surg. 2001;122:39–46.
80. Bentall H, De Bono A. A technique for complete replacement of the ascending aorta. Thorax. 1968;23:338–9.
81. Finkbohner R, Johnston D, Crawford ES, Coselli J, Milewicz DM. Marfan syndrome. Long-term survival and complications after aortic aneurysm repair. Circulation. 1995;91:728–33.
82. Mesana TG, Caus T, Gaubert J, Collart F, Ayari R, Bartoli J, Moulin G, Monties J. Late complications after prosthetic replacement of the ascending aorta: what did we learn from routine magnetic resonance imaging follow-up? Eur J Cardiothorac Surg Off J Eur Assoc Cardiothorac Surg. 2000;18:313–20.
83. Edwards MB, Taylor KM, Shellock FG. Prosthetic heart valves: evaluation of magnetic field interactions, heating, and artifacts at 1.5 t. J Magn Reson Imaging JMRI. 2000;12:363–9.
84. Sawyer-Glover AM, Shellock FG. Pre-mri procedure screening: recommendations and safety considerations for biomedical implants and devices. J Magn Reson Imaging JMRI. 2000;12:92–106.
85. Shellock FG. Biomedical implants and devices: assessment of magnetic field interactions with a 3.0-tesla mr system. J Magn Reson Imaging JMRI. 2002;16:721–32.
86. Treasure T, Pepper J, Mohiaddin R. Atenolol versus Losartan in Marfan's syndrome. N Engl J Med. 2015;372(10):978–9.
87. Golesworthy T, Lamperth M, Mohiaddin R, Pepper J, Thornton W, Treasure T. The tailor of Gloucester: a jacket for the Marfan's aorta. Lancet. 2004;364:1582.

88. Pepper J, Golesworthy T, Utley M, Chan J, Ganeshalingam S, Lamperth M, Mohiaddin R, Treasure T. Manufacturing and placing a bespoke support for the Marfan aortic root: description of the method and technical results and status at one year for the first ten patients. Interact Cardiovasc Thorac Surg. 2010;10:360–5.
89. Pepper J, John Chan K, Gavino J, Golesworthy T, Mohiaddin R, Treasure T. External aortic root support for Marfan syndrome: early clinical results in the first 20 recipients with a bespoke implant. J R Soc Med. 2010;103:370–5.
90. Treasure T, Takkenberg JJ, Golesworthy T, Rega F, Petrou M, Rosendahl U, Mohiaddin R, Rubens M, Thornton W, Lees B, Pepper J. Personalised external aortic root support (PEARS) in Marfan syndrome: analysis of 1–9 year outcomes by intention-to-treat in a cohort of the first 30 consecutive patients to receive a novel tissue and valve-conserving procedure, compared with the published results of aortic root replacement. Heart. 2014;100:969–75.
91. Walker PG, Cranney GB, Scheidegger MB, Waseleski G, Pohost GM, Yoganathan AP. Semiautomated method for noise reduction and background phase error correction in MR phase velocity data. J Magn Reson Imaging JMRI. 1993;3:521–30.
92. Bernstein MA, Zhou XJ, Polzin JA, King KF, Ganin A, Pelc NJ, Glover GH. Concomitant gradient terms in phase contrast MR: analysis and correction. Magn Reson Med Off J Soc Magn Reson Med/Soc Magn Reson Med. 1998;39:300–8.
93. Pitcher A, Cassar TE, Suttie J, Francis JM, Leeson P, Blair E, Wordsworth BP, Forfar JC, Myerson SG, Markl M, Neubauer S, Petersen SE. Visualisation of aortic flow disturbance in Marfan syndrome by 4D phase-contrast CMR. J Cardiovasc Magn Reson Off J Soc Cardiovasc Magn Reson. 2011;13 Suppl 1:201.
94. Bieging ET, Frydrychowicz A, Wentland A, Landgraf BR, Johnson KM, Wieben O, Francois CJ. In vivo three-dimensional MR wall shear stress estimation in ascending aortic dilatation. J Magn Reson Imaging JMRI. 2011;33:589–97.
95. Weigang E, Kari FA, Beyersdorf F, Luehr M, Etz CD, Frydrychowicz A, Harloff A, Markl M. Flow-sensitive four-dimensional magnetic resonance imaging: flow patterns in ascending aortic aneurysms. Eur J Cardiothorac Surg Off J Eur Assoc Cardiothorac Surg. 2008;34:11–6.
96. Geiger J, Markl M, Herzer L, Hirtler D, Loeffelbein F, Stiller B, Langer M, Arnold R. Aortic flow patterns in patients with Marfan syndrome assessed by flow-sensitive four-dimensional MRI. J Magn Reson Imaging JMRI. 2012;35:594–600.
97. Stalder AF, Russe MF, Frydrychowicz A, Bock J, Hennig J, Markl M. Quantitative 2D and 3D phase contrast MRI: optimized analysis of blood flow and vessel wall parameters. Magn Reson Med Off J Soc Magn Reson Med/Soc Magn Reson Med. 2008;60:1218–31.
98. Krittian SB, Lamata P, Michler C, Nordsletten DA, Bock J, Bradley CP, Pitcher A, Kilner PJ, Markl M, Smith NP. A finite-element approach to the direct computation of relative cardiovascular pressure from time-resolved MR velocity data. Med Image Anal. 2012;16:1029–37.
99. Lamata P, Pitcher A, Krittian S, Nordsletten D, Bissell MM, Cassar T, Barker AJ, Markl M, Neubauer S, Smith NP. Aortic relative pressure components derived from four-dimensional flow cardiovascular magnetic resonance. Magn Reson Med Off J Soc Magn Reson Med/Soc Magn Reson Med. 2014;72:1162–9.
100. Hope TA, Kvitting JP, Hope MD, Miller DC, Markl M, Herfkens RJ. Evaluation of Marfan patients status post valve-sparing aortic root replacement with 4D flow. Magn Reson Imaging. 2013;31:1479–84.
101. Geiger J, Arnold R, Herzer L, Hirtler D, Stankovic Z, Russe M, Langer M, Markl M. Aortic wall shear stress in Marfan syndrome. Magn Reson Med Off J Soc Magn Reson Med/Soc Magn Reson Med. 2013;70:1137–44.
102. Kvitting JP, Ebbers T, Wigstrom L, Engvall J, Olin CL, Bolger AF. Flow patterns in the aortic root and the aorta studied with time-resolved, 3-dimensional, phase-contrast magnetic resonance imaging: implications for aortic valve-sparing surgery. J Thorac Cardiovasc Surg. 2004;127:1602–7.

9 Thoracic Aortic Surgery in Marfan Syndrome

Pouya Youssefi and Marjan Jahangiri

Introduction

One of the cardinal features of Marfan Syndrome (MFS) is involvement of the cardiovascular system, with predominant effect on the thoracic aorta. The most life-threatening complication of MFS is aneurysm of the thoracic aorta. This can lead to acute aortic dissection or rupture. The mainstay of surgical treatment of the thoracic aorta in Marfan patients is to prophylactically replace or repair part of the thoracic aorta before dissection or rupture occurs. However, it also encompasses emergency surgical management of acute aortic dissection when this lethal disorder does present itself.

Before the era of open heart surgery, the predominant cause of death in patients with MFS was acute dissection or rupture of the thoracic aorta. This generated an average life expectancy of 45 years of age for Marfan patients. The improvement in current medical and surgical therapy of the thoracic aorta has significantly improved this average life expectancy, extending it up to 70 years [1, 2].

Anatomy of the Thoracic Aorta

Surgery of the aorta is one of the most challenging areas of cardiac surgery. To achieve optimal surgical results, which are a necessity if embarking on surgery for young patients, it is essential to have an exhaustive knowledge of the anatomy of the aorta.

The thoracic aorta can be divided into four anatomical sections: the root, ascending aorta, aortic arch, and descending thoracic aorta. The most common site for aneurysm formation is progressive aortic root dilatation, and this can extend further

P. Youssefi, BSc (Hons) MBBS MRCS(Eng) • M. Jahangiri, FRCS(CTh) (✉)
Department of Cardiothoracic Surgery, St. George's Hospital, London, UK
e-mail: marjan.jahangiri@stgeorges.nhs.uk

© Springer-Verlag London 2016

A.H. Child (ed.), *Diagnosis and Management of Marfan Syndrome*,
DOI 10.1007/978-1-4471-5442-6_9

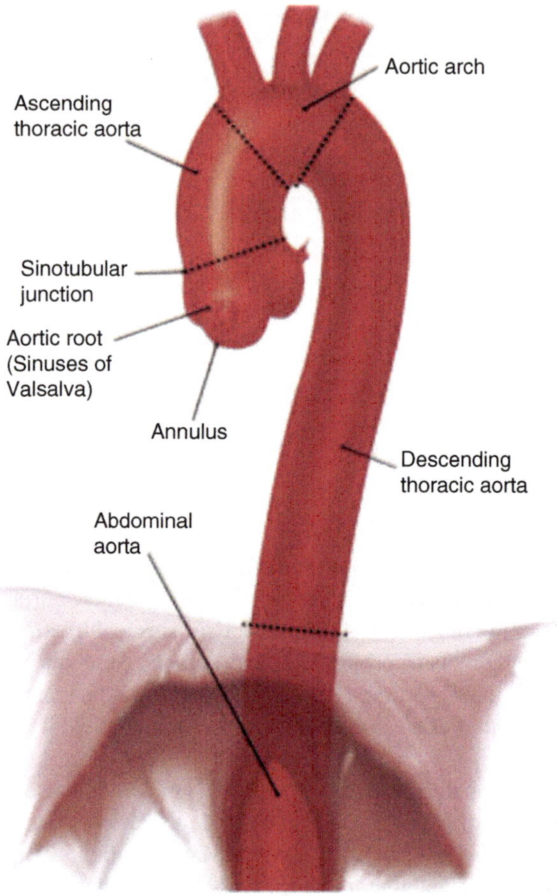

Fig. 9.1 Anatomy of thoracic aorta (Figure from Isselbacher [3])

up into the ascending aorta. Less commonly, the aortic arch and descending aorta can also become aneurysmal in Marfan syndrome patients (Fig. 9.1).

Aortic Root

The aortic root consists of the functional aortic annulus, the aortic valve leaflets with their attachments, and the three bulges in the aortic wall named the sinuses of Valsalva. It is from the sinuses that the two coronary arteries supplying blood to the myocardium arise. The left coronary artery arises from the left coronary sinus, and the right coronary artery arises from the right coronary sinus. The remaining sinus is named the non-coronary sinus. In the same respect, the three aortic valve leaflets are named the left, right and non-coronary leaflets.

The aortic annulus, otherwise named the ventriculo-aortic junction or basal ring, describes the transition zone between the left ventricle and the aortic root. This zone is often described by different specialists in different ways. For the cardiologist and echocardiographer, the annulus relates to the plane passing through the nadir of the semilunar leaflet hinges. For the cardiac surgeon, it corresponds to the leaflet hinge-lines onto which a prosthetic valve is sewn. For an anatomist, the annulus is where the myocardium of the left ventricle ends and the aortic wall begins [4].

If the annulus is thought of as a ring, one half of its circumference is a fibrous portion, and the other half is a muscular portion. The fibrous portion lies beneath the non-coronary sinus and half of the left coronary sinus. It consists of the aorto-mitral continuity, where the base of the anterior leaflet of the mitral valve becomes continuous with the annulus. The muscular portion lies beneath the right coronary sinus and the other half of the left coronary sinus. This consists of the muscular interventricular septum.

At the point where the bulging sinuses of Valsalva end, and the tube-like ascending aorta starts, is named the sino-tubular junction. The circumference of the sino-tubular junction is similar to that of the annulus, and often slightly smaller. This gives the aortic root a structure which allows the aortic valve leaflets to co-apt and close during diastole in a way which prevent regurgitation of blood back into the ventricle. This relation is lost in the Marfan root. As the sinuses dilate and become bulbous, they splay out the commissures and attachments of the valve leaflets. This prevents the leaflets co-apting correctly, and leads to central regurgitation. Enlargement of the sinuses also pushes the coronary artery openings upwards.

Within the lumen of the aortic root, the majority of the leaflet hinge-lines lie above the level of the annulus. The lowest points of the leaflet hinge-lines cross the level of the annulus. The highest points reach to within 1–2 mm of the sino-tubular junction. On the outside of the aortic root, the annulus corresponds to the transition zone between myocardial tissue and the aorta. This is an important zone surgically, as it is the limit of aortic root dissection when performing aortic valve sparing root replacement surgery. Around the left and non-coronary sinus, this zone corresponds to the roof of the left atrium. Around the right coronary sinus, it corresponds to right ventricular outflow tract and myocardium overlying the interventricular septum [5].

The aorta is a dynamic structure, and changes size and shape during the cardiac cycle. There is a 10 % change in diameter of the annulus between systole and diastole, with a relatively greater deformation within the muscular portion compared to the fibrous portion of the annulus [6] (Figs. 9.2, 9.3, and 9.4).

Ascending Aorta

The ascending aorta commences at the junction between the sinuses of Valsalva, and the tubular ascending aorta, named the sino-tubular junction. Here, it is around 3 cm in diameter in a healthy adult. It ascends for a short distance before curving posteriorly and to the left before it becomes the aortic arch. The ascending aorta is contained within the pericardial sac, and is enclosed in a tube of serous pericardium, which it shares with the pulmonary artery. To the right of the ascending aorta lies the superior vena cava, anteriorly in the lower part lies the appendage of the right atrium (which also lies in front of the aortic root), and to the left lies the pulmonary trunk. The right main pulmonary artery travels behind the ascending aorta.

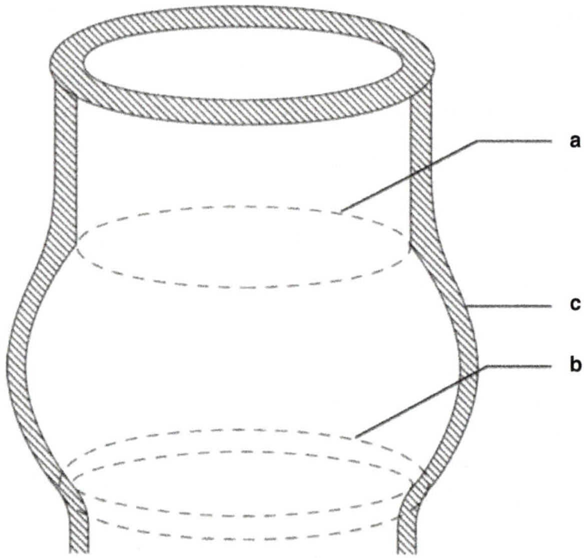

Fig. 9.2 The aortic root: *a* Sinotubular junction, *b* ventriculo-aortic junction, *c* sinuses of Valsalva (Figure from de Kerchove et al. [4])

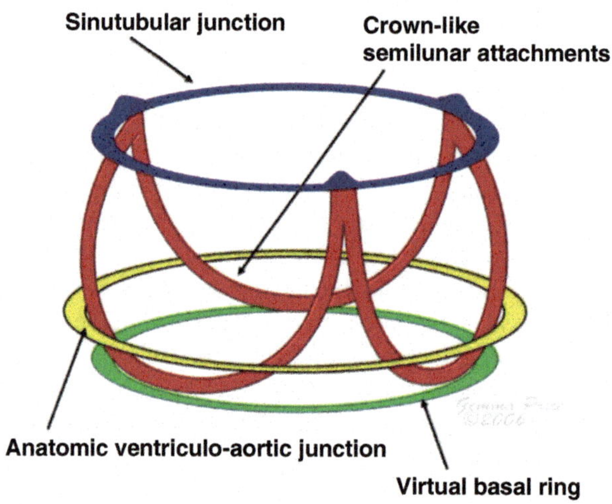

Fig. 9.3 Diagrammatic representation of the aortic root (Figure from Tilea et al. [6]))

Aortic Arch

The aortic arch begins at the superior border of the right second sternocostal joint. The junction between the ascending aorta and the aortic arch is marked by a fold of the pericardial sac. It runs posteriorly and to the left to travel in front of the trachea, and subsequently downward to the left of the body of the fourth thoracic vertebra. It becomes the descending thoracic aorta at the lower border of this vertebra (Fig. 9.5).

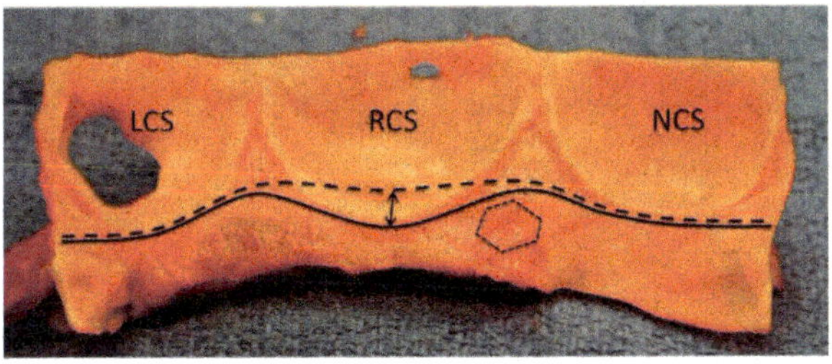

Fig. 9.4 The opened aortic root seen from within the lumen. Continuous *black line* shows the ventriculo-aortic junction, *interrupted black line* shows the limit of proximal aortic root dissection, *double black arrow* shows the segment of myocardium included into the base of the right coronary sinus, *dotted line encircles* the membranous septum, *LCS* left coronary sinus, *RCS* right coronary sinus, *NCS* non-coronary sinus (Figure from de Kerchove et al. [4])

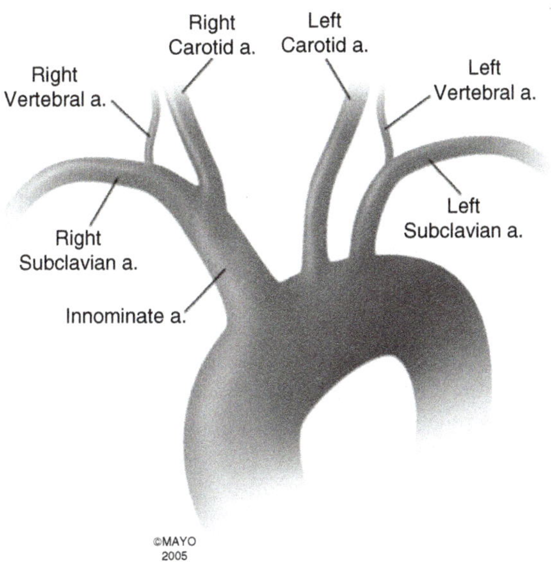

Fig. 9.5 The most common aortic arch branching pattern (Figure from Layton et al. [7])

The aortic arch can be divided into three hypothetical areas: right, central and left. The right part consists of the short length between the pericardial fold and the origin of the brachiocephalic artery (the first of three major head and neck vessels which branch from the aortic arch, also known as the innominate artery). The central part, which is convex in shape, gives rise to the brachiocephalic artery, left common carotid artery, and left subclavian artery. These three branches are crossed anteriorly by the left brachiocephalic vein, which can pose difficulties with exposure during surgery to replace the aortic arch. This vein can when necessary be ligated and divided to improve exposure to the arch vessels.

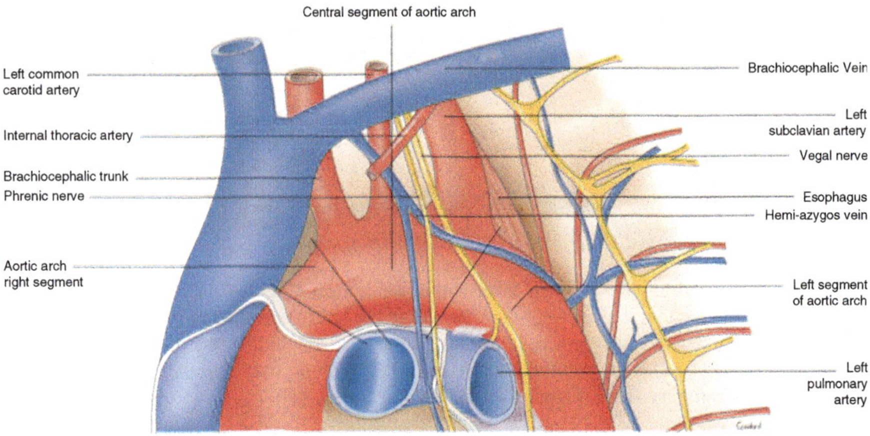

Fig. 9.6 Surrounding anatomy of the aortic arch (Figure from Berdajs et al. [8])

The left vagus nerve runs down from the neck in front of the left common carotid artery to then lie on the surface of the anterior wall of the aortic arch. It then turns to the left and heads towards the ligamentum arteriosum (see below). From here, it descends to pass posterior to the hilum of the left lung. The left phrenic nerve travels initially along a similar path to the vagus nerve, albeit more superficial. It does not directly contact the aortic arch, and runs more anteriorly to pass in front of the hilum of the left lung.

Behind the origin of the left subclavian artery from the aortic arch lies the trachea and the oesophagus. The trachea lies to the right of the oesophagus, and can be found when dissecting the space between the left common carotid artery and left subclavian artery. At this point, on the anterior surface of the trachea, lies the recurrent laryngeal nerve, a branch of the left vagus nerve which must be preserved during dissection of the arch.

The ligamentum arteriosum, the remnant of the ductus arteriosus, lies between the pulmonary trunk and the inferior surface of the aortic arch, just 1–1.5 cm distal to the origin of the left subclavian artery. This is in the left or final part of the aortic arch. The left vagal nerve runs down from the anterior surface of the aortic arch towards the ligamentum arteriosum. Before diving to pass behind the left hilum, it gives off the recurrent laryngeal nerve at the level of the ligamentum arteriosum, which then hooks around the inferior wall of the arch and then passes upward towards the anterior surface of the trachea (Fig. 9.6).

Descending Thoracic Aorta

The aortic arch continues as the descending thoracic aorta just below the aortic isthmus. This is the section of the distal arch that is positioned between the origin of the left subclavian artery and the attachment of the ligamentum arteriosum. During foetal development, this area is significantly narrowed. Just distal to attachment of the ductus arteriosus, the aorta has a fusiform dilatation, called the aortic spindle. The narrowing of the isthmus and the dilatation of the spindle even themselves out, but still persist to a minor degree in the adult. On average, the diameter of the spindle is 3 mm larger than the isthmus in adults.

The descending aorta lies in its proximal section to the left side of the vertebral column. It usually gives off nine pairs of intercostal arteries. Other branches given off include pericardial, bronchial, oesophageal, mediastinal, subcostal and phrenic. By the time it reaches the diaphragm at the level of the twelfth thoracic vertebra, it lies closer to the midline. The aortic hiatus of the diaphragm is traversed by the aorta, azygos vein and thoracic duct.

Indications for Surgery

Emergency Surgery for Aortic Dissection

Acute aortic dissection is a life-threatening complication which can occur in patients with MFS. It occurs when a tear in the inner wall, or intima, of the aorta allows blood to flow between the layers of the wall of the aorta. This forces the layers apart, and blood flowing between the layers of the aortic wall (the false lumen), may compress blow flow within the true lumen of the aorta. This can cause ischaemia of organs perfused by branches of the aorta, leading to possible myocardial infarction, stroke, paraplegia, renal failure, mesenteric ischaemia, and/or limb ischaemia. Rupture of the aorta may also ensue. Dissection downwards towards the aortic root may also result in structural changes to the aortic valve with loss of its suspensory support, thus leading to acute regurgitation. Other complications include pericardial effusion and tamponade from ruptured blood within the pericardium.

Aortic dissection can be classified depending on the anatomical extent of the dissection. A number of different classification systems have been proposed over the years, however the most internationally recognized classification systems now are the Stanford [9] classification and the Debakey [10] classification systems. The key point of classifying an aortic dissection depends on whether the ascending aorta is involved regardless of the location of the tear. If the dissection involves the ascending aorta, it is a Stanford Type A dissection, which corresponds to the Debakey Type I or Type II. Debakey Type II dissections are confined to the ascending aorta, whereas Debakey Type I dissections extend beyond the brachiocephalic artery. Stanford Type B dissections involve the descending aorta and are distal to the left subclavian artery. By far the commonest type of dissection involves the ascending aorta, arch and descending aorta, and this is the most lethal combination (Fig. 9.7).

Type A dissection is an absolute indication for emergency surgery. In the Marfan patient who develops type A dissection, this is an indication to replace the aortic root. This may be with or without preserving the aortic valve depending on its

Classification of aortic dissection

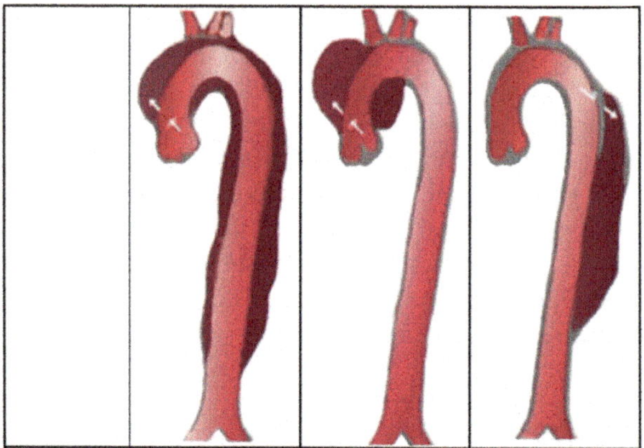

Percentage	60 %	10–15 %	25–30 %
Type	DeBakey I	DeBakey II	DeBakey III
	Stanford A (Proximal)		Stanford B (Distal)

Fig. 9.7 The Stanford and Debakey classifications of aortic dissection

morphology and whether there is significant valvular regurgitation. The standard operation is replacement of the sinuses of Valsalva and as much of the ascending aorta as possible. If the tear extends into the aortic arch (which is rare in patients with MFS), then replacement of the arch will also be necessary.

Acute type B dissection is generally not as life-threatening as acute type A dissection. When taking the general population, early survival is satisfactory using medical management alone, unless distal ischaemic complications or aortic rupture occur [11]. Patients with life-threatening complications of type B dissections require emergency treatment with either endovascular stent-graft treatment, open surgical aortic graft replacement, interventional or surgical flap fenestration, or extra-anatomic surgical bypass. In recent years, there has been a move towards early intervention in the acute setting even in uncomplicated patients. This has been in the form of endovascular stent-graft treatment. However, patients with MFS deserve special consideration in this setting. Stent-grafting in the Marfan patient at this point in time is not recommended, and should only be used when operative intervention is indicated but open repair is deemed too risky and prohibitive [11]. This is because there is limited information regarding the effect of the radial forces that a stent-graft places on the abnormal and weak aorta of patients with MFS. Furthermore, these patients are often young at presentation, and since the long term durability of stent-grafts is unknown, this intervention is not prudent. Open thoraco-abdominal aortic replacement can be safely achieved in experienced centres with acceptable morbidity and mortality, and is still the treatment of choice for Marfan patients with descending aorta pathology.

Elective Surgery

The purpose of elective surgery in patients with MFS is to prevent aortic dissection or rupture. It is difficult to predict with great confidence when an aorta will dissect. There are rarely ever any symptoms or signs to predict impending dissection. Therefore, we still rely on measurement of aortic size to guide timing of intervention.

Natural history studies at Yale University by Elefteriades et al. [12] have looked at the lifetime risk of rupture or dissection. They showed specific "hinge points" in the aortic size at which rupture or dissection occur. In the ascending aorta, these hinge points occur at 6 cm, and in the descending aorta 7 cm. Further analysis showed a 15.6 % yearly risk of rupture, dissection or death in patients with aortic size ≥6.0 cm. It is thought that if planned surgery carries a risk lower than this, the patient should have surgery. This concept has governed cardiovascular guidelines on management of the aorta for many years. The aim of these guidelines is to promote prophylactic surgery before catastrophic complications manifest. In the Marfan population, more stringent guidelines are used due to the increased risk of aortic complications. In the current era, experienced aortic surgeons can perform operations at low risk, and thus the following guidelines are currently used.

Current European Society of Cardiology guidelines [13] on the management of aortic disease, similar to guidelines from North America [14], state that patients with MFS should undergo surgery when the aortic root diameter is 50 mm, with class I level C evidence. Those with a family history of aortic dissection should be treated more aggressively, as tendency for the aorta to dissect runs in families. Therefore, a positive family history of dissection is an indication to operate at a root diameter of 45 mm or above. The rate of change of aortic size is another factor to consider. Progressive enlargement between surveillance imaging is a worrying sign, and thus an increase in size of >3 mm/year is also an indication to operate at a diameter of 45 mm or above. Other indications to operate at this lower size threshold include severe aortic or mitral valve regurgitation. If the patient has symptoms of valvular regurgitation and/or an increase in the size of left ventricle, then the same rules for valve surgery apply. If the patient merits aortic valve replacement, it may be deemed unwise to replace the aortic valve alone and leave the Marfan root in situ. Female patients who plan to become pregnant may also be considered for surgery at a lower size threshold of 40–45 mm, to prevent aortic complications during pregnancy or in the post-partum period.

As well as diameter alone, another measurement which can be used for guidance on timing of surgery is the cross-sectional area of the root in square centimetres, divided by the patient's height in metres. If this value exceeds ten, it may also be considered an indication for surgery. Z-scores taking into account root size, height and weight may also be used to aid in timing of surgery [15].

As for the descending thoracic aorta, elective replacement should be considered if size reaches 50 mm. Replacement of the descending aorta is challenging, and decisions regarding surgery should be made by surgeons experienced in performing these operations [11].

Types of Surgery

Aortic Root Replacement (Bentall Procedure)

In 1967, Bentall and De Bono [16] devised an operation for replacement of the aortic root and ascending aorta by using a Starr-Edwards valve hand-sewn into a tube graft. This was a considerable contribution to the field of cardiac surgery, with an even more significant impact on the life expectancy of patients with MFS. Prior to this operation, the average life expectancy for Marfan patients was around 45 years. With this operation, and the subsequent techniques that ensued (see below), average life expectancy has been quoted as high as 70 years in some studies [1].

The Bentall operation is one which has stood the test of time, and is still the most commonly performed operation for replacement of the aortic root. It remains the gold standard to which all root procedures must be compared. It consists of root replacement with a conduit (Dacron tube graft) and a prosthetic aortic valve (either mechanical or biological). The coronary arteries have to be mobilised, and subsequently re-implanted onto the conduit. When the procedure was first described, it involved a graft inclusion technique whereby the composite valve-graft was placed inside the opened native dilated aortic root, and after completion of the various anastomoses, the native aneurysmal aorta was wrapped around the new root. The aim of this wrap was to contain the bleeding which occurred at the suture lines in the porous Dacron graft of that era. This was satisfactory at the time, and perioperative mortality became as low as 10 %. However, it led to medium and long term problems with pseudoaneurysm formation from bleeding into the native aneurysmal wrap. Repeat operations to deal with these complications posed significant risk.

Subsequent adaptation of the technique has led to the exclusion composite valve-graft replacement. This version of the operation involves excision of the aneurysmal section of aorta right down to the annulus. Without having the inclusion wrap of native aneurysmal aorta around the conduit, the surgeon is able to visualize and deal with all bleeding points before completion of the operation. Newer versions of Dacron grafts are significantly less porous, and this has reduced the rates of bleeding even further.

Setup for the operation involves standard median sternotomy or mini-J sternotomy. The patient is systemically heparinised and monitored with serial ACT (activated clotting time) measurements. For patients where the aneurysm is confined to the aortic root and/or ascending aorta, arterial cannulation of the distal ascending aorta is sufficient to completely excise the aneurysmal section of the aorta. Venous drainage of the patient is carried out by inserting a 2-stage cannula into the right atrial appendage. A vent is inserted into the right superior pulmonary vein and advanced into the left ventricle to reduce myocyte distension and minimise myocardial oxygen demand. Placement of a cross-clamp on the distal ascending aorta allows antegrade infusion of cold blood potassium-rich cardioplegia into the aortic root via a separate cannula, thus arresting the heart in diastole and providing myocardial protection during the ischaemic clamp time. This needs to be repeated every 20 min directly into the coronary ostia whilst the cross-clamp is still on, to prevent the heart from contracting.

The ascending aorta is opened and assessment of the aortic valve is made. Complete dissection of the aortic root and its components is carried out. If the aortic valve is normal in structure, consideration may be given to a valve-sparing root replacement (see below). Otherwise, the valve is excised and the annulus is decalcified if necessary. The coronary arteries are dissected and mobilised on buttons of aortic tissue. The degree of mobilisation of the coronary arteries is important – too little and there may be tension and narrowing once they are re-connected, too much and they kink.

The aneurysmal section of the aorta is excised. The valve is sized using the appropriate valve sizer. Valve sutures with pledgets are placed from the ventricular to the aortic sides of the annulus, in a horizontal mattress fashion. Distance between sutures must be equal to provide a constant tension on the anastomosis and prevent bleeding. Good surgical technique is imperative to follow the curve of the needle through the aortic annulus, as unwanted leverage on the needle will create irregular needle holes leading to bleeding at the end of the operation. The valve sutures are then passed through the cuff of the prosthetic valve at the corresponding points. The valve is parachuted down and subsequently the sutures are tied in turn. The annular suture line is checked for gaps and appropriate repairs made if necessary.

Now that the combined valve-graft conduit is attached to the annulus, the coronary artery buttons can be re-implanted. Hand-held cautery is used to cut a hole the size of the coronary button into the appropriate location on the graft. A 5/0 polypropylene suture is then used to anastomose the coronary buttons to the conduit.

Then the distal anastomosis between the Dacron graft and the distal ascending aorta is performed. After tailoring the conduit graft, this is done with a 4/0 polypropylene running suture, starting at the most posterior point and then working round each side in turn to finish anteriorly. As the most anterior part of the suture line is reached, the vent is turned off and the heart is allowed to slowly fill. Before the anastomosis is tied down, the heart and new composite valve-graft are de-aired through the distal anastomosis. Once the suture is tied down, further de-airing can be continued through a small hole made in the anterior portion of the Dacron graft. Ventilation is recommenced to push air out of the pulmonary vasculature and into the heart, hence aiding in de-airing. Trans-oesophageal echocardiography can be used to assess the de-airing process. The cross-clamp can then be removed. Once the surgeon is happy that the heart has been de-aired thoroughly and myocardial function is restored, cardiopulmonary bypass can be discontinued.

Advantages and Disadvantages

The Bentall procedure allows for use of either a mechanical valve or a bioprosthetic valve (porcine or bovine) in combination with an artificial graft. In the majority of patients with MFS who have this operation, they will be at a relatively young age. Therefore, a mechanical valve will be the most commonly used of the valve types, as bioprosthetic valves generally have a life-span of 10–15 years before decline in

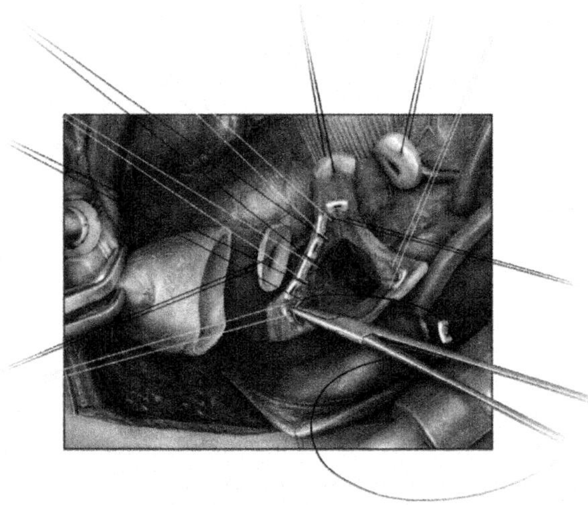

Fig. 9.8 The aortic valve has been excised and the coronary buttons mobilised. Valve sutures with pledgets have been placed in the annulus corresponding to the left coronary sinus (Figure from Girardi [18])

function. Mechanical valves have the theoretical advantage of lasting for the lifespan of the patient, but they require life-long anticoagulation with warfarin. This itself carries a risk of bleeding, which although small in probability, has an incremental effect for every year anticoagulation is used (around 1 %/year) [17]. Life-long warfarin for a young patient should not be taken lightly, and careful discussion with the patient is paramount. Even with anticoagulation, mechanical valves do carry a small risk of thromboembolism (1 %/year) [17].

In young patients unable or unwilling to take warfarin, a bioprosthetic valve may be used. This may be because of a pre-existing bleeding diathesis, liver disease, excess alcohol intake, or simply a life-style choice. It may also be used in young female patients who wish to bear children in the future, as warfarin is associated with a risk of teratogenicity when taken during pregnancy. The implication of using a bioprosthetic valve in young patients is that they will inevitably require further procedures later on in life. Redo operations always carry a higher risk than the first, as the tissues develop dense adhesions making surgery more challenging. But experienced surgeons can still attain satisfactory morbidity and mortality outcomes in these procedures. In recent years, advances in catheter-based valve procedures have led to successful trans-catheter valve-in-valve implantation where a new valve is inserted within a degenerated bioprosthetic valve. This omits the need for redo surgery. However, to date this has been restricted to elderly patients too sick to undergo redo open heart surgery. The long term results and longevity of these valves is unknown. Therefore, they are not recommended for use in young Marfan syndrome patients (Figs. 9.8 and 9.9).

Valve-Preserving Root Replacement

In the early 1990s, it was with the intention of sparing patients the burden of life-long anticoagulation that two different surgeons from both sides of the Atlantic separately devised valve-sparing root replacement (VSRR) operations. Sarsam and

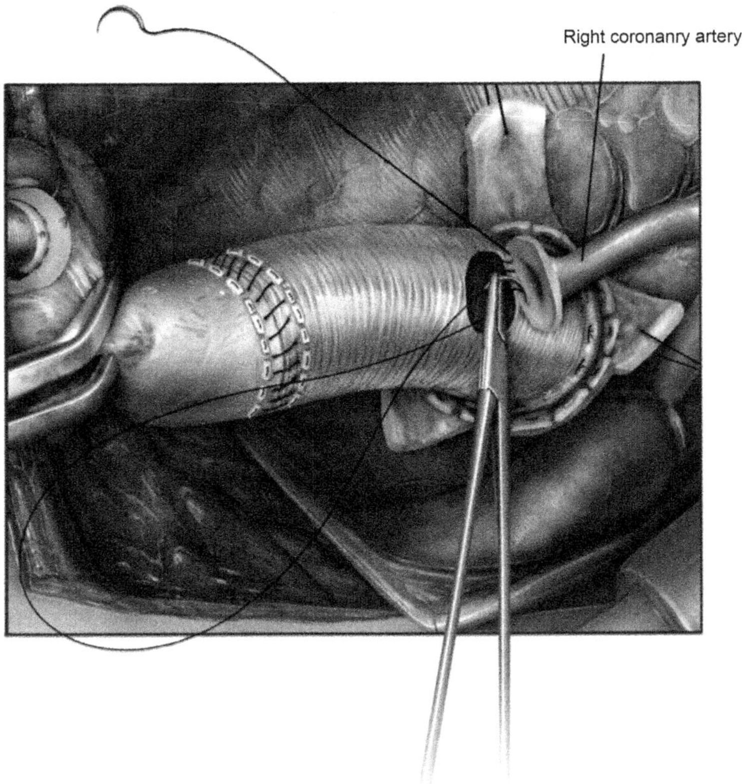

Fig. 9.9 The right coronary button is being anastomosed to the tube conduit (Figure from Girardi [18])

Yacoub [19] and David et al. [20] developed the remodelling and reimplantation procedures respectively, whereby the aneurysmal aortic root could be replaced without replacing the aortic valve. These are more challenging operations compared to the Bentall procedure, requiring the surgeon to craft an aortic root in which the suspensory support of the aortic valve has to be reconstructed without causing any deformity or asymmetry, any small degree of which would cause valvular regurgitation.

Remodelling Technique

The remodelling technique was first described by Professor Sir Magdi Yacoub [19]. The technique consists of radical excision of the sinuses down to the aortic annulus, whilst sparing the valve leaflets, their hinge-points, and the commissures. The integrity of the aortic root is then reconstructed using a artificial tube graft which is manually shaped to form appropriate-sized sinuses. The aortic valve is suspended again in relation to the neo-sinuses created.

The setup of the operation is similar to that of the Bentall procedure described above. The aortic root is dissected free from surrounding structures. Once the ascending aorta is transected, the aortic valve leaflets are assessed for any defects, fenestrations, and for adequate co-aptation. If the surgeon is satisfied that the leaflets are healthy enough to achieve good long-term function and co-aptation, the valve-sparing procedure can be embarked upon. The diseased and enlarged aortic sinuses are excised down to the aortic annulus, leaving only 4-6 mm of aortic wall attached to the aortic annulus. The coronary arteries are dissected and mobilised as with the Bentall procedure.

The next step is to choose an appropriately sized tube graft. This is a critical part of the operation, and an error at this point may make an otherwise skilled attempt at the operation futile. Yacoub first described this measurement by taking horizontal mattress sutures above the top of each commissure and stretching the three commissures in a vertical direction. The valve cusps were observed to see if they would co-apt correctly. Once the cusps were optimally co-apting, the distance between the commissures was measured. This would then represent one-third of the circumference of the tube graft, and would thus provide a guide to the diameter of the graft needed. In subsequent years, this measurement has been described by others as using a tube graft of a diameter 10–15 % smaller than the average length of the valve free margins (or double the height of the leaflets). A simpler technique is to size the annulus using valve sizers and subsequently use a tube graft 1–2 mm larger. Whichever technique is used, most adult patients require grafts of 26–30 mm in diameter. In adolescents and small individuals, a tube graft around 20 mm would be used.

One end of the tube graft is taken and three equidistant vertical lines are cut into it. This divides the circumference of that end of the tube graft into three sections of equal length. The height of the grooves is made to be the height of the commissures (distance between the bottom of the sinus to the top of the commissures). These measurements are made by trans-oesophageal echocardiography prior to the establishment of cardiopulmonary bypass. If this turns out to be larger than necessary, it can easy be trimmed during suturing of the graft to the annulus. Cutting these three grooves creates three extensions of the tube graft which are square at their ends. The sharp edges are rounded. This creates the three neo-sinuses of the tube graft.

The three mattress sutures earlier placed at the top of the three commissures are then passed through the apex of each of the three grooves in the tube graft, and the tube graft is parachuted down to the annulus. Now the Dacron neo-sinuses can be trimmed to size if necessary. Each Dacron neo-sinus is then sutured to the aortic annulus surrounding each sinus using 4/0 polypropylene. We recommend anchoring each neo-sinus in the middle (in the midpoint of each valve cusp). The next step is to sew each neo-sinus by starting at the commissure and working towards the bottom of the sinus. In our experience, this reduces the possibility of valvular regurgitation and disturbance of leaflet mechanism, which can occur near the top of the commissures. These suture lines are technically challenging, as they need to be adequately haemostatic, but at the same time maintaining a perfect symmetry which allows the re-suspended aortic valve to co-apt without any prolapse or regurgitation.

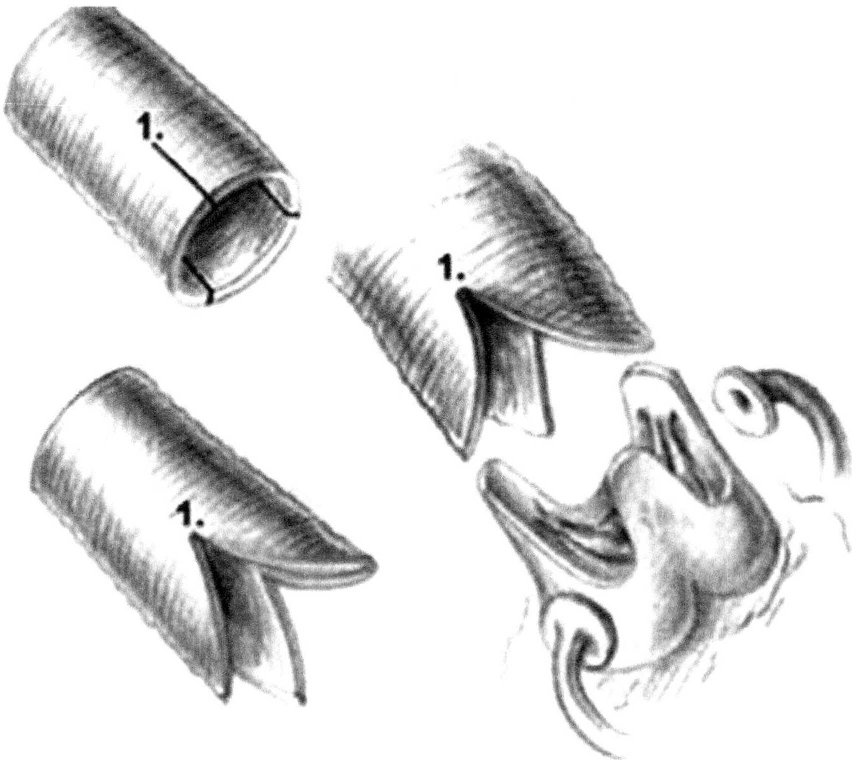

Fig. 9.10 The tube conduit is cut to shape three neo-sinuses (Figure from Hopkins et al. [21])

Subsequently, two circular holes are created at the appropriate location in the neo-sinuses to accommodate the two coronary buttons. These holes are made using hand-held cautery, and the coronary button anastomosis is carried out in the same manner as in the Bentall procedure, as is the remainder of the operation.

De-airing is performed in a standard fashion. Once the heart has been weaned from cardiopulmonary bypass, it is imperative to assess the function of the aortic valve via trans-oesophageal echocardiography. If regurgitation is present, cardiopulmonary bypass needs to be re-established and repair of the valve carried out. If repair is not possible, then the difficult decision needs to be made as to redoing the root replacement with a Bentall procedure. The valve preserving operation is unforgiving with a steep learning curve, and should not be carried out in inexperienced hands (Figs. 9.10 and 9.11).

Reimplantation Technique

The reimplantation technique was first described by Dr Tirone David [20], whereby a Dacron graft is sealed below the annulus of the aortic valve. It involves two suture

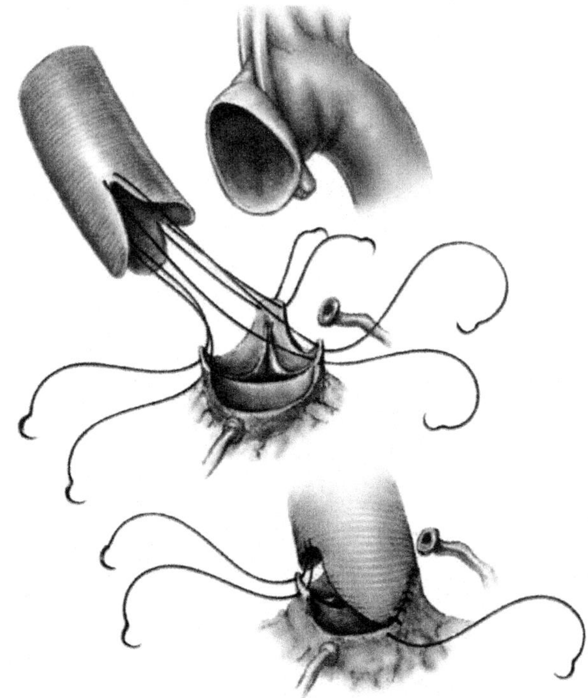

Fig. 9.11 Anastomosis of the tube graft to the aortic root (Figure from Cameron [22])

lines as compared to one suture line in the remodelling procedure. The two suture lines are sub-annular, and intra-aortic. The reimplantation technique has been modified numerous times over the years. The first version was named the David I procedure, and subsequent variations have led to the David V procedure. A further iteration has been the David V – Standford Modification technique. What started out as a technique using a straight tube graft (David I), has proceeded in stages to using an oversized straight tube graft which is then plicated proximally to create neo-sinuses (David V). The intention of these modifications has been to create a larger diameter neo-sinus which is better at allowing unhindered valve leaflet excursion, and preservation of sinus flow vortices. The Stanford Modification involves the use of an appropriate sized second graft (which is smaller than the tube graft used for the root replacement) to anastomose to the larger root graft and in doing so create the new sino-tubular junction.

The setup of the operation is the same as the previously described root operations. The aortic valve is again assessed for function once the ascending aorta has been transected. Again, the aorta is trimmed down to the annulus, leaving 7–8 mm of native aortic wall attached to the annulus. Next, the aortic root is carefully dissected away from surrounding structures, which includes separating it from the pulmonary artery, atria and right ventricular outflow tract. This dissection must extend to just below the level of the annulus. A Hegar dilator is then used to size the tube conduit by being placed through the valve and into the left ventricular outflow tract.

It should fit in comfortably, but not be too tight. This correct size is then added to 11 mm and the resulting number is the size of the tube conduit. This is usually 32–38 mm in adults.

Next, the subannular layer of sutures are placed. This suture line is specific to the reimplantation technique, and is not part of the remodelling procedure. Horizontal mattress sutures are placed in a planar fashion under the annulus with the sutures coming out externally from the aortic root. Each pair of sutures is clipped, ready to be used in the next step. There should be one horizontal mattress suture directly underneath each commissure.

The appropriate sized tube graft is then marked with a pen such that the circumference at one end of the graft is divided into three equal sectors. These lines help to guide where the horizontal mattress sutures underneath each commissure should go. The rest of the mattress sutures are sequentially placed into one end of the tube graft. Once they are all placed, the tube graft is parachuted down to the annulus. The aortic valve and the small rim of aortic wall should fall within the tube graft. The same Hegar dilator which was used to finally size the conduit is again placed through the aortic valve, and the subannular sutures are tied. This prevents narrowing the outflow tract and annulus too much. The three commissural sutures are tied first, followed by the rest.

The three valve commissures are lifted up by placing a polypropylene horizontal mattress suture inside-to-out at the top of each commissure. This allows the three commissures to be anchored to the graft at 120° intervals. A small amount of saline is injected into the root to see if the leaflets co-apt correctly when fluid rests in the sinuses. If leaflet co-aptation is satisfactory, the anchoring sutures are tied down, and each limb of the suture is then used to suture the rim of aortic wall around the valve to the tube conduit in a running fashion. It is important with these sutures to stay close to the base of the valve leaflets, but not too close to impinge on them.

The coronary buttons are then anastomosed to circular holes created at the appropriate locations in the tube graft. In the Modified Stanford technique, a second tube graft smaller in size than the one used for the root is then anastomosed to this tube graft in order to create a crimping effect of the sino-tubular junction.

Advantages and Disadvantages

The main advantage of valve-sparing root replacement over the traditional Bentall procedure is the conservation of the native valve and avoidance of either a mechanical valve which requires life-long anticoagulation, or a bioprosthetic valve which will likely need re-intervention in young patients. With this significant advantage does come some drawbacks too. The valve-sparing operation is technically much more challenging, and few surgeons have a large experience with this operation. Furthermore, it is an operation which has a steep learning curve, and is associated with a four-fold increase in rate of re-intervention on the aortic valve when compared to the Bentall procedure (1.3 %/year vs 0.3 %/year). There is no difference in rates of endocarditis (0.3 %/year vs 0.2 %/year) [23].

Valve-sparing root replacement has emerged as an alternative in patients who have minimal valve involvement. It avoids the needs for life-long anticoagulation

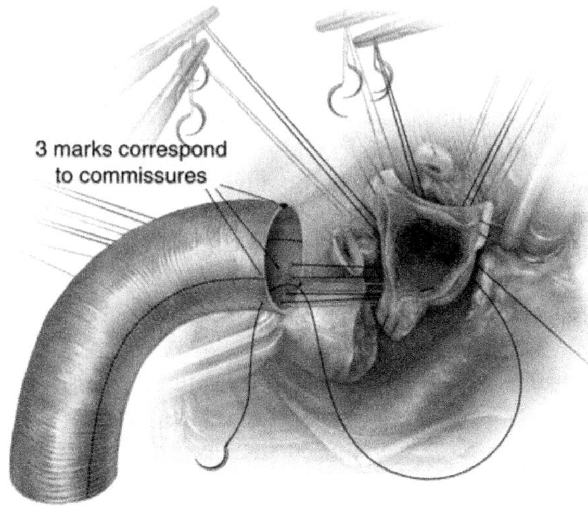

Fig. 9.12 The subannular horizontal sutures are placed through the graft before it is lowered down to the aortic root (Figure from Ikonomidis [24])

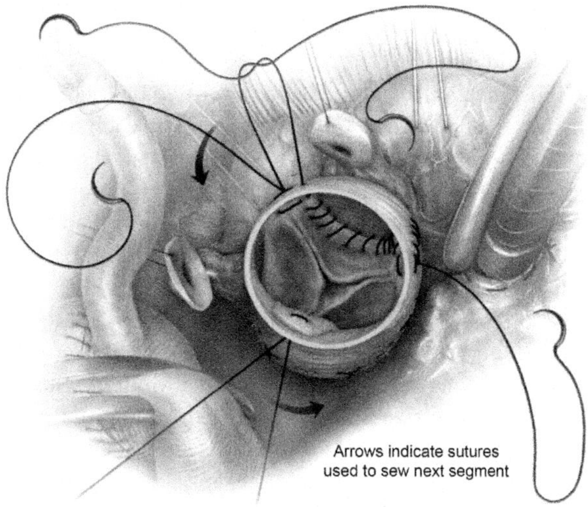

Fig. 9.13 The aortic cuff around the valve is sutured to the graft in running fashion (Figure from Ikonomidis [24])

and late valve-related thromboembolism. The short and medium term results are good in the hands of experienced surgeons. What remains unknown is the truly long-term results (Fig. 9.12 and 9.13).

Replacement of the Aortic Arch

For patients with aneurysms of the aortic arch (either in isolation or as part of an aneurysm starting from the aortic root and extending up into the arch), the head and neck vessels will need to be disconnected and the aneurysmal arch excised [25]. This requires the use of deep hypothermic circulatory arrest. There are however a variety of cerebral perfusion strategies for providing oxygenated blood to the brain during this period of circulatory arrest to reduce the neurological ischaemic burden.

This operation is usually carried out through a median sternotomy, however if more extensive resection of the descending aorta is required, a clamshell thoracotomy (bilateral anterior thoracotomy) may also be utilised to give better exposure to the descending aorta. The patient is heparinised in preparation for cardiopulmonary bypass. A number of arterial cannulation options may be utilised. Here we describe right axillary artery cannulation as it also is part of the cerebral perfusion strategy.

The right axillary artery is exposed through a subclavicular incision. An 8 or 10 mm tube graft is anastomosed end-to-side to the axillary artery. Venous cannulation is carried out through the right atrium. Once cardiopulmonary bypass is established, the patient is cooled down to 18–20 °C. The arch and its branches are dissected out carefully. Once the patient has reached the desired temperature with electroencephalographic silence, flow is reduced and the brachiocephalic artery, left common carotid artery and left subclavian artery are clamped. Flow is resumed at 10 mL/kg to now establish antegrade cerebral perfusion from the right axillary artery through the right common carotid artery and vertebral artery and via the Circle of Willis. A left arm blood pressure between 40 and 60 mmHg is aimed for. The head is topically cooled with ice and intravenous steroids are administered. The electroencephalogram and cerebral oximetry are observed for bilateral flow and adequate cerebral protection.

The aorta can now be transected and the blood volume drained. The three head and neck vessels are divided proximal to their clamps. The aneurysmal section is excised. If the aneurysm only extends to the distal arch, the excised section can be limited to just before the origin of left subclavian artery. The stump of the left subclavian artery would then have to be oversewn.

Alternatives to the technique of cerebral protection described here include selective antegrade cerebral perfusion, whereby individual cannulae are inserted into the divided brachiocephalic, left common carotid and left subclavian arteries once the aorta has been transected. This requires additional individual cannulae and perfusion lines from the cardiopulmonary bypass machine. Another alternative is retrograde perfusion through a venous cannula inserted into the superior vena cava, however there is some evidence questioning the benefits of this technique.

The aortic arch is sized for a suitable tube graft. A number of different grafts are available, including a simple tube graft with a side arm (for subsequent arterial perfusion), and tube grafts with three branches for the head and neck vessels, as well as the side arm. The distal anastomosis is performed with the proximal descending aorta. If there is aneurysmal disease of the descending thoracic and/or abdominal aorta, a 2-stage elephant trunk technique is used [26]. Here, a longer tube graft is used, and it is folded in on itself at the point of desired distal anastomosis. The inverted tube graft is passed down into the descending aorta, and the distal anastomosis is carried out at the inversion fold. Subsequently, the inner part of the inverted graft is pulled up into the surgical field and this will become the neo-arch. The section of the graft remaining in the descending aorta is the so-called "elephant trunk". This will remain in the descending aorta and can be utilised in the second stage of

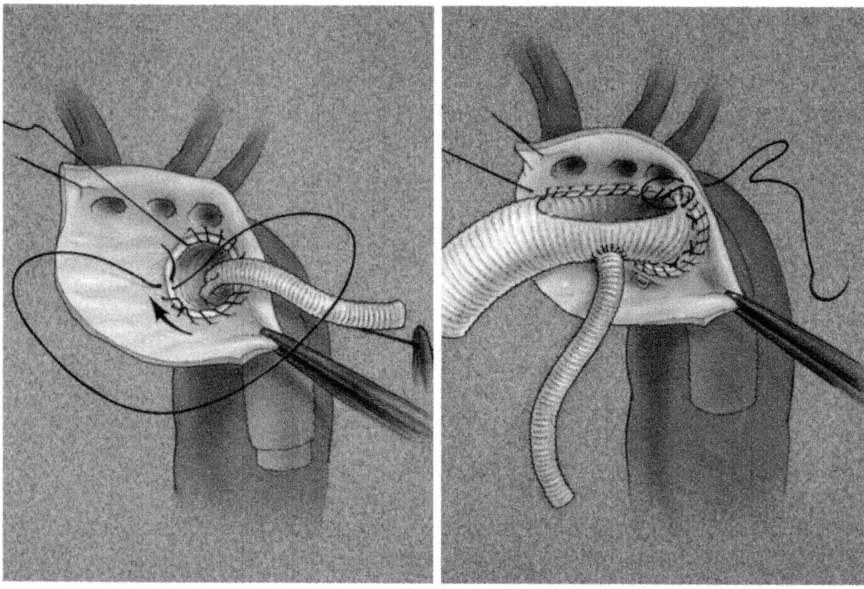

Fig. 9.14 First stage of the elephant trunk technique. The first diagram shows the distal anastomosis to the descending aorta, with the tube graft inverted. The second diagram shows an island anastomosis of the head and neck vessels to the tube graft (Figure from Svensson [25])

the procedure, either for an open procedure to anastomose a second tube graft for replacement of the descending thoracic/thoracoabdominal aorta, or for an endovascular procedure to be used as a landing zone for a covered stent.

Once the distal anastomosis is carried out, the head and neck vessels can be anastomosed as an island [25] or individually [26]. Our preference is island anastomosis where possible. Antegrade cerebral perfusion is converted once again to antegrade whole body perfusion once anastomosis to the head and neck vessels is completed (and a clamp placed on the tube graft just proximal to this). Finally, the proximal anastomosis is made either to the root replacement tube graft in the case of root and arch aneurysm, or to the native ascending aorta in the case of isolated arch aneurysm.

After thorough de-airing, the cross-clamp is removed and the heart allowed to reperfuse for a number of minutes. Once rewarming is complete, the heart can be weaned from cardiopulmonary bypass (Fig. 9.14).

Replacement of the Descending Aorta

The replacement of the descending aorta is carried out through a left thoracotomy, with the left lung deflated [25]. In the case of thoracoabdominal aneurysms, this becomes a thoraco-laparotomy. The descending aorta will need to be cross-clamped for the repair, and therefore the circulation to the lower half of the body will need to be bypassed. Commonly left heart bypass will be used, although a number of other options are available including full cardiopulmonary bypass, deep hypothermic circulatory arrest, and apico-aortic shunt. Left heart bypass has the goal of diverting a portion of oxygenated blood from the left atrium to the aorta distal to the section being replaced. The proximal cannula is usually inserted into the left inferior pulmonary vein or the left atrial appendage. The portion of blood travelling to the ascending aorta, arch and head and neck vessels will be pumped by the left ventricle. The portion of blood diverted from the left atrium to the distal circulation will be driven by a centrifugal pump.

One of the risks of surgery on the descending aorta is that of paraplegia. This can be caused by a combination of factors. Firstly, the blood supply to the spinal cord is variable and different patients have different degrees of collateralisation. Certain intercostal arteries (supplying spinal arteries) may be more important than others. Surgery often involves re-implantation of some intercostal patches or buttons. Cross-clamping the descending aorta has been shown to increase cerebrospinal fluid (CSF) pressure. Since spinal perfusion pressure is the difference between systemic blood pressure and CSF pressure, this effect causes a decrease in spinal cord perfusion pressure, thereby increasing the risk of paraplegia. One way of preventing this is to carry out CSF drainage, thereby maintaining spinal cord perfusion pressure [27].

Outcomes After Surgery

A recent report by the Aortic Valve Operative Outcomes in Marfan Patients Study Group described early 1-year outcomes after root surgery on patients with MFS across 19 surgical centres [28]. They reported a 30-day mortality of 0.6 % for both Bentall procedure and valve-sparing root replacement, with 1-year survival rates of 97 % and 98 % respectively. They did find a higher rate of grade ≥2+ aortic regurgitation in 7 % of the valve-sparing root replacement group. However, consideration should be given to the fact that the majority of these 19 centres performed only a small number of cases per year.

Longer-term results were reported in a meta-analysis by Benedetto et al. [23] who analysed 1385 patients across 11 studies (972 patients had Bentall procedures and 413 had valve-sparing procedures). The mean follow-up was 8.0 years for the Bentall group and 4.7 years for the valve-sparing group, giving a combined total of 1279 patient-years. They reported a re-intervention rate of 0.3 %/year versus 1.3 %/year for the Bentall procedure and valve-sparing procedures respectively. The thrombo-embolic event rates were 0.7 %/year versus 0.3 %/year for the two groups respectively.

Mortality following aortic arch replacement varies between 2 and 17 % [25]. Larger surgical centres performing higher number of operations tend to obtain better results. 30-day mortality for repair of thoraco-abdominal aneurysms are reported as low as 5 % in some series, with a permanent paraplegia rate of 4 % [29].

Anaesthetic Considerations

Pre-operative Assessment

As with all patients undergoing major cardiac surgery, a careful evaluation of medical history, organ system review, and drugs history must be undertaken. Close attention must be paid to symptoms and signs specific to MFS, such as spontaneous pneumothorax, ectopia lentis, dural ectasia, pathological fractures, and scoliosis [30]. A dental assessment must be made in order to reduce the risk of prosthetic endocarditis. Pre-operative examination of the airway is important as the presence of prognathism, a high arched palate, and reduced neck extension may pose difficulties during tracheal intubation.

Intra-operative Management

Positioning of the patient on the operating table must be done carefully. It is important to assess the patient for joint laxity to avoid dislocations and injuries when the patient is asleep. The temporo-mandibular joint may also be at risk during intubation if excessive traction is used. If somatosensory evoked potentials or motor evoked potentials will be used during surgery, then neuromuscular blocking agents and volatile agents are avoided. Propofol infusion will be used for maintenance. A trans-oesophageal echocardiography probe is used for pre-op and post-operative assessment [30].

Pregnancy

Pregnancy is associated with an increased risk of aortic dissection for women with MFS. The majority of these events occur in the third trimester and peripartum period. There also appears to be a higher rate of growth of aorta during pregnancy. Furthermore, the long-term risk of aortic dissection or operative intervention on the thoracic aorta is higher in women with MFS who have had previous pregnancies compared to nulliparous women with MFS [31].

Both the haemodynamic and hormonal changes that take place during pregnancy account for this increased risk of aortic complications. The hyperdynamic and hypervolaemic status of the pregnant mother increase arterial wall stress and shear forces which act on the intima of the aorta. Further changes are made to the histological makeup of the aortic wall due to hormonal changes.

An aortic root dimension ≥40 mm in pregnancy is associated with a 10 % risk of aortic dissection for Marfan patients. More than half of pregnant women with MFS with an aortic root size ≥40 mm will either develop aortic dissection, a life-threatening dilatation, or require surgery during pregnancy [31].

Women with MFS contemplating pregnancy should have a preconception assessment by obstetricians as well as cardiologists. Assessment of the aorta, heart function and valvular function should be carried out with echocardiography and computed tomography (CT) or magnetic resonance imaging (MRI). These assessments will inform the decision as to whether prophylactic surgery is required before conception.

During pregnancy, all women with MFS should be regularly imaged with transthoracic echocardiography every 1–2 months for measurement of aortic root size. MRI is safer than CT if further imaging is required. Medical therapy with beta-adrenergic blockers is recommended to control blood pressure and prevent aortic dilatation. Angiotensin II blockers are contraindicated.

When aortic dissection occurs during pregnancy, it carries a significant risk to mother and foetus (50 % mortality). Type A dissections are much more common in pregnancy. Treatment is urgent repair of the dissection with close and detailed foetal monitoring. During the third trimester, depending on the haemodynamic and metabolic condition of the mother, consideration should be given to urgent caesarean section as well as repair of the dissection.

Elective repair of aortic aneurysms during pregnancy remains a challenge. A multi-disciplinary approach involving foetal medicine, cardiology, cardiothoracic surgery, anaesthetics and paediatrics is required. Surgery during the first trimester is associated with foetal malformations, and in the third trimester there is an increased risk of maternal mortality and preterm delivery. Therefore, any planned surgery during the course of pregnancy should be undertaken during the second trimester. Surgery can be performed without hypothermia and with pulsatile perfusion. Foetal blood flow monitoring can be performed via transabdominal and/or transvaginal Doppler ultrasound [32].

In the post-partum period, the increased risk of dissection continues for a number of months. Beta-blockade is usually continued for 3 months post-partum, and aortic monitoring should be maintained during this period.

Children

Dissection is very rare under the age of 12. It is predominantly mitral valve pathology which is the leading cause of death in young children with MFS. The aortic root behaves differently between early childhood and late teenage years in MFS. The infantile form of MFS is associated with an earlier onset of aneurysm formation. The size threshold for surgical repair is 50 mm, but again surgery is indicated at smaller sizes if there is a family history of aortic dissection, more than mild aortic regurgitation, and a rapidly expanding aneurysm (1 cm/year) [33].

Aortic root replacement in children remains a challenging area due to multiple factors. There is the potential for growth of cardiovascular structures in a young child. There is no long-term follow-up of valve preserving root replacement, however it remains the favoured choice with an aortic annulus greater than 18 mm and a tricuspid undamaged valve. A mechanical Bentall procedure is a good alternative. Homografts are used in small roots with an annulus <18 mm, however they are associated with early valve dysfunction. Pulmonary autotransplantation (Ross procedure) is contraindicated due to deficient wall properties of the pulmonary root [33].

References

1. Milewicz DM, Dietz HC, Miller DC. Treatment of aortic disease in patients with Marfan syndrome. Circulation. 2005;111:e150–7.
2. Michel J-B, Touat Z, Houard X, et al. New concepts in human abdominal aortic aneurysm pathophysiology: comparison with acending aortic and other locations. In: Sakalihasan N, Kuivaniemi H, Michel J-B, editors. Aortic aneurysms. Liege: Les Editions de l'Universite de Liege; 2008. p. 165–85.
3. Isselbacher EM. Thoracic and abdominal aortic aneurysms. Circulation. 2005;111:816–28.
4. de Kerchove L, El Khoury G. Anatomy and pathophysiology of the ventriculo-aortic junction: implication in aortic valve repair surgery. Ann Cardiothorac Surg. 2013;2:57–64.
5. Treasure T. Cardiovascular surgery for Marfan syndrome. Heart. 2000;84:674–8.
6. Tilea I, Suciu H, Tilea B, Tatar C, Ispas M, Serban R. Anatomy and function of normal aortic valvular complex. Calcific Aortic Valve Dis. http://dx.doi.org/10.5772/53403.
7. Layton K, Kallmes D, Cloft H, Lindell E, Cox V. Bovine aortic arch variant in humans: clarification of a common misnomer. Am J Neuroradiol. 2006;27:1541–2.
8. Berdajs D, Turina M. Surgical anatomy of the aorta. In: Operative anatomy of the heart. Springer-Verlag Berlin Heidelberg 2011.
9. Daily PO, Trueblood HW, Stinson EB, Wuerflein RD, Shumway NE. Management of acute aortic dissections. Ann Thorac Surg. 1970;10:237–47.
10. DeBakey ME, McCollum CH, Crawford ES, Morris Jr GC, Howell J, Noon GP, Lawrie G. Dissection and dissecting aneurysms of the aorta: twenty-year follow-up of five hundred twenty-seven patients treated surgically. Surgery. 1982;92:1118–34.
11. Svensson LG, Kouchoukos NT, Miller DC, Bavaria JE, Coselli JS, Curi MA, Eggebrecht H, Elefteriades JA, Erbel R, Gleason TG, Lytle BW, Mitchell RS, Nienaber CA, Roselli EE, Safi HJ, Shemin RJ, Sicard GA, Sundt 3rd TM, Szeto WY, Wheatley 3rd GH. Expert consensus document on the treatment of descending thoracic aortic disease using endovascular stent-grafts. Ann Thorac Surg. 2008;85:S1–41.
12. Elefteriades JA, Farkas EA. Thoracic aortic aneurysm clinically pertinent controversies and uncertainties. J Am Coll Cardiol. 2010;55:841–57.
13. Erbel R, Aboyans V, Boileau C, Bossone E, Bartolomeo RD, Eggebrecht H, Evangelista A, Falk V, Frank H, Gaemperli O, Grabenwoger M, Haverich A, Iung B, Manolis AJ, Meijboom F, Nienaber CA, Roffi M, Rousseau H, Sechtem U, Sirnes PA, Allmen RS, Vrints CJ. 2014 ESC Guidelines on the diagnosis and treatment of aortic diseases: document covering acute and chronic aortic diseases of the thoracic and abdominal aorta of the adult. The Task Force for the Diagnosis and Treatment of Aortic Diseases of the European Society of Cardiology (ESC). Eur Heart J. 2014;35:2873–926.
14. Svensson LG, Adams DH, Bonow RO, Kouchoukos NT, Miller DC, O'Gara PT, Shahian DM, Schaff HV, Akins CW, Bavaria JE, Blackstone EH, David TE, Desai ND, Dewey TM, D'Agostino RS, Gleason TG, Harrington KB, Kodali S, Kapadia S, Leon MB, Lima B, Lytle BW, Mack MJ, Reardon M, Reece TB, Reiss GR, Roselli EE, Smith CR, Thourani VH, Tuzcu EM, Webb J, Williams MR. Aortic valve and ascending aorta guidelines for management and quality measures. Ann Thorac Surg. 2013;95:S1–66.
15. Cameron D. Surgery for congenital diseases of the aorta. J Thorac Cardiovasc Surg. 2015;149:S14–7.
16. Bentall H, De Bono A. A technique for complete replacement of the ascending aorta. Thorax. 1968;23:338–9.
17. Nishimura RA, Otto CM, Bonow RO, Carabello BA, Erwin 3rd JP, Guyton RA, O'Gara PT, Ruiz CE, Skubas NJ, Sorajja P, Sundt 3rd TM, Thomas JD, American College of Cardiology/American Heart Association Task Force on Practice G. 2014 AHA/ACC guideline for the management of patients with valvular heart disease: a report of the American College of Cardiology/American Heart Association Task Force on Practice Guidelines. J Am Coll Cardiol. 2014;63:e57–185.

18. Girardi LN. Composite root replacement with a mechanical conduit. Oper Tech Thorac Cardiovasc Surg. 2008;13:148–60.
19. Sarsam MA, Yacoub M. Remodeling of the aortic valve anulus. J Thorac Cardiovasc Surg. 1993;105:435–8.
20. David TE, Feindel CM. An aortic valve-sparing operation for patients with aortic incompetence and aneurysm of the ascending aorta. J Thorac Cardiovasc Surg. 1992;103:617–21; discussion 22.
21. Hopkins RA. Aortic valve leaflet sparing and salvage surgery: evolution of techniques for aortic root reconstruction. Eur J Cardiothorac Surg Off J Eur Assoc Cardiothorac Surg. 2003;24:886–97.
22. Cameron D, Vricella L. Valve-sparing aortic root replacement with the valsalva graft. Oper Tech Thorac Cardiovasc Surg. 2005;10:259–71.
23. Benedetto U, Melina G, Takkenberg JJ, Roscitano A, Angeloni E, Sinatra R. Surgical management of aortic root disease in Marfan syndrome: a systematic review and meta-analysis. Heart. 2011;97:955–8.
24. Ikonomidis JS. Valve-sparing aortic root replacement—"T. David V" method. Oper Tech Thorac Cardiovasc Surg. 2009;14:281–96.
25. Svensson LG. The elephant trunk procedure: uses in complex aortic diseases. Curr Opin Cardiol. 2005;20:491–5.
26. Roselli EE, Isabella MA. Frozen elephant trunk procedure. Oper Tech Thorac Cardiovasc Surg. 2013;18:87–100.
27. Coselli JS, LeMaire SA, Koksoy C, Schmittling ZC, Curling PE. Cerebrospinal fluid drainage reduces paraplegia after thoracoabdominal aortic aneurysm repair: results of a randomized clinical trial. J Vasc Surg. 2002;35:631–9.
28. Coselli JS, Volguina IV, LeMaire SA, Sundt TM, Connolly HM, Stephens EH, Schaff HV, Milewicz DM, Vricella LA, Dietz HC, Minard CG, Miller DC, Aortic Valve Operative Outcomes in Marfan Patients Study G. Early and 1-year outcomes of aortic root surgery in patients with Marfan syndrome: a prospective, multicenter, comparative study. J Thorac Cardiovasc Surg. 2014;147:1758–66. 1767.e1–4.
29. Coselli JS. Update on repairs of the thoracoabdominal aorta. Texas Heart Inst J Texas Heart Inst St Luke's Episcopal Hospital, Texas Children's Hospital. 2013;40:572–4.
30. Castellano JM, Silvay G, Castillo JG. Marfan syndrome: clinical, surgical, and anesthetic considerations. Semin Cardiothorac Vasc Anesth. 2013;18:260–71.
31. Cox DA, Ginde S, Kuhlmann RS, Earing MG. Management of the pregnant woman with Marfan syndrome complicated by ascending aorta dilation. Arch Gynecol Obstet. 2014;290:797–802.
32. Yates MT, Soppa G, Smelt J, Fletcher N, van Besouw JP, Thilaganathan B, Jahangiri M. Perioperative management and outcomes of aortic surgery during pregnancy. J Thorac Cardiovasc Surg. 2015;149:607–10.
33. Zanotti G, Vricella L, Cameron D. Thoracic aortic aneurysm syndrome in children. Semi Thorac Cardiovasc Surg Pediatr Cardiac Surg Annu. 2008;11:11–21.

10 Abdominal and Thoracoabdominal Aortic Replacement for Marfan Syndrome

Ruwan A. Weerakkody, Ulrich Rosendahl, Anthony L. Estrera, Hazim J. Safi, and Nicholas J. Cheshire

Definitions, Classification and Context

Thoracoabdominal aortic aneurysm (TAAA) refers to aneurysmal disease affecting variable extents of the thoracic and abdominal aorta concurrently. TAAA may occur as a primary pathology or secondary to aortic dissection. The extent of aortic involvement in TAAA is defined by the Crawford classification (Fig. 10.1), which is the basis for stratifying prognosis and also determines the surgical approach [1].

In the general population, TAAA is a rare pathology (incidence: 6/100,000 person years) [2] typically affecting the older patient and associated with the usual risk factors for atherosclerosis. The Marfan syndrome (and other Mendelian causes of aortopathy) form a distinct subset within TAAA overall, with a younger age of onset, where traditional risk factors are not a major component. The natural history and characteristics of the disease in this group are different [3, 4].

Of aortopathies in Marfan syndrome, TAAA is a relatively common presentation (accounting for almost a half of all aortic operations [5]) often occurring after or concurrently with a proximal aortic presentation, most commonly an aortic root aneurysm [6, 7]. Abdominal aortic aneurysms (AAA) are rarely observed in

R.A. Weerakkody, PhD (✉)
Department of Surgery, Imperial College London, London, UK
e-mail: Weerakkody@cantab.net

U. Rosendahl
Department of Surgery, Royal Brompton and Harefield Aortic Centre, London, UK

A.L. Estrera • H.J. Safi
Department of Cardiothoracic and Vascular Surgery, Memorial Hermann Heart and Vascular Institute, University of Texas, Austin, TX, USA

N.J. Cheshire, MD, FRCS(Eng), FRCS(Ed)
Department of Surgery, Imperial College London, London, UK

Department of Surgery, Royal Brompton and Harefield Aortic Centre, London, UK
e-mail: nick.cheshire@imperial.ac.uk

© Springer-Verlag London 2016
A.H. Child (ed.), *Diagnosis and Management of Marfan Syndrome*,
DOI 10.1007/978-1-4471-5442-6_10

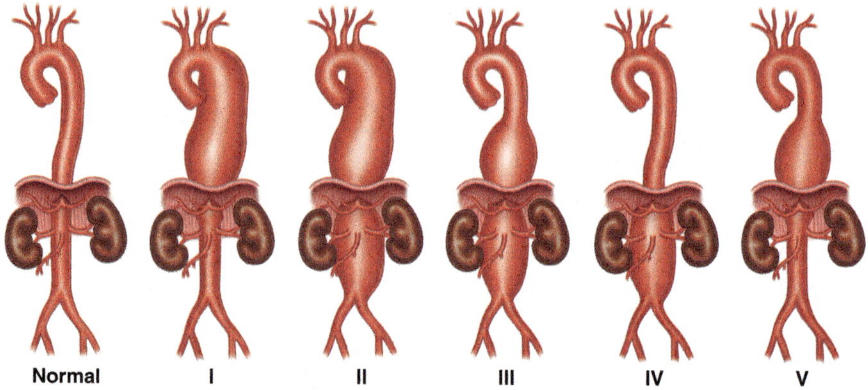

Fig. 10.1 Crawford classification of TAAA extent (from Safi et al., Annals Surgery 2003 [10]). In brief, type I aneurysms extend from the level of the left subclavian artery to the renal arteries; type II, the most extensive and complex to repair, extend from the level of the left subclavian artery to the aortoiliac bifurcation; type III start at or are distal to T6 and affect the lower part of the descending thoracic aorta and the abdominal aorta; and type IV involve the abdominal aorta below the diaphragm but extending up to the diaphragm. Type V is a variant of Type III, more recently defined, involving a lesser extent of the abdominal aorta

isolation in Marfan syndrome, and when they do occur, are observed as part of a TAAA or following prior TAAA repair. Therefore, they will be considered as a subgroup of TAAA for the purposes of this review.

Patient Factors and Selection for Surgery

Owing to the extent of the aorta involved and the corresponding major systemic disruption to blood supply, which is an inevitable aspect of repair, TAAA replacement tends to be associated with a significantly higher burden of mortality and morbidity than other aortic presentations, with few centres worldwide undertaking it. Nevertheless, at the outset, lie the same two questions as for any aneurysm; first, concerning the timing of aortic replacement and second, concerning the best strategies to minimise the surgical risk as far as possible. Both of these attempt to balance the risk from the natural course of the disease (which tends to be aggressive and unpredictable in Marfan syndrome) against the risk of intervention (which is also significant).

Identification of At-Risk Marfan Patients

The best outcomes in aortic surgery in general depend on identifying the disease early and planning an elective repair at the correct time [7,9, 10]. A significant proportion of TAAA overall (13–16 %) follow a prior aortic pathology, and in Marfan syndrome this proportion is a great deal higher (around 50–68 %); a similar proportion of ascending or aortic root operations in Marfan syndrome are followed by subsequent aneurysmal disease in the distal aorta, including TAAA [6–9]. Thus, a close surveillance of known aortic cases in Marfan syndrome is advocated and we would agree with current guidelines that this should involve annual imaging by magnetic resonance angiography (MRA) or computed tomogram angiography (CTA) in a stable postoperative patient and closer surveillance once new pathology is detected [3, 4]. Similarly, surveillance by MRA/CTA of any newly diagnosed Marfan patient and any relatives carrying the familial *FBN1* mutation should be instigated and maintained at appropriate intervals [3].

Specific Considerations in the Marfan Patient

The Marfan patient presenting with TAAA is younger (mean age 39–49 years) and physiologically fitter compared with the majority of TAAA patients (who present at a greater mean age of 68 years and have significant cardiorespiratory comorbidities) [5, 8, 10–12]. The generalised connective tissue dysfunction manifests firstly in a larger extent of aorta involved on presentation. The disease course is more aggressive: Marfan TAAA's demonstrate faster growth rate, earlier rupture and greater propensity to dissection [4, 7, 8, 13]. Furthermore, there is a higher frequency of recurrence, with a tendency for new aneurysm formation in intervening untreated parts of the native aorta or in autologous grafts or patches used for revascularisation of visceral branches of the abdominal aorta [5, 8, 11, 14]. These all suggest that a more durable and a more extensive repair is indicated and indeed some centres advocate a full length aortic repair in any Marfan patient with aortic dissection [15] (Table 10.1).

There appears to be a further group of apparently Mendelian cases of aortopathy who do not meet Ghent criteria or have a *FBN1* mutation. From our own cohort (Ibrahim et al (unpublished)) and others [5, 16], this group appears to be phenotypically intermediate between the proven Marfan group and the sporadic group, or

Table 10.1 Specific considerations in Marfan TAAA patients

Factor	Strategy
Younger age, physiologically fitter	More durable repair (open surgery)
More aggressive/extensive disease & tendency to recurrence	Lower size-threshold for elective repair
	More extensive repair at first presentation
	Open surgery in preference to endovascular options
Generalised connective tissue disorder with tendency for aneurysmal degeneration of intervening (untreated) aorta or autologous grafts/patches	More extensive repair
	Use of pre-fabricated (synthetic) branched grafts as opposed to autologous patches to re-connect visceral/renal vessels

partly overlapping with the Marfan group. Elucidating the spectrum of genetic mutations underlying this group and correlation with phenotype in larger cohorts will allow a more informed or personalised approach to their surgical management; the wider application of high-throughput DNA sequencing technologies will certainly help this in future [17]. However, for the moment, we approach those cases with a strong family history, younger age of onset or phenotypically more aggressive presentation in a similar manner to the Marfan group [3].

Indications for Intervention

A patient with a symptomatic aneurysm of any size should be considered for repair. Symptoms are usually non-specific and include chest, abdominal or back pain or cough. An acute presentation heralds a rapid expansion and possible imminent rupture, requiring emergent investigation and treatment.

For asymptomatic patients (approximately 50 %), aneurysm diameter is used as a guide to predict when the operative risk is exceeded by the risk of rupture, to guide the timing of aortic replacement. It is known that the risk of rupture with respect to aortic diameter is not a linear relationship, and in fact increases steeply above a certain threshold (or "hinge point") [18]. The exact value for the latter is not accurately known either in sporadic TAAA or in the Marfan patient presenting with TAAA. Therefore, a range of size thresholds for intervention have been proposed. Absolute aortic diameter from 5 to 6.5 cm or relative values of twice the normal aortic diameter in the individual patient have been suggested as suitable cut-off points for management [3, 6, 18]. A fast-growing aneurysm (>0.5 cm/year) is also an indication for repair.

In the Marfan syndrome, it is accepted that these thresholds for intervention should be lowered [4, 8, 13]. Any TAAA caused by aortic dissection (Stanford Type B), which in the general population is managed conservatively if uncomplicated, has a poorer prognosis in the Marfan patient, therefore operative intervention is indicated [19]. Furthermore, since it can be argued that the immediate operative risk to the younger, physiologically fitter Marfan patient is lower, earlier intervention is warranted. In summary, we would consider operative intervention in any Marfan patient with an aortic dissection (or family history of dissection), any symptomatic TAAA or an asymptomatic TAAA with maximal diameter >5 cm or growth rate >0.5 cm/year.

Surgical Strategy and Available Modalities

The essential aim is to replace the aneurysm and a variable proportion of surrounding non-aneurysmal aorta with a synthetic graft. The greater extent of involved aorta, and the propensity to recurrent disease means an extensive repair is often warranted at the outset, sometimes involving the whole length of the descending aorta from the termination of the aortic arch in the upper thorax to the aortoiliac bifurcation in the lower abdomen (Fig. 10.2).

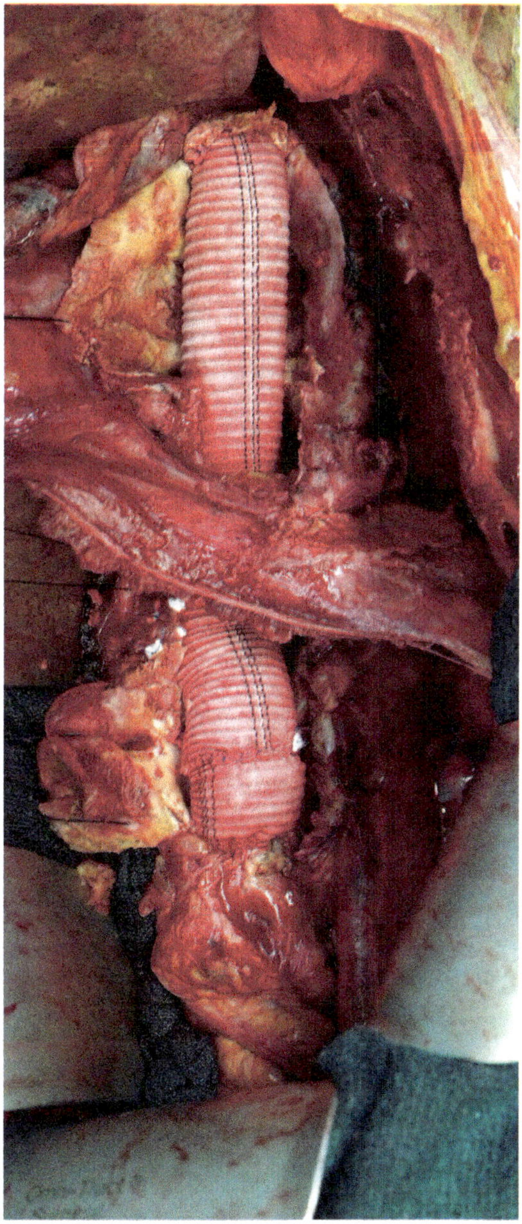

Fig. 10.2 Intraoperative photograph of revascularised thoracoabdominal aorta. A Dacron graft replaces the aorta from the proximal (thoracic) end (top of picture), extending under the diaphragm to the distal abdominal aorta. The continuous *black line* on the Dacron graft starts at the proximal (thoracic) end of the aorta; at the distal (abdominal) end, there is a short extension graft sutured graft to graft. The *black* indicator line is disrupted at this site

The biggest concern in approaching TAAA surgery is in managing the major physiological and metabolic challenge, which arises from disruption of blood supply to most of the thorax, abdomen, all organs therein as well as the lower limbs. These are in addition to the usual challenge of a long general anaesthetic, which carries its own risk of myocardial inhibition, stroke and mortality. Therefore, the aim is to optimise the patient pre-operatively and, during and after the operation, to utilise all necessary means to support physiology and minimise the ischemic insult to key organs (mainly the spinal cord, kidneys and abdominal viscera).

There are three potential modalities available: open surgical replacement, which is carried out via thoraco-laporotomy or endovascular stent graft placement or by a combination of the two (known as the "hybrid" technique). In reality, open surgical replacement is the gold standard in Marfan syndrome and endovascular options are only indicated in special conditions. The focus of this chapter will therefore be on open surgery, followed by a discussion of endovascular techniques.

Preoperative Preparation

Pre-operative optimisation focuses on four critical areas: the heart, neurovascular supply, lungs and kidneys. Though coronary artery disease or strokes are not common in the MFS patient, it is important to rule out left ventricular dysfunction (by echocardiogram and/or exercise stress testing) as well as significant carotid disease (by carotid duplex ultrasonography). Though the main risk factors for pulmonary complications include smoking history or COPD (which may be less common in the Marfan patient compared with other TAAA patients), intra-operative factors such as thoracotomy, diaphragmatic incision, unilateral lung collapse and operative site involving the thorax contribute to the fact that pulmonary complications comprise the most common following TAAA repair. Pulmonary function tests, spirometry and arterial blood gases are carried out with desirable targets of FEV1 >1.0 L, pCO_2 <4.5 kPa and in borderline cases, a period of 1–3 months optimisation and smoking cessation to optimise the patient's condition. The arterial supply to the kidneys is assessed (with a view to pre-operative or intraoperative revascularisation) and pre-operative dialysis is undertaken if necessary.

Open Surgery – Procedural Details and Key Considerations

The operative technique has been described in detail previously [10]. Here we shall briefly outline the key events and issues, which impact on the overall care of the patient.

The approach depends upon the extent of involved aorta. In the most extensive TAAA (Crawford types I and II, Fig. 10.1), which form the majority of TAAA seen in Marfan syndrome, a single long thoraco-laporotomy incision beginning at the tip of the scapula, passing anteriorly through the fourth or fifth intercostal spaces and extending in the midline of the abdomen is used. This allows access to, and adequate exposure of, the whole length of the descending thoracic and abdominal aorta. The left lung is collapsed to allow access to the heart and thoracic aorta. Left heart bypass is instigated. This takes oxygenated blood from the left atrium or a left pulmonary vein and returns it via a pump system, distal to the repair site, usually the femoral artery, ensuring ongoing distal aortic perfusion while the repair proceeds (the brain, head and neck and upper limbs will be perfused proximally via the aortic arch vessels, which are proximal to the repair and therefore not disrupted). The abdominal aorta is approached and exposed by retroperitoneal dissection.

After full exposure, the aorta is sequentially clamped and opened, beginning at the proximal thoracic aorta. A synthetic graft is sewn onto the proximal, normal aorta above the aneurysm. Intercostal vessels (from a critical watershed area of T7–T12) are selectively implanted back into the graft. The proximal aspect of the graft is now in direct connection with the proximal aorta and, once isolated from the rest of the graft by a clamp, allows the re-implanted intercostal vessels to be perfused through it, while the rest of the repair takes place distally. After clamping and opening the abdominal aorta, the visceral vessels (coeliac plexus, superior and inferior mesenteric arteries) and renal arteries are explanted and perfused via separate cannulas from the left heart bypass system. The distal end of the graft is sewn onto the distal abdominal aorta. The visceral and renal arteries are then anastomosed on to the graft. The graft now forms a continuous conduit from the proximal thoracic aorta down to the distal abdominal aorta, with perfusion to the spinal cord and abdominal viscera maintained through their re-implanted vessels.

The process of clamping the aorta interrupts normal blood flow to the branches of the aorta, causing widespread end-organ ischaemia for that duration: this period is known as the "cross clamp time" [20]. The direct effects of extensive end-organ ischemia as well as secondary effects from ischemia-reperfusion injury - which is a process of cytokine and free radical release from reperfused vascular beds, leading to damage to the lungs, heart and possibly the spinal cord - are the major concern in TAAA [20, 21]. The main complication is paraplegia from spinal cord ischemia, which in the past was as high as 30 % [22, 23]. These effects are reduced by minimising cross-clamp time, which itself depends upon the technical proficiency and speed by which the operation is undertaken. However, the ischemic insult during the cross-clamp period can be further significantly mitigated by the use of a number of adjuncts, resulting in improvements in patient outcomes beyond what is achievable by technical factors alone – these adjuncts have been shown, collectively to prevent between 1 in 5 and 1 in 20 permanent neurological deficits, or in other words represent a reduction in risk of 72 % overall [10, 21]. They include measures either to reduce metabolic demand to a minimum level or to maintain blood flow to critical organs during the cross-clamp period: systemic hypothermia (which may be moderate systemic hypothermia at 32–34° Celsius or deep hypothermic circulatory arrest), use of the left-heart bypass circuit to maintain distal perfusion, and selective perfusion of visceral and renal arteries whilst their branches are disconnected from the aorta. Specific measures for the spinal cord include: intraoperative and post-operative CSF drainage [10, 23–26], identification and re-implantation of intercostal vessels of T8–L2 or the artery of Adamkiewicz, which are thought to comprise a critical arterial supply to the spinal cord [10, 21, 27–30], use of intraoperative motor and sensory evoked potentials to assess the adequacy of spinal cord blood supply/reperfusion [10, 31–33], and (in some cases) localised epidural cooling [34]. Certain pharmacological agents such as steroids, mannitol and free-radical scavengers have also been proposed [35]. To prevent pulmonary complications and prolonged post-operative ventilatory requirements, care is taken to minimise lung trauma and protect the phrenic nerves throughout the procedure.

Post-operative Management

Immediately post-operatively the patient is managed on the intensive care unit with haemodynamic parameters maintained to optimise perfusion and oxygen delivery and minimise fluctuations in blood pressure, particularly periods of hypotension (which compromise spinal cord perfusion). Mean arterial pressure is maintained between 90 and 100 mmHg, haemoglobin concentration at >10 g/dL, cardiac index at >2 L/min, CSF pressure <10 mmHg (as spinal cord blood flow is counteracted by CSF pressure). The spinal drain remains in situ for 2–3 days postoperatively. Careful attention is paid to the development of respiratory complications. Once stabilised, the patient convalesces on the general ward and is rehabilitated to their usual life-routine. Beta-blockers are continued indefinitely post-operatively and moderate exercise limitation is advised (to avoid major haemodynamic stresses such as from contact sports and isometric exercises e.g. weight lifting).

Endovascular and Hybrid Open/Endovascular Options as an Alternative to Open Surgery

Whereas in open surgery, the diseased segment is effectively removed and replaced with a synthetic graft, the endovascular technique involves placing a stent-graft within the existing aorta, to bypass the aneurysmal section. It is introduced in its collapsed state across a wire, via a peripheral artery – usually the femoral artery-guided into the correct position and deployed to its full diameter under fluoroscopy. The graft-size is preselected so that, at maximum diameter, it anchors itself to the normal-diameter aorta proximal and distal to the aneurysmal segment, by radial force alone. For extensive aneurysm, custom-designed grafts also allow fenestrations or branches to allow perfusion of key aortic branch vessels, which would otherwise be excluded by the stent. Alternatively, the Hybrid technique, involves a limited operation to revascularise key branches (visceral and renal arteries) by creating a bypass from an unaffected peripheral branch before inserting the stent [36–42].

Overall, this modality, as a result of its minimally invasive approach, has the advantage of lower anaesthetic risk and lower short-term mortality and morbidity [43, 44]. However, in the Marfan patient its routine use is precluded by a higher rate of technical failure and limited durability resulting from a faster growing aorta. This can predispose to "endoleak" (leakage between the stent and native aorta) and tendency to recurrent disease in the intervening untreated aorta [45, 46]. Biomechanically and pathologically, one might also question the compatibility of a stent graft with the Marfan aorta: evidence of reduced aortic compliance [47], early elastolysis and loss of smooth muscle cell to elastic lamella connections [48, 49] and an earlier predisposition to dissection and aneurysmal dilatation all suggest that the application of a stent graft which relies on radial force for anchoring may adversely interact with an already compromised aortic structure. The most severe adverse events encountered include retrograde dissection and aortic perforation, but more frequently, endoleak and the need for multiple further corrective procedures are the main concern [8].

In specific instances however, owing to the much lower anaesthetic risk, this can be a useful alternative and we have utilised endovascular or hybrid techniques as a 'last ditch' measure in a systemically unstable patient who is unlikely to survive open surgery [42, 50]. Such procedures may form the basis for a more definitive repair once the patient is stabilised.

Outcomes for TAAA Replacement

The reported post-operative outcomes for open surgical replacement of TAAA in Marfan syndrome from experienced centres are good. Outcomes in TAAA patients overall, including Marfan syndrome have improved significantly since these procedures were first undertaken. This partly reflects the experience of the centres from which these outcomes are reported. Centres undertaking a higher volume of procedures show better patient outcomes particularly in relation to TAAA (a concept known as volume outcome relationship) [51]. The major outcome measures in TAAA surgery are early mortality and spinal cord ischaemia in the short term (conventionally measured within 30 days of the operation) and, in the long term, all cause mortality/survival and the need for re-intervention.

When considering short-term mortality, figures are comparable or lower in Marfan TAAA patients (0–6.5 %) [5, 8, 11, 12] compared with TAAA overall (5–14 %) [8, 10, 11, 52, 53]. In a direct comparison of TAAA operations for 31 (mainly Marfan) patients with connective tissue disorder versus 226 patients without, Dardik et al. found that 30 day mortality was almost half in the connective tissue disorders group compared with the wider group (Table 10.2). This probably reflects the lower age and lower burden of major cardiorespiratory comorbidity in those with Marfan syndrome compared with the older sporadic group.

On the other hand, rates of symptomatic spinal cord ischaemia (presenting with either a temporary or permanent paraplegia) are probably higher in the Marfan group, reflecting the fact that the Marfan group has a greater extent of aorta involved – over 50 % of Marfan TAAA patients present with the Crawford type II TAAA (the most extensive form) [5, 8, 11]. Extent of aortic disease, specifically presenting with Crawford type II TAAA is probably the major risk factor for the development of post-operative spinal cord ischemia (conferring between a 4 and 20-fold greater risk, compared with other types and is also the most responsive to protection by the use of intra-operative adjuncts) [10, 25]. In the same study, multivariate analysis also revealed the importance of comorbid risk factors for the development of spinal cord ischaemia post-operatively including: age, smoking, renal dysfunction and history of cerebrovascular accident [10]. In a smaller comparative

Table 10.2 Outcomes for Marfan TAAA replacement

Study	Le Maire 2006	Dardik 2002	Mommertz 2008	Kaltat 2007	Pacini 2013
Patient group	Marfan	Marfan	Marfan	Marfan	Marfan Endovascular (meta-analysis)
No.	178	28	22	19	54
Details	From a larger cohort of 398 aortic operations in Marfan patients	From a larger cohort of 31 patients with inherited connective tissue disorder (28 Marfan, 3 Ehlers Danlos) and 226 sporadic cases	From a larger cohort of 206 TAAA cases	Cohort of 22 Marfan patients with TAAA, 19 surgically operated	Systematic review and meta-analysis of 12 studies presenting data for endovascular treatment in Marfan patients
Male	62 %	61 %	–	64 %	75 %
Mean age	39	48.6	40	38	41
<u>**Pathology**</u>					
I	19 %	26 %	27 %	11 %	
II	57 %	52 %	50 %	79 %	
III	14 %	29 %	18 %	11 %	
IV	10 %	6 %	5 %		
Other	9 %[a]		36 %[d]		
Dissections	71 % (65 % chronic)	52 %	100 %	100 %	100 % (79 % chronic)
Emergency	7 %	7 %	9 % (rupture)	26%[e]	32 % (urgent & emergency)
<u>**Short term outcomes (within 30 days)**</u>					
Mortality	3 %	6.50 %	0 %	0 %	2 %
Spinal cord ischemia	4 %	19.4%[b]	0 %	0 %	2 %
Re-operation rate (technical failure)	5 %		5 %	15.7%[f]	30 %[g]
Other	Lung 22 %, Cardiac 11 %, Renal 8 % Stroke 1 %	Lung 10 % Cardiac (MI) 6 % Renal 13 % Stroke 0	Lung 14 % Cardiac 9 % (MI=0), Renal 0 %	Lung:11 % Renal-support 0 % Stroke:5 %	
Length of stay (ICU stay) in days		14 (6.4)		19(8)	13

Table 10.2 (continued)

Study	Le Maire 2006	Dardik 2002	Mommertz 2008	Kaltat 2007	Pacini 2013
Long term outcomes					
Mean follow-up period	5 years	5 years	38 months	56 months	30 months
Survival	98 %	>54%[c]	100 %	90 %	88 %
Re-operation rate	2 %				18 %

Summary outcome data from major series reporting open TAAA repair for Marfan syndrome (columns 1–4) compared with meta-analysis of all available endovascular outcomes in Marfan TAAA (column 5). I–IV refer to Crawford classification of TAAA

[a]Completion/reverse elephant trunk

[b]Though no sign diff in paraparesis rate, multivariate analysis showed presence of CTD as possible predictor of paraparesis post op (OR 1.2–70, p=0.03)

[c]This series showed no significant difference in long term survival in Marfan patients compared with sporadic patients

[d]Arch aneurysms concurrent with TAAA

[e]This includes two ruptures

[f]One SMA thrombosis

[g]25 % early endoleak rate and 5 % conversion to open surgery

study, Dardik et al showed a small but statistically significant increased risk of spinal cord ischemia in patients with connective tissue disorder compared to those without [11].

In terms of long-term survival and outcome after TAAA replacement, no significant difference in long-term survival between MFS and non-MFS patients has been observed. Long-term survival is affected by a number of factors including age, smoking, renal dysfunction, emergency presentation, and anatomy, specifically Crawford type II TAAA. The use of adjuncts, which aim to maintain perfusion during aortic clamping are protective. These data suggest that early detection and elective treatment of TAAA is beneficial, particularly in the face of more extensive aortic involvement and more aggressive natural history as seen in the Marfan syndrome.

Whilst giving excellent results in non-MFS sporadic cases, outcomes of endovascular techniques in Marfan syndrome show a high rate of technical failure in terms of endoleak and high corresponding re-intervention rates [45, 46]. Pacini et al undertook a systematic review of 54 Marfan patients with aortic dissections from 12 publications. In this metanalysis, short term mortality was low (2 %). Early endoleak (within 30 days of the procedure) occurred in 22 % of patients overall and in 30 % of chronic dissections [46], significantly higher than rates reported for non-MFS patients (which are between 7 and 12 %) [43, 54]. It has been suggested that early endoleak is not as prevalent when the proximal aspect of the stent is overlapped with an existing synthetic graft, although existing evidence as a whole does not support this notion [45, 46]. In the long term (over a mean duration of 2.5 years after operation) this group had endoleak and reintervention rates of 18 % each (compared with

1–9 % endoleak rate in non-MFS aortas) [42, 43, 50, 54, 55] and a 12 % mortality, with a mean age of death of 41 years. Overall, current outcomes support the surgical approach to TAAA replacement, which uses early open surgery as the first option and endovascular strategies in specific conditions where open surgery is precluded.

Conclusions

TAAAs are the most extensive and some of the most surgically complex of aortopathies. In Marfan syndrome, they are further complicated by a more aggressive pathology including faster growth rate and greater propensity to dissection in the MFS patient. This requires early detection and surveillance, which in the future, will be aided by the more widespread application of new genomic technologies, allowing more detailed genotype-phenotype correlation and risk-stratification. Early elective replacement and an extensive repair at first presentation minimises recurrence and the need for further procedures. Open surgery, though in the past marred by very high mortality and morbidity, is now the gold standard for treatment as technical developments over the past three decades have allowed good long-term outcomes and durability. When carried out at experienced centres this has allowed Marfan syndrome patients to experience comparable outcomes to TAAA patients overall. Endovascular options have very limited scope in this group but may be a useful alternative in very specific situations where open surgery is not possible.

References

1. Crawford ES, et al. Thoracoabdominal aortic aneurysms: preoperative and intraoperative factors determining immediate and long-term results of operations in 605 patients. J Vasc Surg. 1986;3(3):389–404.
2. Bickerstaff LK, et al. Thoracic aortic aneurysms: a population-based study. Surgery. 1982;92(6):1103–8.
3. Hiratzka LF, et al. 2010 ACCF/AHA/AATS/ACR/ASA/SCA/SCAI/SIR/STS/SVM guidelines for the diagnosis and management of patients with thoracic aortic disease: executive summary. J Am Coll Cardiol. 2010;55(14):1509–44.
4. Milewicz DM, Dietz HC, Miller DC. Treatment of aortic disease in patients with Marfan syndrome. Circulation. 2005;111(11):e150–7.
5. LeMaire SA, et al. Spectrum of aortic operations in 300 patients with confirmed or suspected Marfan syndrome. Ann Thorac Surg. 2006;81(6):2063–78; discussion 2078.
6. Crawford ES, Cohen ES. Aortic aneurysm: a multifocal disease. Presidential address. Arch Surg (Chicago, Ill.: 1960). 1982;117(11):1393–400.
7. Finkbohner R, et al. Marfan syndrome. Long-term survival and complications after aortic aneurysm repair. Circulation. 1995;91(3):728–33.
8. Mommertz G, et al. Thoracoabdominal aortic aneurysm repair in patients with Marfan syndrome. Eur J Vasc Endovasc Surg. 2008;35(2):181–6.
9. Girdauskas E, et al. Distal aortic reinterventions after root surgery in Marfan patients. Ann Thorac Surg. 2008;86(6):1815–9.
10. Safi HJ, et al. Distal aortic perfusion and cerebrospinal fluid drainage for thoracoabdominal and descending thoracic aortic repair: ten years of organ protection. Ann Surg. 2003;238(3):372–80; discussion 380–1.

11. Dardik A, et al. Durability of thoracoabdominal aortic aneurysm repair in patients with connective tissue disorders. J Vasc Surg. 2002;36(4):696–703.
12. Kalkat MS, et al. Presentation and outcome of Marfan's syndrome patients with dissection and thoraco-abdominal aortic aneurysm. Eur J Cardiothorac Surg. 2007;32(2):250–4.
13. Gott VL, et al. Replacement of the aortic root in patients with Marfan's syndrome. N Engl J Med. 1999;340(17):1307–13.
14. Kawamoto S, et al. Thoracoabdominal aorta in Marfan syndrome: MR imaging findings of progression of vasculopathy after surgical repair. Radiology. 1997;203(3):727–32.
15. Omura A, et al. Early and late results of graft replacement for dissecting aneurysm of thoracoabdominal aorta in patients with Marfan syndrome. Ann Thorac Surg. 2012;94(3):759–65.
16. Albornoz G, et al. Familial thoracic aortic aneurysms and dissections--incidence, modes of inheritance, and phenotypic patterns. Ann Thorac Surg. 2006;82(4):1400–5.
17. Weerakkody R, et al. Genetic analysis of aneurysm and dissection of the descending thoracic aorta using next-generation sequencing. Br J Surg. 2014;101:8–9, 2p. Suppl.: 2 Special Issue: SI.
18. Elefteriades JA. Natural history of thoracic aortic aneurysms: indications for surgery, and surgical versus nonsurgical risks. Ann Thorac Surg. 2002;74(5):S1877–80; discussion S1892–8.
19. Umana JP, Miller DC, Mitchell RS. What is the best treatment for patients with acute type B aortic dissections--medical, surgical, or endovascular stent-grafting? Ann Thorac Surg. 2002;74(5):S1840–3; discussion S1857–63.
20. Safi HJ, et al. Effect of extended cross-clamp time during thoracoabdominal aortic aneurysm repair. Ann Thorac Surg. 1998;66(4):1204–9.
21. MacArthur RG, et al. Organ protection during thoracoabdominal aortic surgery: rationale for a multimodality approach. Semin Cardiothorac Vasc Anesth. 2005;9(2):143–9.
22. Safi HJ, et al. Progress and future challenges in thoracoabdominal aortic aneurysm management. World J Surg. 2008;32(3):355–60.
23. Hollier LH, et al. Risk of spinal cord dysfunction in patients undergoing thoracoabdominal aortic replacement. Am J Surg. 1992;164(3):210–3; discussion 213–4.
24. Acher CW, et al. Combined use of cerebral spinal fluid drainage and naloxone reduces the risk of paraplegia in thoracoabdominal aneurysm repair. J Vasc Surg. 1994;19(2):236–46; discussion 247–8.
25. Safi HJ, et al. Cerebrospinal fluid drainage and distal aortic perfusion: reducing neurologic complications in repair of thoracoabdominal aortic aneurysm types I and II. J Vasc Surg. 1996;23(2):223–8; discussion 229.
26. Svensson LG, et al. Experience with 1509 patients undergoing thoracoabdominal aortic operations. J Vasc Surg. 1993;17(2):357–68; discussion 368–70.
27. Zoli S, et al. Predicting the risk of paraplegia after thoracic and thoracoabdominal aneurysm repair. Ann Thorac Surg. 2010;90(4):1237–44; discussion 1245.
28. Shiiya N, et al. Spinal cord protection during thoracoabdominal aortic aneurysm repair: results of selective reconstruction of the critical segmental arteries guided by evoked spinal cord potential monitoring. J Vasc Surg. 1995;21(6):970–5.
29. Safi HJ, et al. Importance of intercostal artery reattachment during thoracoabdominal aortic aneurysm repair. J Vasc Surg. 1998;27(1):58–66; discussion 66–8.
30. Ross SD, et al. Preservation of intercostal arteries during thoracoabdominal aortic aneurysm surgery: a retrospective study. J Thorac Cardiovasc Surg. 1999;118(1):17–25.
31. Jacobs MJ, et al. The value of motor evoked potentials in reducing paraplegia during thoracoabdominal aneurysm repair. J Vasc Surg. 2006;43(2):239–46.
32. Webb TH, Williams GM. Thoracoabdominal aneurysm repair. Cardiovasc Surg. 1999;7(6):573–85.
33. Williams GM, et al. Preoperative selective intercostal angiography in patients undergoing thoracoabdominal aneurysm repair. J Vasc Surg. 2004;39(2):314–21.
34. Black JH, Davison JK, Cambria RP. Regional hypothermia with epidural cooling for prevention of spinal cord ischemic complications after thoracoabdominal aortic surgery. Semin Thorac Cardiovasc Surg. 2003;15(4):345–52.

35. Wisselink W, et al. Ischemia-reperfusion injury of the spinal cord: protective effect of the hydroxyl radical scavenger dimethylthiourea. J Vasc Surg. 1994;20(3):444–91; discussion 449–50.
36. Donas KP, et al. Early and midterm outcome of a novel technique to simplify the hybrid procedures in the treatment of thoracoabdominal and pararenal aortic aneurysms. J Vasc Surg. 2009;50(6):1280–4.
37. Watanabe Y, et al. Successful endografting with simultaneous visceral artery bypass grafting for severely calcified thoracoabdominal aortic aneurysm. J Vasc Surg. 2002;35(2):397–9.
38. Kotsis T, et al. Treatment of thoracoabdominal aortic aneurysms with a combined endovascular and surgical approach. Int Angiol. 2003;22(2):125–33.
39. Svensson LG, et al. Elephant trunk procedure: newer indications and uses. Ann Thorac Surg. 2004;78(1):109–16; discussion 109–16.
40. Flye MW, et al. Retrograde visceral vessel revascularization followed by endovascular aneurysm exclusion as an alternative to open surgical repair of thoracoabdominal aortic aneurysm. J Vasc Surg. 2004;39(2):454–8.
41. Fulton JJ, et al. Endovascular stent-graft repair of pararenal and type IV thoracoabdominal aortic aneurysms with adjunctive visceral reconstruction. J Vasc Surg. 2005;41(2):191–8.
42. Bianchini Massoni C, et al. Follow-up outcomes of hybrid procedures for thoracoabdominal aortic pathologies with special focus on graft patency and late mortality. J Vasc Surg. 2014;59(5):1265–73.
43. Riambau V, et al. Final operative and midterm results of the European experience in the RELAY Endovascular Registry for Thoracic Disease (RESTORE) study. J Vasc Surg. 2011;53(3):565–73.
44. Nienaber CA, et al. Strategies for subacute/chronic type B aortic dissection: the Investigation of Stent Grafts in Patients with type B Aortic Dissection (INSTEAD) trial 1-year outcome. J Thorac Cardiovasc Surg. 2010;140(6 Suppl):S101–8; discussion S142–46.
45. Cooper DG, et al. Treating the thoracic aorta in Marfan syndrome: surgery or TEVAR? J Endovasc Ther. 2009;16(1):60–70.
46. Pacini D, et al. Endovascular treatment for type B dissection in Marfan syndrome: is it worthwhile? Ann Thorac Surg. 2013;95(2):737–49.
47. Metafratzi ZM, et al. The clinical significance of aortic compliance and its assessment with magnetic resonance imaging. J Cardiovasc Magn Reson. 2003;4(4):481–91.
48. Dingemans KP, et al. Ultrastructural pathology of aortic dissections in patients with Marfan syndrome: comparison with dissections in patients without Marfan syndrome. Cardiovasc Pathol. 2006;15(4):203–12.
49. Pereira L, et al. Pathogenetic sequence for aneurysm revealed in mice underexpressing fibrillin-1. Proc Natl Acad Sci U S A. 1999;96(7):3819–23.
50. Resch TA, et al. Combined staged procedures for the treatment of thoracoabdominal aneurysms. J Endovasc Ther. 2006;13(4):481–9.
51. Karthikesalingam A, et al. Volume-outcome relationships in vascular surgery: the current status. J Endovasc Ther. 2010;17(3):356–65.
52. Coselli JS, et al. Morbidity and mortality after extent II thoracoabdominal aortic aneurysm repair. Ann Thorac Surg. 2002;73(4):1107–15; discussion 1115–6.
53. Coselli J, Bozinovski J, LeMaire SA. Open surgical repair of 2286 thoracoabdominal aortic aneurysms. Ann Thorac Surg. 2007;83:S862–4.
54. Thrumurthy SG, et al. A systematic review of mid-term outcomes of thoracic endovascular repair (TEVAR) of chronic type B aortic dissection. Eur J Vasc Endovasc Surg. 2011;42(5):632–47.
55. Kische S, et al. Endovascular treatment of acute and chronic aortic dissection: midterm results from the Talent Thoracic Retrospective Registry. J Thorac Cardiovasc Surg. 2009; 138(1):115–24.

Ophthalmic Abnormalities in Marfan Syndrome

11

Aman Chandra and David G. Charteris

The ocular manifestations of Marfan Syndrome (MFS) are varied. They include myopia, corneal flattening, ectopia lentis (EL), and retinal detachments. The prevalence of these in MFS is unclear, though a recent survey of the UK Marfan Trust, suggested that 30 % of patients with MFS had EL, and 15 % had had retinal detachments [1]. We will discuss the most important of these features below.

Ectopia Lentis (Lens Subluxation/Dislocation)

Ectopia Lentis (EL) is the most diagnostic ophthalmic abnormality in Marfan syndrome [2]. Alternate conditions may cause EL [3, 4], thus careful genetic investigations must be undertaken to definitively diagnose or exclude MFS in the presence of EL [5]. The subluxation is due to weaknesses of the lens .zonular fibres secondary to abnormal fibrillin. Fibrillin-1 is a critical structure in these zonules, and thus it is unsurprising that these are affected in MFS. Subluxation of the lens is usually bilateral and symmetrical. Occasionally, complete dislocation of the lens into the vitreous cavity or into the anterior chamber can also occur. The subluxation of the lens usually occurs in the first two decades and, in general, is stable once an individual reaches their twenties. The subluxed lens itself can however develop a cataract, which can lead to visual impairment. Occasionally a subluxed or dislocated lens

A. Chandra, MRCSEd, FRCOphth, PhD (✉)
Department of Ophthalmology, Southend University Hospital, Southend-on-Sea, Essex, SSO ORY, United Kingdom
e-mail: aman.chandra@southend.nhs.uk

D.G. Charteris, MD, FRCS, FRCOphth
Vitreo-Retinal Unit, Moorfields Eye Hospital, City Road, London EC1V 2PD, UK
e-mail: david.charteris@moorfields.nhs.uk

© Springer-Verlag London 2016

A.H. Child (ed.), *Diagnosis and Management of Marfan Syndrome*,
DOI 10.1007/978-1-4471-5442-6_11

will become unstable resulting in fluctuating vision [6, 7]. Furthermore, anterior subluxation of the lens may compromise the drainage angle of the eye, resulting in raised intraocular pressure and secondary glaucoma.

Often visual acuity will remain relatively good, despite subluxation of the lens. Optical correction with appropriate glasses or contact lenses (often to correct around the lens itself in the 'aphakic' part of the pupil) will be sufficient to maintain adequate vision.

If the vision becomes significantly impaired by a cataract, if there is troublesome fluctuation of vision caused by the instability of the lens, or if an individual is intolerant to aphakic glasses or to contact lenses then surgical correction should be considered [3]. The current surgical technique for lens dislocation/subluxation in Moorfields Eye Hospital is the operation of vitreolensectomy. This uses an approach through the pars plana of the eye using automated ultrasonic fragmentation and cutting to remove the dislocated lens and the vitreous gel. Removal of both the lens and the vitreous gel minimises the chances of subsequent retinal detachment, which has been a significant complication of previous forms of surgery for lens dislocation in Marfan syndrome. At the same time that this procedure is performed a detailed examination of the retina is undertaken and laser or cryotherapy is applied to surround any areas of lattice retinal degeneration or retinal tears which might predispose to retinal detachment. This form of surgery can also be applied to eyes which have EL and a concomitant retinal detachment; the detachment itself can be repaired simultaneously often using intraocular expansile gas or silicone oil tamponade.

Our results using this technique at Moorfields Eye Hospital [8] demonstrated that only two of a total of 40 eyes did develop a retinal detachment following such a procedure and these were successfully managed with further retinal surgery. Following the surgery itself, correction with contact lenses is often adequate (many individuals will have been contact lens wearers prior to the surgery). For certain individuals a lens implant may be considered. This procedure differs from that employed in standard cataract surgery where the lens capsule and lens zonular fibres are intact. Where vitreolensectomy has been performed a lens implant may be sutured into the posterior chamber, captured in the sclera, clipped to the iris, or placed in the anterior chamber [9]. Surgical correction following removal of the lens can be undertaken simultaneously with the vitreolensectomy procedure, or as a secondary procedure at a later date.

Myopia

Myopia is more common in Marfan syndrome patients and is regarded as a minor diagnostic feature of MFS [2]. However, myopia itself is very common, and for this reason we do not feel that it serves any diagnostic utility in MFS.

In many cases myopia is of low to moderate degree in MFS and can easily be corrected with glasses or contact lenses. Where there has been substantial subluxation or dislocation of the crystalline lens the Marfan patient may be rendered hypermetropic (long-sighted) and occasionally the refraction may be somewhat unstable. The above refractive errors can often be adequately corrected with glasses or contact lenses. Occasionally, however, particularly where there is a large difference in refraction between the eyes, vitreolensectomy may be performed to correct a refractive error.

Retinal Detachment

As outlined above, retinal detachment can occasionally occur as a complication of surgery to remove a lens which is dislocated or subluxed. This complication is now much less common using the modern viteolensectomy approach. Retinal detachment may occur in the absence of prior lens surgery, with our survey suggesting this to be the case in up to 80 % of RD cases in MFS [1]. Surgical management of this may involve removal of the lens by a vitreolensectomy procedure if EL is concomitant. Other manoeuvres would include a combination of laser or cryotherapy, intraocular gas injection (occasionally silicone oil may be used as a tamponade) and a silicone plastic explant placed around the eye. Generally such techniques will be successful, although in 30–40 % of cases detachment surgery will require subsequent procedures to stabilise the retina [1].

In a small percentage of cases the detachment will be caused by a giant retinal tear (defined as a retinal tear greater than 25 % of the circumference of the eye). Again, this will require vitrectomy procedure and may require silicone oil to be used as the tamponading agent.

Other Ophthalmic Problems

Strabismus (squint) is more common in Marfan syndrome individuals [10] and may in some cases be associated with amblyopia. Abnormalities of the anterior chamber can rarely be associated with raised ocular pressure (and sometimes glaucoma [11]) and occasionally dislocation of the lens into the anterior chamber can produce acute glaucoma. This type of lens dislocation can result in an acutely painful eye and requires urgent ophthalmic management. Finally, the cornea of patients with MFS is reported to be thinner and flatter than the normal population [12]. It is therefore not advisable for these patients to consider corneal refractive surgery.

General Ophthalmic Management in Marfan Syndrome

It is advisable that an ophthalmologist examines individuals with MFS or a family history of MFS at an early age. Regular checks of visual acuity and refractive error should also be carried out to detect any development of lens abnormalities in children. An optometrist or an ophthalmologist may carry these out. It is probably advisable that children refrain from sports where there is excessive head contact or deceleration, such as boxing or bungee jumping, but most sports such as football and athletics are acceptable. Parents should maintain a degree of awareness for any loss of vision that the child may experience and seek prompt ophthalmic advice should this occur.

References

1. Chandra A, Ekwalla V, Child A, Charteris D. Prevalence of ectopia lentis and retinal detachment in Marfan syndrome. Acta Ophthalmol. 2014;92(1):e82–3.
2. Loeys BL, Dietz HC, Braverman AC, Callewaert BL, De Backer J, Devereux RB, et al. The revised Ghent nosology for the Marfan syndrome. J Med Genet. 2010;47(7):476–85.
3. Chandra A, Charteris D. Molecular pathogenesis and management strategies of ectopia lentis. Eye (Lond). 2014;28(2):162–8.
4. Chandra A, Aragon-Martin JA, Hughes K, Gati S, Reddy MA, Deshpande C, et al. A genotype-phenotype comparison of ADAMTSL4 and FBN1 in isolated ectopia lentis. Invest Ophthalmol Vis Sci. 2012;53(8):4889–96.
5. Chandra A, Patel D, Aragon-Martin JA, Pinard A, Collod-Beroud G, Comeglio P, et al. The revised ghent nosology. Reclassifying isolated ectopia lentis. Clin Genet. 2014;87(3):284–7.
6. Nelson LB, Maumenee IH. Ectopia lentis. Surv Ophthalmol. 1982;27(3):143–60.
7. Cross HE, Jensen AD. Ocular manifestations in the Marfan syndrome and homocystinuria. Am J Ophthalmol. 1973;75(3):405–20.
8. Hubbard AD, Charteris DG, Cooling RJ. Vitreolensectomy in Marfan's syndrome. Eye (Lond). 1998;12(Pt 3a):412–6.
9. Wagoner MD, Cox TA, Ariyasu RG, Jacobs DS, Karp CL. Intraocular lens implantation in the absence of capsular support: a report by the American Academy of Ophthalmology. Ophthalmology. 2003;110(4):840–59.
10. Izquierdo NJ, Traboulsi EI, Enger C, Maumenee IH. Strabismus in the Marfan syndrome. Am J Ophthalmol. 1994;117(5):632–5.
11. Izquierdo NJ, Traboulsi EI, Enger C, Maumenee IH. Glaucoma in the Marfan syndrome. Trans Am Ophthalmol Soc. 1992;90:111–7; discussion 118–22.
12. Heur M, Costin B, Crowe S, Grimm RA, Moran R, Svensson LG, et al. The value of keratometry and central corneal thickness measurements in the clinical diagnosis of Marfan syndrome. Am J Ophthalmol. 2008;145(6):997–1001.

Spinal Deformity in Marfan Syndrome (MFS)

12

Nanjundappa S. Harshavardhana
and Mohammed H.H. Noordeen

Introduction

Marfan syndrome (MFS) was first described by the French physician Dr. Antonine Marfan in 1896 when he described a 5.5 year old girl named Gabrielle who had tall stature, long and slender limbs, with an asthenic build (dolichostenomelia) [1]. It is one of the most common inherited connective tissue disorders and is transmitted as an autosomal dominant trait characterised by complete penetrance, but with variable expressivity. The disorder is attributed to a mutation involving the Fibrillin (FBN-1) gene located on the long arm of chromosome 15 (i.e. 15q21) that shows striking pleotropism with clinical variability [2]. A family history of MFS with an affected first degree relative is usually present in 75 % of the instances. Up to 25 % of affected patients may not have a family history and they may represent a de novo mutation of FBN-1 [3]. The incidence of MFS is estimated to be 1–3 per 10,000 in the population and it affects both sexes equally often [4]. The diagnosis is largely clinical and is characterised by cardinal features that mainly affect three major systems, that is,

- The skeletal,
- The ocular, and
- The cardiovascular.

N.S. Harshavardhana, MS, Dip SICOT, EBOT (✉)
Department of Spinal Surgery, Spinal Deformity Unit (SDU),
Royal National Orthopaedic Hospital, Brockley Hill,
London, UK
e-mail: nharsha@outlook.com

M.H.H. Noordeen, MA, BM, MCh Ortho, FRCS(Tr&Orth)
Department of Trauma and Orthopaedic Surgery, Spinal Deformity Unit (SDU),
Royal National Orthopaedic Hospital, Brockley Hill,
London, UK
e-mail: hnoordeen@aol.com

© Springer-Verlag London 2016

A.H. Child (ed.), *Diagnosis and Management of Marfan Syndrome*,
DOI 10.1007/978-1-4471-5442-6_12

The genetic association was first established by Dietz et al. in 1991 when they detected a mutation of the FBN-1 gene. It shares overlapping clinical features with congenital contractural arachnodactyly (i.e. Beal's syndrome), which is caused by a mutation involving the FBN-2 gene [5]. In fact, it is believed that Dr. Marfan's original description of the affected girl indicates that she probably had this condition and would no longer meet the current diagnostic criteria of MFS. The differential diagnosis includes:

- Mitral valve prolapse syndrome,
- Weill-Marchesani syndrome,
- Loeys-Dietz syndrome,
- Shprintzen-Goldberg syndrome,
- Homocystinuria,
- Ehlers-Danlos syndrome,
- MASS (mitral, aortic, skin & skeletal) manifestation phenotype, and
- Beals syndrome.

Fibrillin-1 is an extracellular matrix glycoprotein that is essential for fibrinogenesis and is present in connective tissues, including bone. The mutations increase the susceptibility to proteolysis leading to the fragmentation of microfibrils, which causes changes in cell-to-cell signaling through the latent transfer binding protein. The abnormalities of fibrillin also cause a loss of inhibitory effect on transforming growth factor beta (TGF-β) which affects the microfibril structure systemically, resulting in the dysfunctional signaling of TGF-β that is implicated in the pathophysiology of MFS. Similarly increased TGF-β activation and signaling, secondary to mutations involving the TGFBR1 and TGFBR2 genes located on chromosomes 9 and 3, are also observed in patients with other Marfan-related disorders [6].

Children born with this condition are normal at birth with normal mentation, but the clinical manifestations become more evident with increasing age. The natural history is premature mortality, usually secondary to a cardiovascular event. Since the 1970s, with advances in cardiac sciences, surgeries focused on the aortic valvular area have significantly increased the longevity of these patients to near normal in contemporary era [7].

Diagnosis

MFS is characterised by cardinal skeletal features that include tall stature with thin habitus and long slender digits (arachnodactyly). The most common skeletal manifestation is scoliosis, which is seen in at least 60 % of the patients [8]. Chest cage deformities, i.e. pectus excavatum/ carinatum, are also common. They typically have arm span to height ratio of >1.05 with a decreased upper segment to lower segment (US:LS) ratio. Pes planus and protrusio acetabuli are also not uncommon.

The Ghent nosology has incorporated the clinical features of seven systems, and determines whether major/minor criteria and systemic involvement are present. The major criteria are infrequent in other CTD and have high specificity. Nevertheless, debate persists to this day as to whether the Ghent nosology is too stringent and excludes truly affected MFS cases [9]. Further details of testing for MFS and the merits and limitations of these criteria are discussed in more detail in other chapters. The overall consensus, however, is to let the geneticist (rather than the clinician) apply the stringent Ghent nosology in the clinical diagnosis of MFS.

Scoliosis in MFS

The axial skeleton is the most commonly affected part of skeletal system in MFS. The reported incidence of scoliosis in established diagnosis of MFS varies from 40 to 60 % [10]. In 1939, the first reported series, published by Fahey et al., had 45 scoliosis patients from 132 MFS cases [11]. Subsequently, Sinclair et al. (1960), Wilner et al. (1964), and Scheier et al. (1967) observed scoliosis of mild to moderate severity [12–14]. Ford et al. (1968), in their review of MFS, found at least 13 % of patients had severe scoliosis which required aggressive bracing, fusion, or both [15]. Sliman et al. (1971) were the first to observe striking similarities and unique differences between the scoliosis of MFS vs. idiopathic etiology, and they concluded that MFS scoliosis has a poorer prognosis [16]. Robins et al. (1975) reported a 44 % incidence of scoliosis (35 out of 64 MFS patients with scoliosis) and observed poor response to treatment with a Milwaukee brace (MB) [17]. Spinal fusion with Harrington instrumentation yielded a 41 % correction with an average loss of 7° over 2.3 years of follow-up [17]. Sponseller et al evaluated 113 patients with MFS from their hospital database and found that 82 of them were skeletally immature. 52 out of 82 patients had scoliosis, and all but two (i.e. 50 out of 82) had scoliosis which was convex to the right [18]. The incidence of scoliosis in their series was 60 %. The thoracic spine was the most common region affected, followed by the thoracolumbar junction. Though these curves resembled the idiopathic curve type/pattern, certain unique features were evident. MFS patients had a higher incidence of having double thoracic or triple major curves. In addition, on the sagittal plane, there was a loss of thoracic kyphosis (TK) with reversal to thoracic lordosis in the most severe cases [18]. This, coupled with pectus excavatum, resulted in a reduced AP diameter of the chest with resultant mechanical compression of the large airways, which predisposed these patients to recurrent chest infections. Fewer patients had hyperkyphosis (i.e. TK of >50°) which was seen in 40 %.

The scoliosis in MFS differs significantly from idiopathic scoliosis by having rapid progression with a poor response to non-operative treatment. Furthermore, vertebral morphology is affected significantly, which makes operative treatment challenging. The key findings in vertebral bodies and posterior elements in children with MFS scoliosis include [19]:

- Narrow pedicles,
- Vertebral and sacral scalloping,
- Wide transverse processes,

- Thin laminae, and
- Low bone mineral density (BMD).

There is a high prevalence of lumbosacral transitional vertebra, and the presence of spondylolysis/spondylolisthesis is also not uncommon. Sponseller et al studied the sagittal plane deformity in MFS and proposed a classification to describe it. The two main sub-groups identified were (i) Transitional vertebra at or above L2, and (ii) Transitional vertebra below L2. Further sub-types for these two main sub-groups are illustrated in Table 12.1 [18]. They emphasised evaluating the sagittal profile in choosing fusion levels for scoliosis correction to avoid junctional problems (i.e. proximal junctional kyphosis [PJK] and distal junctional kyphosis [DJK]).

Table 12.1 The Sagittal profile classification in Marfan syndrome [21]

Type I	Normal transitional zone (at or above L2)	Normal kyphosis (20°–50°)	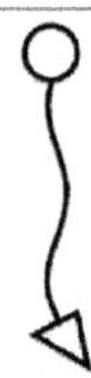
		Hypokyphosis (≤19°)	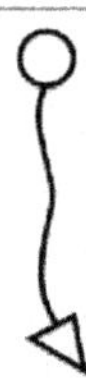
		Hyperkyphosis (≥51°)	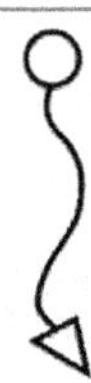
Type II	Abnormal transitional zone (below L2)	Long kyphosis	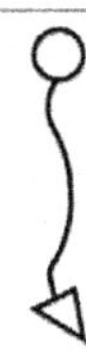
		Reversal of direction	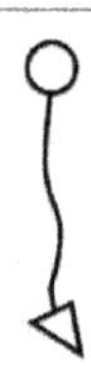

Multi-planar deformities (i.e. kyphoscoliosis) with chest cage deformation secondary to pectus excavatum/carinatum pose unique challenges and are often fraught with life-threatening risks. Multi-disciplinary input with the involvement of a cardiologist, respiratory physician, paediatrician, thoracic surgeon, in addition to a spinal surgical team is desired to optimise surgical results and outcomes.

Increasingly, medical rapid prototyping technology (RPT) based on three-dimensional printing principles is used to replicate 1:1 scale models, which helps to better illustrate the underlying deformity, counsel patients and parents, and plan the surgical correction prior to intraoperative correction [20]. Evidence exists which confirms this to be a standard of care in complex spinal deformity vertebral column resection (VCR) surgeries [21]. One such case example of an RP model in a patient with complex multi-planar congenital spinal deformity along with its three-dimensional computed tomography reconstruction (i.e. 3D CT) scan is illustrated in Fig. 12.1.

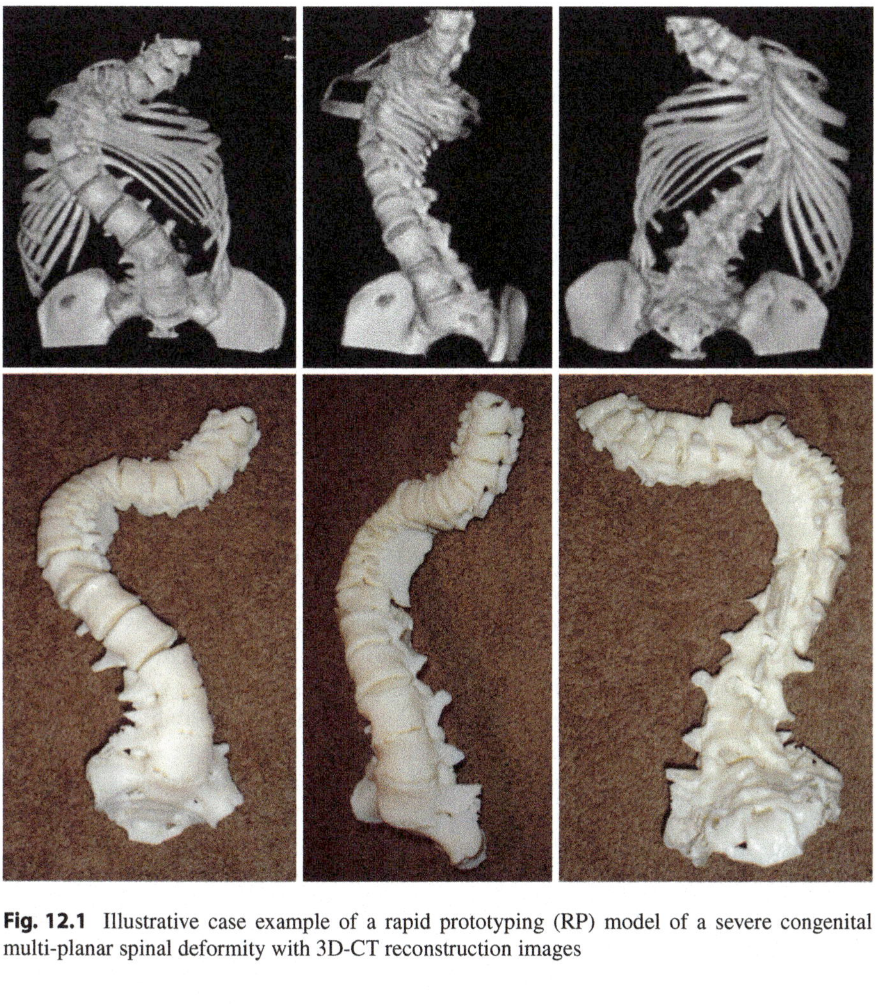

Fig. 12.1 Illustrative case example of a rapid prototyping (RP) model of a severe congenital multi-planar spinal deformity with 3D-CT reconstruction images

The appendicular skeleton is also involved, producing leg length inequality (LLE), angular deformities of the lower extremities, pes planus, and flexion contracture at the elbows. Protrusio acetabuli was also found to be common [22] (See the rheumatological manifestations of MFS and the surgical management of pectus excavatum/carinatum in other chapters of this book).

Cervical Spine

Patients with MFS have a loss of normal cervical lordosis or reversal of lordosis with cervical kyphosis on sagittal evaluation. The incidence of cervical kyphosis was 16 % (i.e. one in six) and at least 36 % of the patients had basilar impression (i.e. cranial setting) [23]. In addition, they also have increased atlanto-axial movement on flexion-extension movement, particularly in children, who are at a risk of developing atlanto-axial rotatory subluxation in up to 20 % of the instances. Ligamentous laxity with some degree of muscle hypotonia is believed to be the causative factor behind these manifestations. Surprisingly, the incidence of cervical stenosis was rare and no more than 2–3 % [23]. The incidence of neck pain was similar to age- and sex-matched controls without MFS. The overall risk of neurological complication in MFS is rare, and routine screening radiographs of the neck in all patients with MFS, prior to a general anaesthetic, is not recommended. Patients with MFS ought to refrain from playing contact sports (to protect the aorta and the lens of the eye) and any sports that cause high impact loading of the cervical spine (in particular, diving, weight lifting, and American football) [23].

Dural Ectasia

Dural ectasia (DE) refers to the widening of the thecal sac and nerve root sleeves in the caudal portion of the spine. There is a high incidence of DE in MFS (56–92 %) and DE is not necessarily pathognomic of MFS [24]. Other conditions where it is commonly present include neurofibromatosis, Ehlers-Danlos syndrome, tumors, trauma, congenital scoliosis, and ankylosing spondylitis. In fact DE is the second most common manifestation of MFS after aortic dilation/dissection. The Ghent nosology recommends screening for DE, indicating its presence as high in importance for the diagnosis of MFS. CT and MRI scans detect DE with high sensitivity and specificity. The receiver operator characteristics (ROC) curve demonstrates a large area for both CT (0.863) and MRI (0.910), with the MRI being superior in addition to the added advantage of eliminating irradiation [25]. An index case example of MFS with dural ectasia as seen on T_2 weighted coronal and sagittal MRI images is illustrated in Fig. 12.2. One of the most widely used criteria for describing DE in MFS is the one proposed by Ahn et al., and it is summarised in Table 12.2. It comprises major and minor criteria and they recommended a volumetric *gold*

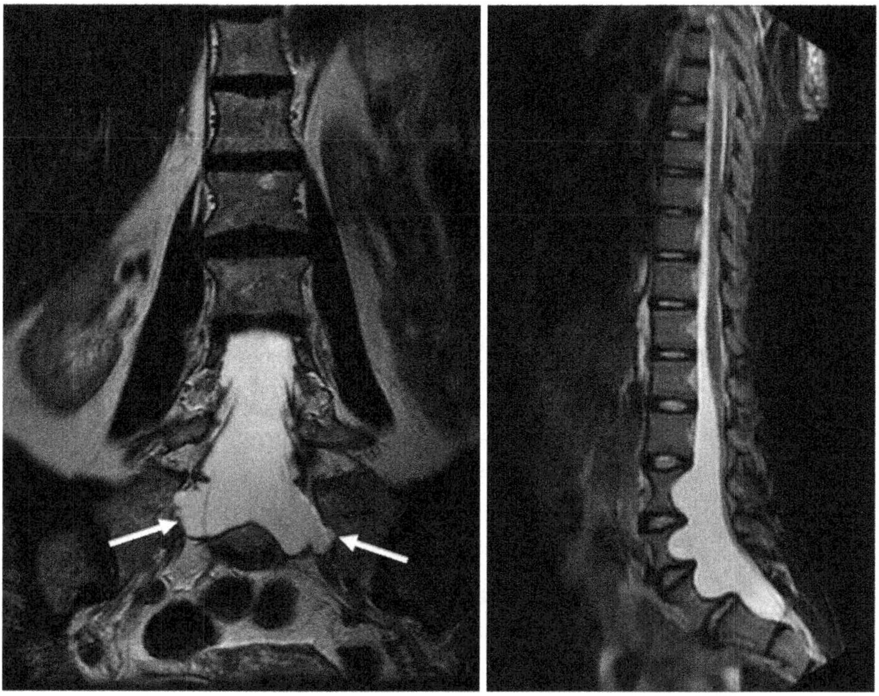

Fig. 12.2 A T_2 weighted MRI scan of the lumbar spine showing dural ectasia in a patient with Marfan syndrome. The lateral extensions of dura around the S_1 nerve root sleeves are indicated in *white arrows*

Table 12.2 The Ahn criteria for the description of dural ectasia in Marfan syndrome [28]

Major criteria	Minor criteria
1. Width of dural sac below L5 > width above L4	1. L5 nerve root sleeve diameter >6.5 mm
2. Anterior sacral meningocoele	2. S1 scalloping >3.5 mm

Dural ectasia exists if one major or two minor criteria are present

standard criteria for the diagnosis of DE to be a volume of >7 cm^3 (i.e. more than two standard deviations [SD] above the mean for normal controls) when measured from the caudal to inferior end plate of the L_5 vertebra [25].

DE develops owing to hydrostatic pressure exerted upon inherently weakened dura and it is invariably present below L_5 owing to this vertebra having the greatest fluid pressure in the most caudal portion of the spine. Its incidence increases as the patient ages [26]. DE most commonly causes intractable back pain or severe headaches, and neurological deficit necessitating decompression surgery. Patients can also be completely asymptomatic, and incidentally detected DE on advanced imaging can be seen in up to 40 % of MFS children. The natural history of DE is unknown and a diagnostic criterion to aid in the evaluation of DE in children is yet to be developed.

Spondylolisthesis

Patients with MFS have twice the incidence of spondylolisthesis compared to the general population (5–6 % vs. 2–3 %) [27]. The spondylolisthesis of MFS tend to be of an usually higher Myereding grade, with at least twice the slip angle (i.e. 30 %), in comparison to normal cohorts (whose average slip angle is 15 %). The slip angle further increased to an average of 60 % with the presence of scoliosis. Patients with bilateral pars defects had a high risk of progression owing to the vertebral body and sacral scalloping with DE. Symptomatic spondylolisthesis mandates the extension of instrumentation/inclusion of the pelvis in spinal fusion, which is fraught with complications such as pseudoarthrosis, dural leak, risk of arachnoiditis, and pseudomeningocoele. To this day, there is no published case series that has reported the surgical results of spondylolisthesis in MFS. Winter (1982) and Taylor (1987) have published case reports recommending either decompression with in-situ postero-lateral fusion or decompression with reduction and circumferential 360° fusion as treatment strategies [28, 29].

Bone Mineral Density (BMD) and Protrusio Acetabuli

There is a component of low BMD, especially in adult males with MFS who had an average T score of −1.54 (osteopenia) [30]. The BMD in adolescents and females was surprisingly found to be within normal limits, for reasons unknown, in a series of 51 patients (30 adults and 21 children) studied by Giampietro et al. [30]. Further evidence is needed to define the role of anti-osteoporotic medications (bisphosphonates, selective estrogen receptor modulators [SERM], etc) before their routine prescription for MFS. The incidence of protrusio acetabuli in MFS was reported to be at least 30 % and was independent of BMD of the hip and pelvis [31]. Protrusio acetabuli was purely a radiographic finding that did not correlate with the clinical symptoms and its presence alone was not felt to be an indication to either justify or recommend surgery.

Treatment of Scoliosis in MFS

The scoliosis of MFS closely resembles that of idiopathic scoliosis and the management in this chapter is therefore discussed along those lines. As in idiopathic scoliosis, management is covered under the following three sub-groups depending on age at the manifestation of scoliosis [32]:

(i) Infantile: from birth up to 3 years
(ii) Juvenile: between 3.1 and 9.9 years
(iii) Adolescent/Adult scoliosis: age ≥10 years.

Some professionals group the infantile/juvenile forms as one single entity and discuss them under the broad category 'early-onset scoliosis' (EOS), which is the manifestation of spinal deformity in children aged ≤9.9 years [33]. The treatment of scoliosis in this chapter is therefore covered under two broad sub-groups, namely, (1) Early-onset scoliosis, and (2) Adolescent/adult scoliosis, with an emphasis on its surgical management with practical operative tips.

Early-Onset Scoliosis (EOS) in MFS (Infantile and Juvenile Sub-types)

Infantile scoliosis is the most severe form of MFS and almost all patients have an affected first degree relative diagnosed with MFS. It presents with severe deformity and often a kyphoscoliosis that progressed rapidly. In a series of 14 MFS patients with infantile scoliosis, Sponseller et al observed 13 of them had a family history of MFS [34]. The authors studied eight boys and six girls and observed that all had motor developmental delay. Longevity was significantly reduced, with mean survival of 13 years, and four patients died due to cardiac problems before their tenth birthday. Nine patients were treated by bracing and it was ineffective in all (i.e. 0 % success with a brace), despite wearing it for an average of 11 h/day for a mean of 3.3 years. The most common curve pattern was a double major curve (right thoracic and left lumbar) and 12 patients were treated with surgery. The curve magnitude ranged from 60° to 80° at the time of surgery. Instrumented posterior spinal fusion (PSF) was performed using Luque wires in five and a Harrington rod in four patients. Posterior instrumentation with Luque wires and a Harrington rod without fusion was performed in the remaining three patients. Anchor dislodgement and rod breakages were a rule, rather than an exception, and revision surgery was needed in five patients. They reported a modest 20 % mean correction of scoliosis at the 5 year follow-up, with the mean longevity being 13 years (range: 7–25 years). The overall results of bracing for MFS are poorer than those for idiopathic scoliosis, and the results of one reported study were 17 % [35].

Conventional growing rods (CGR) had been the mainstay in the surgical management of EOS in MFS in the past. Dual rods, inserted subcutaneously, subfascially, or submuscularly were the standard of care until the end of the last decade. They could be inserted by making two tiny skin incisions, and then anchored to the proximal spine (or rib) anchors and spine (or pelvis) anchors distally, followed by rail-roading the growth rod linked with extensible domino or tandem connectors, which would be lengthened under general anaesthesia on a regular four to six monthly basis. Sponseller et al reported a series of ten patients treated with three single and seven dual growing rods and observed a mean curve correction of 51 % [36]. The mean age at surgery was 5.3 years and the mean duration of treatment with CGR was 5.25 years. Dual rods produced better correction than single rods, with reduced incidence of implant-related complications (anchor dislodgements and rod breakages). Definitive spinal fusion was performed on five patients after a mean of 5.5 years, following CGR insertion.

Magnet-driven growing rods (MdGR) are novel implants recently approved by USFDA and NICE for EOS and are the currently recommended standard of care for all etiologies of EOS, with a remaining growth potential of at least 3 years [37]. They eliminate the need for invasive lengthenings under anaesthesia by office-based expansions and are reported to improve pulmonary function, especially in neuromuscular and syndromic scoliosis at 2 years [38]. There are at least five published studies reporting their early clinical results which are all very encouraging [39–43]. There are no published case reports to this day in the English language highlighting their use in MFS. The senior author (MHHN) has now inserted MdGR in a few MFS patients. Two such case examples of EOS secondary to MFS, treated by single and dual MdGR insertions, in two and a half and seven year old boys are illustrated in Figs. 12.3 and 12.4 respectively. A detailed description of our preferred surgical technique is as described below:

Surgical Technique

The patient was placed in prone position under general anaesthesia with endotracheal intubation on a Montreal mattress with adequate padding of all the pressure points. Special care was taken to avoid hyperextension of the upper extremities, which carried the risk of causing brachial plexopathy [44]. Pre-operative planning was undertaken to determine the anchor/instrumentation vertebrae guided by the curve characteristics. Our preference is to use a spine – spine anchor construct with all pedicle screw anchors for distal fixation and hybrid fixation for proximal anchors (pedicle screws and transverse process [TP] hooks). We prefer to have six points of proximal fixation and at least four distal fixation points in all cases. Abnormal lumbo-sacral transition or large dural ectasia with vertebral/sacral scalloping may warrant instrumentation to the pelvis and the use of iliac bolt fixation (our preferred method of pelvic fixation) or S2-Ala screws. Two separate skin incisions were made in the midline at the proximal thoracic spine (usually T2–T5 vertebra) and at the distal thoracolumbar/lumbar spine, exposing the predetermined fusion levels. Pedicle screws of appropriate length and diameter were inserted into the T3 and T4 vertebrae bilaterally by free-hand technique. Two down-going transverse process hooks were inserted into T2 and remained flush to the bone at all times in order to minimise the risk of apical pneumothorax. Two more pedicle screws were then inserted into the previously determined vertebrae as distal fixation anchors. A flexible rod template was used to measure the length of the rod needed and the MdGR was cut to the desired length. Care was taken to ensure that the actuator area containing the magnet remained straight at all times, which is crucial for the integrity of the magnetic coil system. Appropriate sagittal contouring dictated by the curve profile/patient characteristic was then given to the MdGR to facilitate the ease of insertion. The functioning of the magnetic coil was tested with the handheld device before its final insertion.

A 24G chest tube was then used to rail-road the rod submuscularly in a caudo-cranial fashion on the concave side and then it was attached to the fixation anchors, starting with the pedicle screws distally. The rod was attached to the hybrid construct cranially (hooks and pedicle screws). The posterior elements were then decorticated and mixed with bone marrow aspirate obtained at the time of the pedicle screw insertions. 10–20 mg of silicated calcium phosphate (SiCaP) granules were

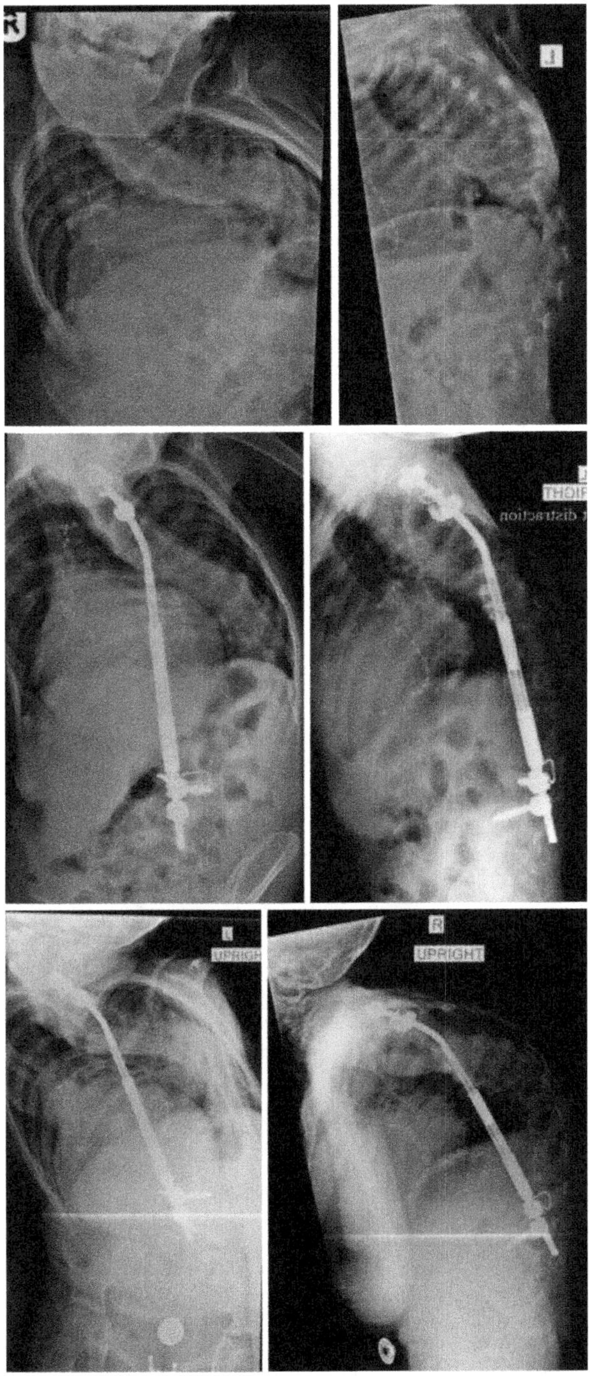

Fig. 12.3 A 2.5 year old Marfan syndrome boy with infantile kyphoscoliosis treated with a single submuscular insertion of a magnet-driven growing rod (MdGR). Preoperative, 1 year, and three and half years postoperative radiographs are shown

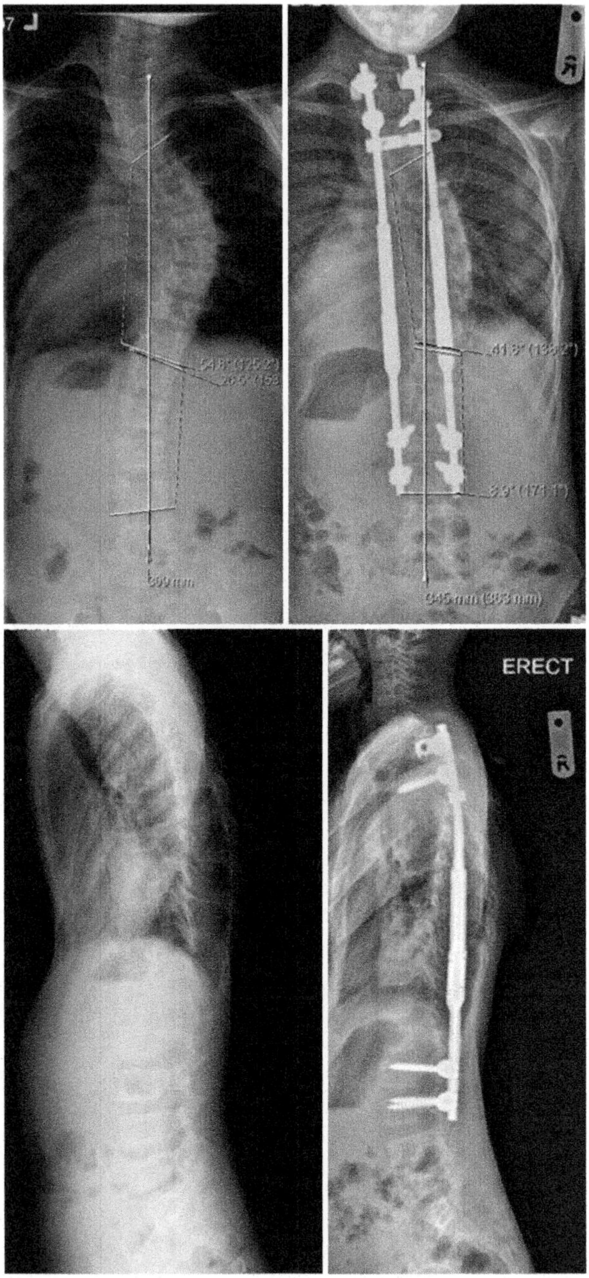

Fig. 12.4 A 7 year old Marfan syndrome boy with juvenile scoliosis and pectus excavatum treated with a novel magnet driven growing rod (MdGR) implant – dual rod insertion. Preoperative and postoperative PA and lateral radiographs are shown

mixed with native/host bone and then laid over both the proximal and distal fixation anchors. An index case, from a 7 year old child with juvenile MFS, illustrating our above technique with the use of a dual MdGR and having a T2–L3 fixation is shown in Fig. 12.4. Our preference is to use a dual rod construct whenever possible. We have used single rods (SR) in a few rigid multi-planar curves (especially those with severe kyphosis/kyphoscoliosis). SR are also particularly helpful for severe sagittal plane deformities, which provide flexibility with a creative design configuration and tension-free soft tissue/skin closure.

Post-operative Care and Rehabilitation

A chest radiograph is taken during recovery to ensure that the lung tissue is well expanded and rule out a spontaneous pneumothorax or secondary to TP hook insertion. The child should be allowed to sit-up, with head end elevated to 30°–40° with effect from day one and erect with effect from post-op day two. We let most of the children begin mobilisation from post-op on day two and they are discharged on day three or four. We do not routinely use orthosis following MdGR insertion, and we begin serial lengthening at 3 months post-op, and at two to three monthly intervals thereafter. Simple stretching exercises and school PT can be resumed at 3 months postoperatively. Contact sports and horse-riding are prohibited for at least 6 months. The initial 3 months of close observation with minimal physical activity ensures adequate arthrodesis at the anchor sites prior to commencing regular/serial distractions. All lengthenings are performed in office, wherein a hand-held magnetic wand is used to locate the precise area of the magnetic coil. Low-dose chest x-rays or ultrasound (USG) are performed after each distraction to confirm that the spine has indeed lengthened and we document the distraction achieved in millimetres [45].

Traditional teaching in the past was to refrain from performing spinal surgery in patients aged <4 years, owing to the severe cardiac involvement, as large curve magnitude combined with poor cardiac reserve precluded one from undertaking surgical correction safely [34]. The rationale that such children would succumb spontaneously to cardiac failure was used to justify such a stand. Serial casting, though an option as a delaying tactic or time-buying strategy, is discouraged because of the restrictive effect it imposes on the lungs and its burden on cardiac physiology. However, with advances in infantile cardiac surgeries, this is being successfully challenged. One such case example of a 2.5 year old boy with neonatal MFS, presenting with severe kyphoscoliosis which was treated by a novel magnet-driven growing rod (MdGR) and operated on by the senior author with a follow-up of 3.5 years, is illustrated in Fig. 12.3. The top row depicts the preoperative radiographs (PA and Lateral) showing a left thoracic infantile scoliosis of ≥70°. A mean 22.3 mm length gain was achieved at one year post-op (middle row radiographs) following a single submuscular MdGR insertion. However, despite satisfactory curve containment in the coronal plane, there was a worsening of sagittal balance with thoracic hyperkyphosis at 3.5 years postoperatively (bottom row radiographs).

Such a phenomenon appears to be a rule than an exception, irrespective of the surgical option exercised. Early definitive spinal fusion is not recommended, as it causes a disproportionately short upper segment with a truncal height of <220 mm resulting in thoracic insufficiency syndrome (TIS) [46].

Adolescent and Adult Scoliosis in MFS

Surgical correction of scoliosis is eventually needed in at least 10–15 % of MFS patients [17, 18]. Definitive spinal fusion is usually performed when the patient has attained skeletal maturity/completed growth (i.e. Risser Gr. ≥IV). A preoperative MRI/CT scan is mandatory to evaluate for posterior element defect/dural ectasia to minimise the risk of durotomy during surgical exposure. Selective fusion of either the thoracic or thoraco-lumbar/lumbar curve is not recommended and long fusion tends to be the rule.

Unlike with idiopathic scoliosis, the surgical correction of MFS is associated with higher intraoperative blood loss, and the use of intraoperative anti-coagulants (i.e. έ-amino caproic acid (EACA) or tranexemic acid) with an intraoperative cell-saver is recommended to minimise the blood loss. A higher incidence of inadvertent durotomy (8 %), pseudoarthrosis rate (21 %), deep infection (8 %), loss of correction achieved with time (30 %), laminar fractures (8 %) and implant failure (anchor dislodgement or rod breakage) is also reported [47, 48]. The ligamentous laxity and attenuated muscle tone pose unique sagittal plane challenges. MFS patients have a higher risk of developing proximal junctional kyphosis (PJK) or distal junctional kyphosis (DJK). Meticulous attention during surgical exposure with retention of the midline soft tissue structures (i.e. the supraspinous and interspinous ligaments) and inclusion of the first lordotic disc (on standing sagittal radiographs) in the instrumentation/construct minimises such events (i.e. PJK and DJK). Instrumentation to the pelvis may be inevitable in the presence of dural ectasia with vertebral scalloping.

Our preference is to correct the scoliosis using a low implant density index (IDI) construct (i.e. IDI of ≤1.5) with either all pedicle screws or a hybrid construct employing a combination of cantilever, translation, and derotation (CTD) techniques adhering to the Noordeen adolescent idiopathic scoliosis (AIS) curve classification algorithm to aid in the selection of fusion levels [49]. Our algorithm identifies three main curve patterns which are further subdivided into two sub-types (depending on the position of the shoulder on the convexity of the curve – i.e. up or down in relation to its counterpart on the concavity) yielding six different curve patterns as illustrated in Fig. 12.5. As a rule, we do not perform or recommend

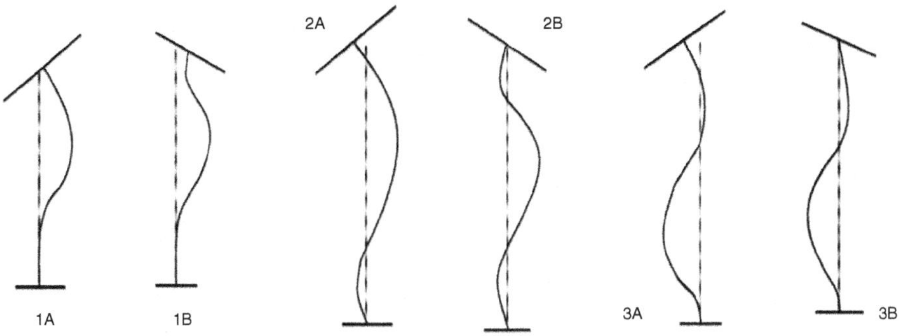

Fig. 12.5 The Noordeen AIS curve classification algorithm: six types of AIS curves. *1* structural thoracic curve. *2* structural thoracic & thoraco-lumbar/lumbar curve. *3* structural thoraco-lumbar/lumbar curve. Sub-types *A* convex shoulder is *up*. *B* convex shoulder is *down*

selective fusion of scoliosis in MFS. An index case example of such a correction in a 15 year old boy is illustrated in Fig. 12.6. We do not routinely use BMP or harvest an iliac crest bone graft (ICBG) to achieve arthrodesis. The gold standard ICBG is fraught with complications including, but not exclusively limited to, donor site morbidity, iliac wing fractures, prolonged hospital stay, iliac hematoma, etc. Our preference is to use silicated calcium phosphate (SiCaP) granules mixed with local autologous bone (spinous process and decorticated posterior elements) to achieve fusion. The use of a low IDI construct minimises implant costs associated with scoliosis correction without compromising clinical results or causing a loss of correction with time.

Practical Operative Tips to Improve Safety and Outcomes [48]

- Positioning the patient in the Trendelenburg position to minimise ballooning of the distal dura
- Avoiding the use of sublaminar wires to minimise the risk of inadvertent durotomy in the current era of pedicle screws which are '*gold standard*' anchors for surgical correction
- Aiming to achieve 50–60 % curve correction to avoid curve decompensation which could potentially result in excessive correction (i.e. >75 %)
- Avoid using laminar hooks as anchors (as there is a risk of laminar fractures and steel stenosis)
- Anaesthetic induction under the supervision of a cardiac anaesthetist with post-operative care in a cardiac ICU/cardiac floor, instead of a general orthopaedic or surgical floor.

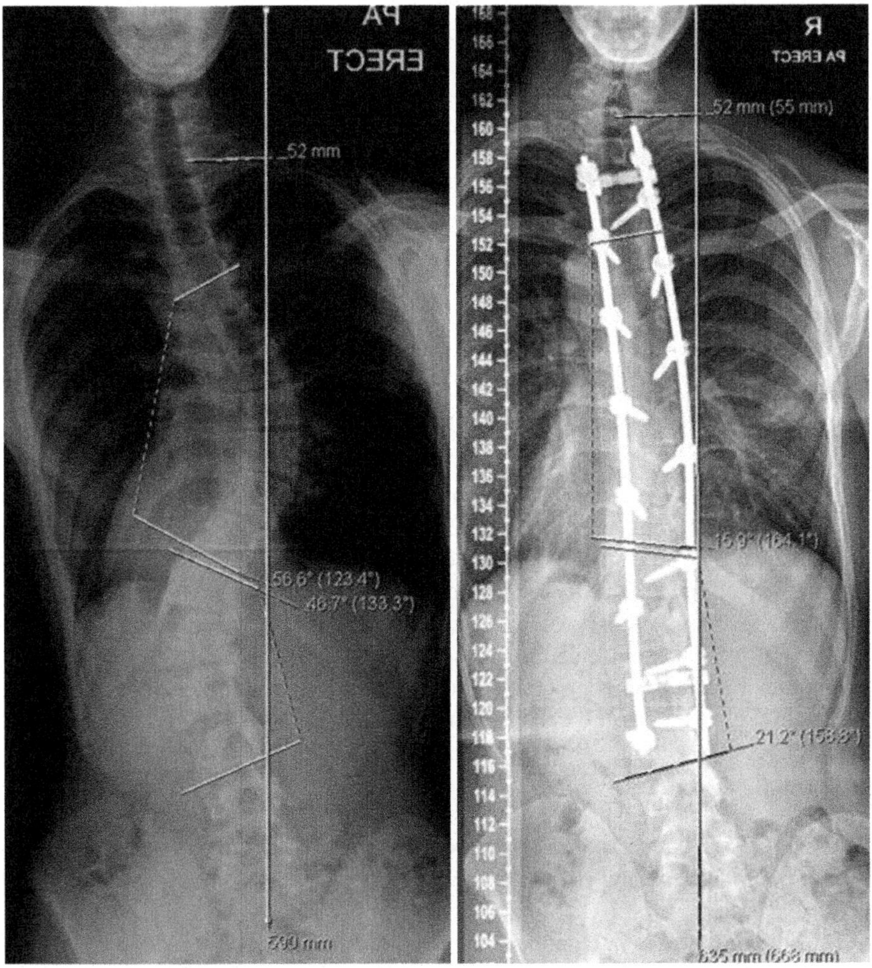

Fig. 12.6 A 15 year old Marfan syndrome boy with adolescent scoliosis treated with posterior instrumented spinal fusion using a low implant density index (IDI) construct. Preoperative and postoperative radiographs are shown

Conclusion

In summary, MFS is a systemic connective tissue disorder with scoliosis as one of its skeletal manifestations. Though the curve type and pattern mimics idiopathic scoliosis, distinct characteristics exists that differentiate MFS scoliosis from idiopathic scoliosis. Curves <20° largely remain unchanged and children should be observed until skeletal maturity for progression of the deformity. Bracing plays a small role, since scoliosis is usually resistant to bracing with poorer results, and it is indicated for curves with a Cobb angle of 21°–40° in the juvenile age group. Serial casts and braces may delay the need for growing rod insertion/growth guided procedures in infantile scoliosis or neonatal MFS, which is often most severe and extremely difficult to treat. Curves >40° usually progress, which ultimately warrants surgical management. Understanding the vertebral morphological differences of the scoliotic spine in MFS is of paramount importance when planning and executing surgical correction.

Neonatal MFS produces some of the most severe multi-planar spinal deformities with significant cardio-pulmonary compromise. These patients usually live up to young adulthood and beyond with advances in cardiac care and pharmacotherapeutic treatment with β-blockers and Angiotensin converting enzyme (ACE) inhibitors [50]. Advances in growing rod technology with magnet-driven growing rods (MdGRs) are a boon to such vulnerable young children, since they eliminate the need for repetitive anesthesia and serve as an internal brace, guiding the curve correction with growth. Early definitive spinal fusion is not recommended, for it leaves an individual with a short trunk, manifesting with thoracic insufficiency syndrome (TIS) [46].

Juvenile scoliosis in MFS is best treated by bracing for moderate curves, and then growth guided procedures for those with severe/progressive curves (i.e. Growing rods: magnet-driven or conventional/Shilla technique/Luque-Trolley instrumentation, etc). MdGRs are increasingly becoming the standard of care for most aetiologies of early-onset scoliosis (EOS) and MFS is no exception. They have an added advantage of facilitating minimal absence from school, with normal psychological maturation, scholastic performance, with one-off surgery and serial office-based lengtheni.ng.

Patients with MFS needing scoliosis surgery have a higher risk of curve decompensation with excessive correction, incidental durotomy, and perioperative complications, compared to surgically treated idiopathic scoliosis patients [47, 48]. Dural ectasia (DE) may pose significant challenges and warrant instrumentation to the pelvis in select cases, owing to poor bone stock or vertebral scalloping which has a higher complication rate (i.e. pseudoarthrosis and implant failure).

Co-existent chest cage deformities may warrant surgery to increase the AP diameter of the chest and normalise the space available for the lungs (SAL) by using a Nuss bar for pectus excavatum [51]. The Nuss bar may cause a worsening of the kyphosis with paraparesis, warranting a high-risk vertebral column resection (VCR), and treating surgeons should be aware of this potential scenario [52]. The surgical correction of scoliosis in MFS should be undertaken at specialist centers with multi-modal intraoperative neuro-monitoring (IONM) in a safe manner. A preoperative work-up with CT/MRI/DEXA scans and medical optimisation and attention to detail improves the surgical outcome and final results.

Acknowledgements The authors would like to acknowledge Dr. JH Perra, MD, FACS – Attending spinal surgeon; Twin Cities Spine Center and Gillette Children's Specialty Healthcare – Minneapolis, MN, U.S.A for providing us with the pictures of the rapid prototyping (RP) model and 3D-CT images of a congenital spinal deformity (Fig. 12.1).

Conflict of Interest (CoI)

1. NS Harshavardhana: No relationships
2. Mohammed H. H. Noordeen:
   Ellipse Tech, Inc. – Consultant and stockholder
   K2M – Consultant
   Stryker Spine – Research and educational support (no period)

Authorship Contribution Statement The two authors (i.e. NSH and MHHN) jointly wrote and made substantial contributions in drafting the outline for the chapter. The clinical case example radiographs are from patients operated upon by MHHN. Both the authors read and approved the final draft of the submitted manuscript. We take full responsibility for the contents of this publication, attesting to both its accuracy and integrity, and we agree to be accountable for all aspects of the work.

References

1. Marfan AB. Un cas de déformation congénitale des quatre membres, plus prononcée aux extrémités caractérisée par l'allongement des os avec un certain degré d'amincissement. Bull Mem Soc Med Hop Paris. 1896;13:220–6.
2. Dietz HC, Pyeritz RE, Hall BD, et al. The Marfan syndrome locus: confirmation of assignment to chromosome 15 and identification of tightly linked markers at 15q15–q21.3. Genomics. 1991;9:355–61.
3. Dietz HC, Cutting GR, Pyeritz RE, et al. Marfan syndrome caused by a recurrent de novo missense mutation in the fibrillin gene. Nature. 1991;352:337–9.
4. Gray JR, Bridges AB, Faed MJ, et al. Ascertainment and severity of Marfan syndrome in a Scottish population. J Med Genet. 1994;31:51–4.
5. Frédéric MY, Monino C, Marschall C, et al. The FBN2 gene: new mutations, locus-specific database (Universal Mutation Database FBN2), and genotype-phenotype correlations. Hum Mutat. 2009;30:181–90.
6. Sakai H, Visser R, Ikegawa S, et al. Comprehensive genetic analysis of relevant four genes in 49 patients with Marfan syndrome or Marfan-related phenotypes. Am J Med Genet A. 2006;140:1719–25.
7. Silverman DI, Burton KJ, Gray J, et al. Life expectancy in the Marfan syndrome. Am J Cardiol. 1995;75:157–60.
8. Pyeritz RE, Francke U. The Second International Symposium on the Marfan syndrome. Am J Med Genet. 1993;47:127–35.
9. Dean JC. Marfan syndrome: clinical diagnosis and management. Eur J Hum Genet. 2007;15:724–33.
10. Keech MK, Wendt VE, Read RC, et al. Family studies of the Marfan syndrome. J Chronic Dis. 1966;19(1):57–83.
11. Fahey J. Muscular and skeletal change in arachnodactyly. Arch Surg. 1939;39:741–60.
12. Sinclair RJG, Kitchin AH, Turner RWD. The Marfan syndrome. Quart J Med. 1960;29:19–46.
13. Wilner HI, Finby N. Skeletal manifestation in the Marfan syndrome. JAMA. 1964;187:490–5.
14. Scheier H. Prognose und Behandlung der Skoliose. Stuttgart: Thieme publishers; 1967. pp. 15–21.
15. Ford J. Scoliosis in Marfan syndrome. Los Amigos Hospital (UCLA School of Medicine): Resident research reports; 1968.
16. Sliman NA. A propos de 16 cas de scoliosis. Marfan Tunisie Med. 1971;2:93–101.

17. Robins PR, Moe JH, Winter RB. Scoliosis in Marfan's syndrome: its characteristics and results of treatment in thirty-five patients. J Bone Joint Surg Am. 1975;57(3):358–68.
18. Sponseller PD, Hobbs W, Riley 3rd LH, Pyeritz RE. The thoracolumbar spine in Marfan syndrome. J Bone Joint Surg Am. 1995;77(6):867–76.
19. Demetracopoulos CA, Sponseller PD. Spinal deformities in Marfan syndrome. Orthop Clin North Am. 2007;38(4):563–72.
20. Sanghera B, Naique S, Papaharilaou Y, Amis A. Preliminary study of rapid prototype medical models. Rapid Prototyping J. 2001;7(5):275–84. What happened to the colon?.
21. Guarino J, Tennyson S, McCain G, et al. Rapid prototyping technology for surgeries of the pediatric spine and pelvis: benefits analysis. J Pediatr Orthop. 2007;27(8):955–60.
22. Grahame R, Pyeritz RE. The Marfan syndrome: joint and skin manifestations are prevalent and correlated. Br J Rheumatol. 1995;34:126–31.
23. Hobbs WR, Sponseller PD, Weiss AP, Pyeritz RE. The cervical spine in Marfan syndrome. Spine. 1997;22(9):983–9.
24. Oosterhof T, Groenink M, Hulsmans FJ, et al. Quantitative assessment of dural ectasia as a marker for Marfan syndrome. Radiology. 2001;220:514–8.
25. Ahn NU, Sponseller PD, Ahn UM, et al. Dural ectasia in the Marfan syndrome: MR and CT findings and criteria. Genet Med. 2000;2(3):173–9.
26. Pyeritz RE, Fishman EK, Bernhardt BA, Siegelman SS. Dural ectasia is a common feature of the Marfan syndrome. Am J Hum Genet. 1988;43(5):726.
27. Sponseller PD. Chapter 103 – Spinal deformities in Marfan syndrome. ridwell KH, De Wald R, editors. The textbook of spinal surgery. 3rd ed. Philadelphia: Lippincott, Williams & Wilkins; 2012.
28. Winter RB. Severe spondylolisthesis in Marfan's syndrome: report of two cases. J Pediatr Orthop. 1982;2(1):51–5.
29. Taylor LJ. Severe spondylolisthesis and scoliosis in association with Marfan's syndrome. Case report and review of the literature. Clin Orthop Relat Res. 1987;221:207–11.
30. Giampietro PF, Peterson M, Schneider R, et al. Assessment of bone mineral density in adults and children with Marfan syndrome. Osteoporos Int. 2003;14(7):559–63.
31. Sponseller PD, Jones KB, Ahn NU, et al. Protrusio acetabuli in Marfan syndrome: age-related prevalence and associated hip function. J Bone Joint Surg Am. 2006;88(3):486–95.
32. James JIP. The etiology of scoliosis. J Bone Joint Surg (Br). 1970;52:410–9.
33. Lenke LG, Dobbs MB. Management of juvenile idiopathic scoliosis. J Bone Joint Surg (Am). 2007;89 suppl 1:55–63.
34. Sponseller PD, Sethi N, Cameron DE, Pyeritz RE. Infantile scoliosis in Marfan syndrome. Spine. 1997;22(5):509–16.
35. Sponseller PD, Bhimani M, Solacoff D, Dormans JP. Results of brace treatment of scoliosis in Marfan syndrome. Spine. 2000;25(18):2350–4. No italics for title of journal?.
36. Sponseller PD, Thompson GH, Akbarnia BA, et al. Growing rods for infantile scoliosis in Marfan syndrome. Spine. 2009;34(16):1711–5.
37. The MAGEC system for spinal lengthening in children with scoliosis. NICE medical technology guidance (MTG18). https://www.nice.org.uk/guidance/mtg18. Accessed 8, 2015.
38. Yoon WW, Sedra F, Shah S, et al. Improvement of pulmonary function in children with early-onset scoliosis using magnetic growth rods. Spine. 2014;39(15):1196–202.
39. Cheung KM, Cheung JP, Samartzis D, et al. Magnetically controlled growing rods for severe spinal curvature in young children: a prospective case series. Lancet. 2012;379(9830):1967–74.
40. Akbarnia BA, Cheung K, Noordeen H, et al. Next generation of growth-sparing techniques: preliminary clinical results of a magnetically controlled growing rod in 14 patients with early-onset scoliosis. Spine. 2013;38(8):665–70.
41. Dannawi Z, Altaf F, Harshavardhana NS, et al. Early results of a remotely-operated magnetic growth rod in early-onset scoliosis. Bone Joint J. 2013;95-b(1):75–80.
42. Akbarnia BA, Pawelek JB, Cheung KMC, et al. Traditional growing rods versus magnetically controlled growing rods for the surgical treatment of early-onset scoliosis: a case-matched 2-year study. Spine Deform. 2014;2(6):493–7.

43. Hickey BA, Towriss C, Baxter G, et al. Early experience of MAGEC magnetic growing rods in the treatment of early onset scoliosis. Eur Spine J. 2014;23 Suppl 1:S61–5.
44. Schwartz DM, Drummond DS, Hahn M, et al. Prevention of positional brachial plexopathy during surgical correction of scoliosis. J Spinal Disord. 2000;13(2):178–82.
45. Stokes OM, O'Donovan EJ, Samartzis D, et al. Reducing radiation exposure in early-onset scoliosis surgery patients: novel use of ultrasonography to measure lengthening in magnetically-controlled growing rods. Spine J. 2014;14(10):2397–404.
46. Karol LA, Johnston C, Mladenov K, et al. Pulmonary function following early thoracic fusion in non-neuromuscular scoliosis. J Bone Joint Surg Am. 2008;90(6):1272–81.
47. Gjolaj JP, Sponseller PD, Shah SA, et al. Spinal deformity correction in Marfan syndrome versus adolescent idiopathic scoliosis: learning from the differences. Spine. 2012;37(18):1558–65.
48. Jones KB, Erkula G, Sponseller PD, Dormans JP. Spine deformity correction in Marfan syndrome. Spine. 2002;27(18):2003–12.
49. Harshavardhana NS, Noordeen MH. Surgical results with the use of Silicated Calcium Phosphate (SiCaP) as bone graft substitute in Posterior Spinal Fusion (PSF) for Adolescent Idiopathic Scoliosis (AIS). Scoliosis. 2015;10(27):1–12.
50. Shores J, Berger KR, Murphy EA, Pyeritz RE. Progression of aortic dilatation and the benefit of long-term beta-adrenergic blockade in Marfan's syndrome. N Engl J Med. 1994;330:1335–41.
51. Nuss D, Kelly RE, Croitoru DP, et al. A 10-year review of a minimally invasive technique for the correction of pectus excavatum. J Pediatr Surg. 1998;33(4):545–52.
52. Sugrue PA, O'Shaughnessy BA, Blanke KM, et al. Rapidly progressive Scheuermann's disease in an adolescent after pectus bar placement treated with posterior vertebral-column resection: case report and review of the literature. Spine. 2013;38(4):E259–62.

Rheumatological Aspects of Marfan Syndrome

13

Anne H. Child and Rodney Grahame

Introduction

Locomotor symptoms are frequent and troublesome in the Marfan syndrome [1, 2]. Close involvement with rheumatologists and orthopaedic surgeons may be indicated to manage painful joint hypermobility and its complications in early to mid-life, and, with increased longevity, degenerative joint disease in later years. Seventy per cent of children experience symptoms of arthralgia, back pain and ligament laxity and injury [1]. The earliest complaints of the child are often knee pain or ankle pain necessitating rest and analgesia. These symptoms, if not appreciated by parents and teachers, may lead to the belief that the child is not trying to participate in family outings or school sporting activities. It is important to allow the child to participate to the extent of his or her ability, but to permit rest, or to terminate the family outing, if the child cannot keep up. Taking a pushchair on family outings makes it a more pleasant activity for all concerned. Allowing the child to act as a referee or a goal keeper or play the least demanding role on the team at school is helpful. Weak ankles and knees, combined with poor eyesight may make the children appear clumsy in sporting activities, and they soon lose interest. It is important to wear sports shoes with ankle support, and even arch supports and heel cups, to render the gait more controlled. Ankle and knee supports may be worn to stabilise these joints, which are prone to recurrent sprains, and in some cases patellar dislocation. In severe cases, surgical fusion of the ankle, or shortening of the patellar ligaments may be helpful. Patients should be taught to gently reduce recurrent

A.H. Child, MD, FRCP (✉)
Cardiovascular and Cell Sciences Research Institute, St George's, University of London, London, UK
e-mail: achild@sgul.ac.uk

R. Grahame, CBE, MD, FRCP, FACP
Rheumatology Unit, Hospital of St John and St Elizabeth, London, UK
e-mail: r.grahame@ucl.ac.uk

© Springer-Verlag London 2016

A.H. Child (ed.), *Diagnosis and Management of Marfan Syndrome*,
DOI 10.1007/978-1-4471-5442-6_13

dislocations of patellae, fingers and toes. These joints gain stability with passing years. Wrist or finger splints may help to stabilise the loose wrist, thumb or fingers, and render writing neater. If the hand tires, especially during examinations, extra time should be given. Using fat pens or pencils, which may be built up, makes the handwriting more legible. For older children, the use of a laptop computer, or even a tape recorder to record lessons, may avoid the need for handwritten notes.

Preventive Measures

Back and neck pain may be eased by ensuring correct posture. Some patients find learning the Alexander method of correct posture at all times, very helpful. Stretching exercises may be taught by a physiotherapist, and sitting for long periods of time should be avoided. It is essential that the chair and desk are of adequate height for the tall child and adult, so that they do not stoop. It is important that computer screens and keyboards are at the correct height to avoid neck and eye strain.

Medical and Surgical Management

Flat, long, thin feet, often with hammer toes, require very careful shoe fitting with orthotics, and for the largest and most difficult feet, hand-made shoes may be the only solution. Surgery for hammer toes can be helpful, but frequently this deformity recurs after surgery, so it may be best just to purchase shoes with extra depth to allow room for the toes. Men with Marfan syndrome are especially prone to spondylolisthesis, and should avoid gaining weight in middle age, and heavy lifting at all ages. In approximately 5 % of all families, there is a tendency to early osteoarthritis, and the hip joint may need replacing by the age of 50. Protrusio acetabulae is known to occur with increased frequency [3–5].

Because of the overgrowth of ribs, pectus deformities may result, and even without this, a tendency to costochondritis, especially in rapidly growing adolescents, may lead to worries about chest pain coming from the heart. This is best treated with reassurance, non-steroidal anti-inflammatory medication, review of possible triggering events such as playing tennis, and if all else fails, intra-articular injection with steroids. In general, steroid injections should be used as a last resort, as they suppress collagen production. Certainly repeated injections are discouraged.

Physiotherapists and occupational therapists may be of great assistance, provided that they are informed that they are not dealing with normal joints. Exercises alone will not markedly strengthen genetically weak ligaments or muscles, although they are helpful to maintain optimum strength. Manipulation of the spine and other painful joints should be gentle.

When prescribing medication for acute or chronic joint complaints, in the Marfan patient, the physician should be aware that most patients, although tall, have very little subcutaneous fat. Therefore, a low dose may be appropriate. In addition, gastric irritation with anti-inflammatory medication should be guarded against, with simultaneous Losec and non-steroidal [anti-inflammatory] medication. Several NSAIDs may have to be tried, starting with the mildest before the most effective one is found.

Should the patient come to surgery, it must be remembered that healing is often delayed, as indicated by a tendency to scar, or to heal with papyraceous scar. Sutures need to be strong, and left in somewhat longer than for the average patient. Antibiotic cover should also be provided to prevent endocarditis, and an experienced anaesthetist should be utilised, as with all surgery, since the combination of high narrow palate, reduced neck extension, and floppy larynx may give rise to difficulty in intubation.

Occupation and Choice of Sports

Fibrillin-1 is an important constituent of bone, cartilage, periosteum, as well as tendons and ligaments and muscle itself. It has a special function in providing insertion of ligaments into bone. This explains the frequency of disability due to pain, dislocation or laxity in the central or peripheral skeleton, as well as skeletal muscle underdevelopment or hypotonia. Muscles tend to be slim and weak, and do respond to regular exercise, but muscle building exercises such as heavy weightlifting should be discouraged, as it is not realistic to expect muscle hypertrophy. It is better to choose sporting activities which are suited to the long, lean frame, such as cycling, basketball or badminton. Occupational choice may also be limited by physical ability, and patients should be encouraged to prolong their academic studies, and enter an occupation which is physically undemanding. Fibrillin deficiency in muscles and ligaments may also play a role in the easy fatigability which affects children and adults alike. Depression tends to occur if the working day takes all the energy a patient has to give. It is better to save some energy for social or leisure pursuits. Similarly, some patients experience an increase in fatigability from the age of 50 onward, necessitating early retirement if they are in a demanding occupation. Informed choice of a less demanding occupation may prolong the working life of the patient.

References

1. Grahame R, Pyeritz RE. The Marfan syndrome: joint and skin manifestations are prevalent and correlated. Br J Rheumatol. 1995;34:126–31.
2. Magrid D, Pyeritz RE, Fisherman EK. Musculo-skeletal manifestation of the Marfan syndrome. Am J Rheumatol. 1992;155:99–104.
3. Wenger DR, Ditkoff TJ, Herin JA, Maulding DM. Protrusio acetabulae in Marfan syndrome. Clin Orthop. 1980;147:134–8.
4. Fast A, Otremsky Y, Pollack D, Floman Y. Protrusio acetabulae in Marfan syndrome: report of two patients. J Rheumatol. 1984;11:549–51.
5. Kuhlman JE, Scot Jr WW, Fisherman EK, Pyeritz RE, Siegelmann SS. Acetabular protrusion in the Marfan syndrome. Radiology. 1987;164:415–7.

The Role of Physiotherapy in Marfan Syndrome

14

Rosemary J. Keer

Introduction

Marfan syndrome is frequently associated with a variety of musculoskeletal abnormalities which have the potential to produce symptoms throughout life. Joint hypermobility is one of the most common musculoskeletal features, affecting 85 % of children and 56 % of adults [1]. Hypermobility caused by ligamentous laxity can lead to poor joint control, rendering the individual prone to pain, recurrent joint sprains and strains, including subluxation and dislocation. The finger, ankle and patellofemoral joints are affected most frequently in the Marfan population. In a small percentage this can progress to early onset osteoarthritis. Scoliosis is also common, being present in 60 % of individuals with Marfan syndrome [2]. This can lead to progressive deformity, particularly during the growth spurts and be associated with back pain and restricted ventilatory capacity.

Managing these symptoms requires a close working relationship between rheumatologists, orthopaedic surgeons, podiatrists, occupational therapists and physiotherapists to help relieve symptoms and prevent complications.

Initially, physiotherapy aims to reduce pain and improve joint control and stability, progressing onto the ultimate aim of injury prevention and enabling the patient to self manage their condition confidently.

R.J. Keer, MSc, MCSP, MACP
Department of Hypermobility Unit, Hospital of St John & St Elizabeth, London NW8 9NH, UK
e-mail: rosemary.keer@hje.org.uk

© Springer-Verlag London 2016

A.H. Child (ed.), *Diagnosis and Management of Marfan Syndrome*,
DOI 10.1007/978-1-4471-5442-6_14

Education and Advice

Education on joint care is an important part of a therapeutic intervention where the emphasis is on educating and empowering the patient to avoid harmful postures and activities which can overstretch and strain hypermobile joints while encouraging exercise and activity to maintain good joint health [3].

Individuals diagnosed with Marfan syndrome (and their families) really appreciate being given the time to talk about the problems associated with their diagnosis. There are often questions around whether they will harm their joints, or body, by being physically active and they may have been given the impression that they are fragile and need to protect their joints. A balance needs to be found between protecting joints in the short term and progressing on to exercise and activity which will ensure good joint function in the long term.

Posture

Good postural habit is important in everyone, but is particularly important in individuals with hypermobile joints as it reduces the stress and strain on the soft tissues of the body, helps to prevent injury and is the most efficient way to support the body during both static and dynamic activities [3].

Individuals with hypermobile joints often rest at the end of range-of-motion in many of their joints, partly as it gives a feeling of more stability and partly as it requires less effort [4]. Favourite postures, for both children and adults, include slumped sitting, standing with 'locked' knees, hanging on the hip and resting on the lateral border of the feet. These and other similar postures can be considered potentially 'harmful' if adopted habitually as it puts prolonged stress on ligamentous tissue in a stretched position rather than using low level muscle co-contraction to support a joint. Education and practice in maintaining joints in a more neutral position will involve improving joint awareness, proprioception, postural alignment and muscle function. An individually tailored postural re-education programme showed good improvement in pain and quality of life in hypermobile individuals [5]. Instruction in the Alexander technique can be very helpful and has been shown to be effective in reducing low back pain [6].

Advice should be specific and often involves ergonomic considerations such as ensuring that the desk and chair set-up both at school and in the office are at the correct height and distance. For children it may involve advice regarding school work; using chunky pens and laptops to reduce symptoms from prolonged writing, carrying school books and participation in sports. For the mother it may involve analyzing and then advising on posture during standing, bending and lifting, all essential activities with young children.

If a scoliosis is present it is prudent to monitor progress throughout childhood paying particular attention to good postural habits. Physiotherapy can be successful in treating scoliosis [7] through exercise designed to improve posture, spinal biomechanics, muscle balance and breathing, although bracing and surgery may be required in more severe cases.

Joint Control

Exercise has been shown to be effective in managing the symptoms of joint hypermobility and helping to prevent problems in the future.

In the initial stages following injury, it may be necessary to rest the area, use an external support and take analgesia to allow the acute pain and swelling to subside. Gentle manual therapy may be helpful to restore normal movement. Attention then turns to improving static and dynamic control of hypermobile joints throughout the full range of movement.

Normal movement relies on the integration of proprioception and motor control. Proprioception is the ability to sense joint position and movement to ensure joints are correctly positioned and have suitable muscle tone for the activity. Proprioceptive acuity is frequently decreased in hypermobile individuals, possibly due to an impairment of segmental musculoskeletal reflexes which is thought to have important implications for stability around the knee in particular, and be part of the explanation for the sensation of the knee 'giving way' [8].

Motor control and joint stability can be improved with a programme of exercises which enhance proprioception and produce effective co-contraction of muscles around a joint. These exercises performed regularly over a 6–8 week period have been shown to significantly reduce pain, reduce hyperlaxity and improve quality of life in hypermobile individuals [9, 10]. Closed kinetic chain exercises are most effective in this respect and can include standing on one leg, mini squats, single leg knee bend and four-point kneeling. These can be made more challenging by progressing on to more dynamic balance activities using a balance (wobble) board, foam rollers and the Swiss ball. Proprioception can be further enhanced by increasing sensory input via the skin through 'hands on' movement facilitation, wearing tight fitting clothing and neoprene gloves and the application of tape during specific exercise or functional rehabilitation sessions.

Once the patient is familiar with, and has adopted better postural control and more effective stability strategies, it is important that the exercise programme is integrated into everyday life. This means practising good joint control when standing, sitting, sitting to standing, walking, and particularly during any provocative or challenging physical situations the individual may have.

Open chain exercises can be added later to be more functionally specific and exercises in general are progressed to encourage an increase in overall physical activity by improving muscle strength and endurance. Generalized muscle weakness is a characteristic of Marfan syndrome and while muscle hypertrophy is unrealistic [11] it is important to optimise muscle strength and endurance.

Exercise and manual therapy may exacerbate pain and this can quickly lead to non compliance. Exercises should as far as possible be pain free. Pain in this context means that too much stress is being placed on soft tissues, possibly causing microinjury of the connective tissue, and is distinct from training pain which is to be expected with more vigorous exercise. The exercise may need to be modified in terms of range, number of repetitions or position to ensure correct muscle activation and adequate control. The 'form' and level of the exercise are of paramount importance to ensure that there is no undue stress on hypermobile tissues which have been further weakened by injury or deconditioning. Initially, exercise should be considered 'easy', performed with a relaxed breathing pattern, with good body awareness and postural control, and with repetitions reduced to single figures if necessary. Hydrotherapy, making use of water as a supportive medium, can be a successful way to get a deconditioned individual, who has difficulty weight-bearing due to pain, starting to strengthen and move again.

Stretching

People with hypermobile joints are often discouraged from stretching for fear that they may overstretch and injure their joints. Frequently though, hypermobile individuals report that they positively benefit from stretching and it can be used as a means to ease out muscular tensions and spasms. As long as stretching is not forced and the individual is aware of their vulnerable areas and has a good understanding of how to care for their joints, gentle stretching can be very beneficial and is not necessarily to be avoided.

External Support

Supporting joints externally in the form of splints and braces is generally discouraged in favour of strengthening muscles to provide more effective support. However, there are times when judicious use is very helpful. Providing support to a joint during the acute phase of an injury, such as a strain or sprain, can facilitate recovery by unloading injured tissues and encouraging more normal movement. In the longer term, well fitting splints which stabilise joints, yet allow good function, can help the individual with lax joints to sustain an activity for longer and can be particularly beneficial in the hand, promoting better writing, typing and participation in music and recreational activities. Tape, applied to the skin to support joints during exercise, has been found to improve proprioception and help to prevent injury, although extra care should be taken when applying and removing tape due to the risk of skin fragility. In addition, it has been reported that close fitting, contour controlled underwear and lycra exercise clothing has been helpful in improving perceived joint stability and reducing pain and can be used on a regular basis.

The typical long, slender foot with flat arch and hammer toes will benefit from sensible, good fitting footwear with a strong heel counter, firm fastenings over the mid foot and cushioning materials to absorb load. Some individuals may require functional foot insoles or orthotics for additional support.

Physical Activity and Physical Fitness

Children and adults are encouraged to take part in regular physical activity to maintain good health and wellbeing. Decreased sports activity is frequently encountered in Marfan syndrome as pain, laxity and dislocation as well as poor muscle development can impact on an individual's ability to excel. The challenge is to find activities and sports which are safe, enjoyable and maximise condition. As a rule, it is recommended that exercise is non-contact, non competitive and of low intensity. Weightlifting is actively discouraged as it is unrealistic to expect muscle hypertrophy and any exercise which encourages breath holding is detrimental [12]. Generally exercise should be low impact, low resistance and aim for endurance rather than strength. Exercise in water, including swimming (good technique is essential to prevent strain of the cervical and lumbar spine), T'ai Chi, Pilates and dance are recommended, as well as walking (leisurely), cycling, golf, bowling, basketball, badminton and jogging. Exercising on the Wii fit has recently been shown to improve balance and lower limb strength and could be a very enjoyable way to exercise for some [13]. During any activity, attention to maintaining good posture and joint control is paramount and individuals should incorporate all they have learnt about their limitations into their chosen activity or sport and follow the principles of pacing.

References

1. Dean JCS. Marfan syndrome: clinical diagnosis and management. Eur J Hum Genet. 2007;15:724–33. doi:10.1038/sj.ejhg.5201851.
2. Al-Kaissi A, Zwettler E, Ganger R, Schreiner S, Klaushofer K, Grill F. Musculoskeletal abnormalities in patients with Marfan syndrome. Clin Med Insights Arthritis Musculoskelet Disord. 2013;6:1–9. doi:10.4137/CMAMD.S10279.
3. Keer RJ, Simmonds JV. Joint protection and physical rehabilitation of the adult with hypermobility syndrome. Curr Opin Rheumatol. 2011;23:131–6. doi:10.1097/BOR.0b013e328342d3af.
4. Keer R, Butler K. Physiotherapy & occupational therapy in the hypermobile adult. In: Hakim AJ, Keer RJ, Grahame R, editors. Hypermobility, fibromyalgia and chronic pain. Edinburgh: Churchill Livingstone; 2010. p. 143–61.
5. Booshanam DS, Cherian B, Joseph CP, et al. Evaluation of posture and pain in persons with benign joint hypermobility syndrome. Rheumatol Int. 2011;31:1561–5. doi:10.1007/s00296-010-1514-2.
6. Woodman JP, Moore NR. Evidence for the effectiveness of Alexander Technique lessons in medical and health-related conditions: a systematic review. Int J Clin Pract. 2012;66:98–112. doi:10.1111/j.1742-1241.2011.02817.x.
7. Lipscomb KJ, Clayton-Smith J, Harris R. Evolving phenotype of Marfan's syndrome. Arch Dis Child. 1997;76:41–6.
8. Ferrell WR, Ferrell PW. Proprioceptive dysfunction in joint hypermobility syndrome and its management. In: Hakim AJ, Keer RJ, Grahame R, editors. Hypermobility, fibromyalgia and chronic pain. Edinburgh: Churchill Livingstone; 2010. p. 96–104.
9. Barton LM, Bird HA. Improving pain by the stabilization of hyperlax joints. J Orthop Rheumatol. 1996;9:46–51.
10. Ferrell WR, Tennant N, Sturrock RD, et al. Proprioceptive enhancement ameliorates symptoms in the joint hypermobility syndrome. Arthritis Rheum. 2004;50:3323–8.

11. Child AH, Grahame R. Rheumatological aspects of Marfan syndrome. In: Child A, Briggs MJ, editors. The Marfan syndrome, a clinical guide. London: British Heart Foundation; 2002. p. 54–5.
12. Turk UO, Alioglu E, Nalbantgil D, Nart D. Catastrophic cardiovascular consequences of weight lifting in a family with Marfan syndrome. Turk Kardiyol Dern Ars. 2008;36:32–4.
13. Nitz JC, Kuys S, Isles R, Fu S. Is the Wii Fit a new-generation tool for improving balance, health and well-being? A pilot study. Climacteric. 2010;13:487–91.

Pulmonary Manifestations of Marfan Syndrome

15

Anne H. Child and Anita K. Simonds

Introduction

While the cardiovascular features of Marfan syndrome most frequently require medical intervention, it is recognised that pulmonary complications occur in up to 10 % of patients [1, 2]. Lung involvement may present in infancy or childhood [3], Complications may arise in adolescence or adult life that have serious consequences and are potentially fatal [4, 5].

Clinical Features

Lung Function in Marfan Syndrome

Abnormalities of fibrillin result in connective tissue friability and laxity. These features can lead to chest wall deformity [6] or, within the lung, flaccidity of small airways and terminal bronchioles, predisposing to premature airway closure, obstruction and air trapping. The function of larger airways can also be abnormal and when this occurs in association with thoracic kyphoscoliosis, central airway obstruction can occur. As a result MFS patients may have mildly abnormal lung function. This is usually manifest as abnormalities of FEV1 and FVC [7, 8], although the literature is divided about this issue. Streeten et al. reported 79 cases of

A.H. Child, MD, FRCP (✉)
Cardiovascular and Cell Sciences Research Institute, St George's, University of London, London, UK
e-mail: achild@sgul.ac.uk

A.K. Simonds, MD, FRCP
NIHR Respiratory Biomedical Research Unit, Royal Brompton & Harefield NHS Foundation Trust, Sydney Street, London SW3 6NP, UK
e-mail: a.simonds@rbht.nhs.uk

© Springer-Verlag London 2016

A.H. Child (ed.), *Diagnosis and Management of Marfan Syndrome*,
DOI 10.1007/978-1-4471-5442-6_15

Table 15.1 Predicted sitting and standing values (%) for FEV1 and FVC, in an index case of Marfan syndrome

FEV1: % of predicted value		FVC: % of predicted value		FEV1/FVC ratio: % of predicted value	
Standing	Sitting	Standing	Sitting	Standing	Sitting
63	87	83	95	78	92

The use of sitting height corrects for the contribution of leg length to increased total height (The upper body segment remains within normal limits)

Marfan syndrome and found there to be little or no abnormality in patients with no other complications of the condition [8]. Notwithstanding this, abnormal body proportions make the interpretation of lung function difficult. If sitting height was used to predict spirometric values (it is possible to pre-calculate predicted FEV1 and FVC from 'upper segment length') the previously observed abnormalities in lung function were in part corrected [8]. This finding is explained by correction for the relative increases in leg length as a proportion of total height (Table 15.1). For those patients with kyphoscoliosis a typical restrictive ventilatory effect is found, in keeping with the chest wall deformity.

Corsico et al. [9] reviewed lung function tests of 64 Italian MFS patients including spirometry, lung volumes and diffusing capacity. Fourteen percent reported previous pneumothorax. Two of the 19 patients who had CT scans were diagnosed with emphysema; both were non-smokers. Seven of these 19 had subpleural apical blebs. Only 37 % of patients had normal lung function; 19 % showed a restrictive pattern and 44 % an obstructive pattern or an isolated diffusion impairment or an isolated hyperinflation. All patients with pneumothorax history showed an obstructive pattern and diffusion impairment. Particular attention should be paid to prevent pneumothorax.

Pneumothorax and Bullous Lung Disease

A number of reports have been published showing an increased occurrence of pneumothorax in Marfan syndrome (especially in males) compared to normal control populations. Various studies have cited the incidence at between 4 and 14 % [10–12].

Furthermore, pneumothoraces are more likely to recur in these patients and there are a number of reports of bilateral disease. Both radiological and autopsy studies have shown pulmonary bullae (often apical) in patients, particularly in those who have had a pneumothorax [13]. Familial pneumothorax is rare and its association with Marfan syndrome is exceptional [14, 15].

The combination of bullae, obstructive spirometry, and impaired carbon monoxide gas transfer in keeping with mild emphysema has been reported [13]. A consistent pattern of distal acinar emphysema was noted in a retrospective series of five patients [16]. Some individuals are simply noted to have bullae on radiological assessment. These findings of bullous lung disease and emphysema may occur independent of smoking. Histologically the elastic fibres in lung biopsy specimens show degenerative changes, and although these are not as severe as those seen in the samples from patients with cutis laxa, the samples from Marfan syndrome patients with emphysema are easily distinguishable from those of normal controls, suggesting that degenerative change in the lung is the likely explanation for these changes rather than congenital cystic changes per se [17]. The management of pneumothorax in Marfan is along similar lines to idiopathic spontaneous pneumothorax. However, given the increased incidence of recurrent disease following tube drainage (with or without pleurodesis), it is recommended that early definitive surgical intervention is performed in these patients [11]. There are no specific features in the management of emphysema in a patient with Marfan syndrome although smoking should be strongly discouraged.

Chest Wall Deformity

Kyphoscoliosis is a feature of Marfan syndrome, the incidence quoted varying between 40 and 75 %. The progression of this skeletal abnormality is often more severe than in the idiopathic type, and double and triple curves are more common. Respiratory complications of a severe restrictive type occur, particularly when the deformity is associated with vertebral inversion or pectus excavatum, both of which are common features [18, 19]. Surgical correction remains the treatment of choice to prevent progressive deformity and secondary respiratory failure. While scoliosis surgery may not actually improve lung function, it may prevent worsening. Some patients at the severe end of the respiratory spectrum may require non-invasive ventilation (NIV) in the perioperative period if having major cardiac surgery, such as valve replacement.

Bronchiectasis and Bronchial Sepsis

The association of bronchiectasis with Marfan syndrome is less clear than for cystic lung disease although there are a number of anecdotal case reports in both children [20] and adults [2, 5]. Wood et al., in their survey of 100 adult patients, found two cases of bronchiectasis, three with recurrent lower respiratory infections and three cases of tuberculosis [12]. Plain chest X-ray is inadequate to diagnose bronchiectasis, but CT detects airway abnormalities characteristic of the condition. Recently [21], 79 Korean MFS patients (47 M:32 F) were evaluated using CT imaging, and airway dilations indicative of bronchiectasis (10/79, 13 %) were commonly found, although the extent of dilatation was not severe, and was frequently confined to a single lobe. Bronchiectasis was evident in three patients (4 %), with underlying bronchiectasis or bronchioloectasis. Four patients (5 %) had previous histories of treatment of pulmonary tuberculosis. No patient was diagnosed with non-tuberculous mycobacteria. Management of bronchiectasis in MFS is the same as for other patients with chronic bronchial sepsis.

Interstitial Lung Disease

As is true for bronchiectasis there are only sporadic reports of lung fibrosis in MFS. There are four cases of upper lobe fibrosis amongst the cases described by Wood et al. [12], and Lipton et al. reported a case of pneumothorax in a patient with bilateral honeycomb lung [22]. These few cases suggest a possible association between interstitial lung disease and the connective tissue defects seen in Marfan syndrome.

Obstructive Sleep Apnoea (OSA)

Sleep apnoea exhibits increased frequency in Marfan syndrome and is not predicted by classic risk factors. Obstructive and central sleep apnoeas may relate to cardiovascular disease variables [23]. Kohler et al. performed sleep studies in 61 patients with Ghent criteria positive MFS and in 26 matched control subjects [24]. In MFS patients, aortic root diameter was measured by echocardiography. Results showed that more patients with MFS than controls had OSA (15.8 % compared with 11.5 %). Mean aortic root diameter was significantly greater in patients with OSA compared to those without OSA ($p<0.0001$). They concluded that the prevalence of OSA is higher in MFS, and OSA may be a risk factor for aortic root dilatation.

Anaesthesia

There is at least one case report of perioperative tracheal obstruction in a patient with floppy central airways, despite intubation, during manipulation of the spine [25]. Intubating Marfan syndrome patients may be difficult, so an experienced anaesthetist should be present (See Chaps. 3 on page 13 and 16 on page 181).

Conclusion

Patients with Marfan syndrome have a higher incidence of respiratory disease than expected. The connective tissue defect underlies both the skeletal and lung parenchymal abnormalities. Various changes occur in the lung, ranging from normal or mildly obstructed physiology to emphysema. The commonest reported manifestations are pneumothorax and cystic changes in the lung. Kyphoscoliosis is a feature of MFS and is often progressive. The management of this skeletal complication is along similar lines to the idiopathic variety although extra care should be taken managing the airway during anaesthesia. The diagnosis of Marfan syndrome (or a forme fruste of it), should be considered in patients presenting with recurrent pneumothoraces or with a family history of pneumothorax. Awareness of both the connective tissue disorder and the cardiovascular complications of the condition should influence the management of pneumothorax in Marfan syndrome.

References

1. McKusick VA. Heritable disorders of connective tissue. 4th ed. Oxford: CV Mosby, Blackwell Scientific Publications; 1972.
2. Foster ME, Foster DR. Bronchiectasis and Marfan's syndrome. Postgrad Med J. 1980;56(660):718–9.
3. Dominguez R, Weisgrau RA, Santamaria M. Pulmonary hyperinflation and emphysema in infants with the Marfan syndrome. Pediatr Radiol. 1987;17:365–9.
4. Takanami I, Morota A, Shikata J. A case report of spontaneous pneumothorax in Marfan syndrome and an immunohistochemical study of type 1 collagen in lung tissue. Japan J Thoracic Dis. 1991;29:1186–9.
5. Saito H, Lijima K, Dambara T, Shiota J, Hirose S, Uekusa T, et al. An autopsy case of Marfan syndrome with bronchiectasis and multiple bullae. Japan J Thoracic Dis. 1992;30:1315–21.
6. Katz H. Thoracic manifestations in Marfan syndrome (arachnodactyly). Q Bull Sea View Hosp. 1952;13:95–106.
7. Fuleihan FJD, Suh SK, Shepard RH. Some aspects of pulmonary function in the Marfan syndrome. Bull John Hopkins Hosp. 1963;113:320–9.
8. Streeten EA, Murphy EA, Pyeritz RE. Pulmonary function in the Marfan syndrome. Chest. 1987;9:408–12.
9. Corsico AG, Grosso A, Tripon B, Albicini F, Gini E, Mazzetta A, Di Vincenzo EM, Angesi ME, Tsana Tegomo E, Ronzoni V, Arbustini E, Cervieri I. Pulmonary involvement in patients with Marfan syndrome. Panminerva Med. 2014;56(2):177–82.
10. Hall JR, Pyeritz RE, Dudgeon MDG, Haller A. Pneumothorax in the Marfan syndrome; prevalence and therapy. Ann Thorac Surg. 1984;37:500–5.
11. Dwyer EM, Troncale F. Spontaneous pneumothorax and pulmonary disease in the Marfan syndrome. Ann Intern Med. 1965;62:1285–92.
12. Wood J, Bellamy D, Child A, Citron KM. Pulmonary disease in patients with Marfan syndrome. Thorax. 1984;39:780–4.
13. Turner JA, Stanley NN. Fragile lung in Marfan syndrome. Thorax. 1976;31:771–5.
14. Yellin A, Shiner RJ, Lieberman Y. Familial multiple bilateral pneumothorax associated with Marfan syndrome. Chest. 1991;100:577–8.
15. Suzuki T, Akiba T, Miyake R, Marushima H, Morikawa T. Familial spontaneous pneumothorax in two adult siblings with Marfan syndrome. Ann Thorac Cardiovasc Surg. 2010;16(5):362–4.
16. Dyhdalo K, Farver C. Pulmonary histologic changes in Marfan syndrome: a case series and literature review. Am J Clin Pathol. 2011;136(6):857–63.
17. Sayers CP, Goltz RW, Mottiaz J. Pulmonary elastic tissue in generalised elastocytosis (cutis laxa) and Marfan syndrome; a light and electron microscopic study. J Invest Dermatol. 1975;65:451–7.
18. Savini R, Cervellati S, Beroaldo E. Spinal deformities in Marfan syndrome. Ital J Orthop Traumatol. 1980;6:19–40.
19. Kelly RE, Goretscky MJ, Obermeyer R, Kuhn MA, Redinger R, Haney TS, Moskowitz A, Nuss D. Ann Surg. 2010;252(6):1072–81.
20. Teoh PC. Bronchiectasis and spontaneous pneumothorax in Marfan syndrome. Chest. 1977;72:672–3.
21. Hwang HS, Yi CA, Yoo H, Yang JH, Kim ~D-K, Koh W-J. The prevalence of bronchiectasis in patients with Marfan syndrome. Int J Tuberc Lung Dis. 2014;18(8):995–7(3).
22. Lipton RA, Greenwald A, Seriff NS. Pneumothorax and bilateral honeycombed lung in Marfan syndrome. Am Rev Respir Dis. 1971;104:924–8.
23. Rybczynski M, Koschyk D, Karmeier A, Gessler N, Sheikhzadeh S, Bernhardt AM, Habermann CR, Treede H, Berger J, Robinson PN, Meinertz T, von Kodolitsch Y. Frequency of sleep apnea in adults with the Marfan syndrome. Am J Cardiol. 2010;105(12):1836–41. Erratum in: Am J Cardiol. 2010;106(5):755.

24. Kohler M, Blair E, Risby P, Nickol AH, Wordsworth P, Forfar C, Stradling JR. The prevalence of obstructive sleep apnoea and its association with aortic dilatation in Marfan's syndrome. Thorax. 2009;64(2):162–6.
25. Kai Y, Yamaoka A, Irita K, Zaitsu A, Takahashi S. Transient tracheal obstruction during surgical correction of scoliosis in a patient with Marfan syndrome. Japan J Anaesthesiol. 1995;44:868–73.

Dental Aspects of Marfan Syndrome

16

Lucy N. Hyde

Clinical Manifestations

The clinical findings in the oral region display the same great variability in expression as is shown throughout the rest of the body in Marfan patients. Important characteristics include a long, narrow face and skull (dolichocephaly), often with mandibular prognathism, prominent supraorbital ridges, sunken eyes and frontal bossing [1, 2].

The most common oral sign is a high, arched palate. This can be a very striking feature, the difference from normal being demonstrated in Figs. 16.1 and 16.2. Collapse of the upper dental arch, and in some cases severe malocclusion and open bite, tend to be associated with the high palate. Weakened capsular ligaments and hyperextensibility of muscles can contribute to habitual dislocations or subluxations of the temporomandibular joint (TMJ) and TMJ dysfunction [1–3]. The teeth tend to be affected more by crowding than by developmental abnormalities; though rare cases of supernumeraries, congenital absence, incomplete development, crown dysplasia, enamel hypoplasia, dentinogenesis imperfecta and multiple odontogenic cysts have been reported. It has also been suggested that the teeth tend to be long and narrow [1]. Other uncommon features mentioned in the literature are cleft palate and bifid uvula, enlarged maxillary sinuses and hypoplasia of the mandible. There is also a possibility that the fibrillin defect could contribute to slight relapse after orthodontic treatment and greater periodontal problems [1].

L.N. Hyde, BDS
Marfan Trust, Cardiovascular and Cell Sciences Research Institute,
St George's, University of London, London, UK
e-mail: lucy.hyde@hotmail.co.uk

© Springer-Verlag London 2016

A.H. Child (ed.), *Diagnosis and Management of Marfan Syndrome*,
DOI 10.1007/978-1-4471-5442-6_16

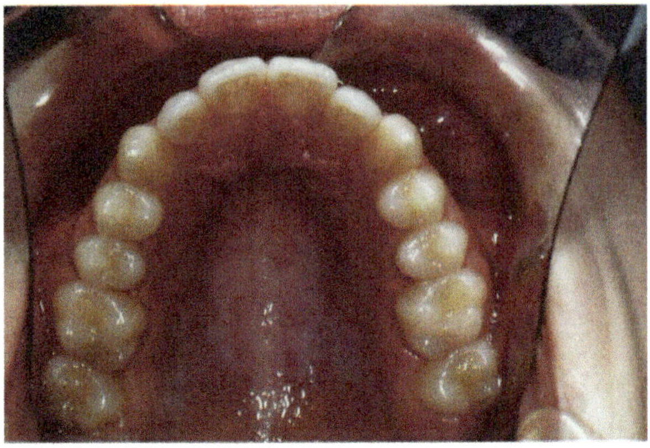

Fig. 16.1 A normal palate

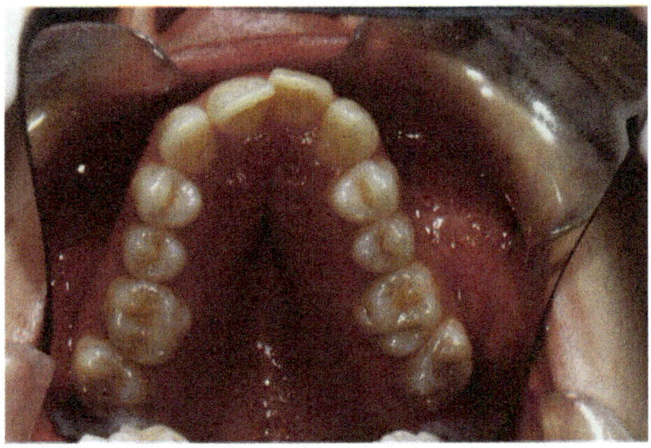

Fig. 16.2 Palate of a patient with Marfan syndrome

Dental Management

In addition to good oral hygiene and regular routine dental treatment, some patients may need orthodontic and possibly oral surgical care. Careful planning from an early age can lead to successful aesthetic results [4]. The prevention of bacterial endocarditis is all-important because of the high incidence of heart valve involvement and abnormalities of the great vessels in Marfan syndrome. There is also an increase of special risk patients who have had cardiac surgery or a previous attack of bacterial endocarditis. Nice guidelines for antibiotic prophylaxis are periodically updated in the British National Formulary and the Dental Practitioners Formulary [5]. It is important to prevent endocarditis before and after surgery. Free endocarditis cards are available from the British Heart Foundation. The possibility of a bleeding tendency has been noted in some affected individuals, and this should be taken into consideration when planning any surgical intervention.

General Anaesthesia

Patients with Marfan syndrome are recognised to have an increased morbidity and mortality risk associated with general anaesthesia. The contributing factors to this are cardiovascular abnormalities, impaired respiratory function, scoliosis, the potential to develop endocarditis and a tendency to spontaneous pneumothorax. Rarely, difficulty with intubation has been reported due to limited neck extension, a high palate and a narrow trachea [6]. Pre-operative assessment should include a through medical examination with a chest x-ray, electrocardiogram and an echocardiogram. Any treatment must be carried out in conjunction with the patient's cardiologist [2, 7].

There is a significant incidence of sleep apnea in Marfan syndrome, which should be assessed with sleep studies. Treatment may include ENT surgery for enlarged adenoids or septal devation, as well as intermittent positive pressure breathing at night [8, 9].

Conclusion

In summary, the dentist must be aware of all the problems associated with treating a patient with Marfan syndrome. Prevention of tooth decay, regular check-ups and careful forward planning all reduce the need for more elaborate and potentially dangerous procedures. The classical marfanoid appearance of the face and mouth can be recognised by a dentist, and could be the first vital step towards diagnosis of the underlying condition. If the diagnosis is suspected, the patient should be referred for echocardiography and genetic counselling through the family practitioner.

References

1. Scott DC. Frontier dentistry part 3 – Marfan syndrome – an oral perspective. Ont Dent. 1982;59(4):54–7.
2. Crosher R, Holmes A. Marfan syndrome: dental problems and management. Dent Update. 1988;15(3):120–2.
3. Fitzpatrick BN, Chapman PJ. The Marfan syndrome. Aust Dent J. 1966;11(5):301–4.
4. Gazit E, Lieberman NI. Severe maxillary constriction in a patient with Marfan syndrome: report of a case. ASDC J Dent Child. 1981;48(4):292–3.
5. Nally F. The Marfan syndrome – report of two cases. Oral Surg Oral Med Oral Pathol Oral Radiol Endod. 1966;22(6):715–24.
6. Verghese C. Anaesthesia in Marfan syndrome. Anaesthesia. 1984;39:917–22.
7. Hirota Y, et al. Systemic management of Marfan syndrome during dental treatment: a case report. Anesth Pain Control Dent. 1993;2(3):162–70.
8. Kohler M, Pitcher A, Blair E, Risby P, Senn O, Forfar C, Wordsworth P, Stradling JR. The impact of obstructive sleep apnea on arotic disease in Marfan's syndrome. Respiration. 2013;86(1):39–44.
9. Rybczynski M, Koschyk D, Karmeier A, Gessler N, Sheikhzadeh S, Bernhardt AM, Habermann CR, Treede H, Berger J, Robinson PN, Meinertz T, von Kodolitsch Y. Frequency of sleep apnea in adults with Marfan syndrome. Am J Cardiol. 2010;105(12):1836–41.

ENT Aspects of Marfan Syndrome

17

Anne H. Child and Joanna Rowntree

The clinical findings in the ear, sinuses, nose and throat display the same great variability in expression as found throughout the rest of the body in Marfan syndrome [1]. Important skeletal characteristics which contribute to ENT problems include a long narrow face and skull (dolichocephaly), often associated with mandibular prognathism, high arched palate, crowded teeth, prominent supra-orbital ridges, deep-set eyes and frontal bossing [2]. The ears are often large, simple, low-set and posteriorly rotated. Ear canals can be narrow and angulated upward and forward. Unilateral hearing loss is not uncommon, although the cause is obscure, possibly due to ossicular malformation during development, but most likely due to recurrent or chronic otitis media in childhood.

The nose is long, often beaked and asymmetrical, with narrow cavities and frequently deviated septum, which may lead to complete blockage of one side of the nose. Mouth breathing may result. In addition, sinuses may be narrow and underdeveloped with narrow drainage channels, therefore recurrent sinusitis is a common problem.

Sleep apnoea is a common associated feature, requiring referral for sleep studies [3, 4]. Frequent unexplained nosebleeds may be a feature in childhood and adolescence, probably due to vascular wall fragility.

A.H. Child, MD, FRCP (✉) • J. Rowntree
Cardiovascular and Cell Sciences Research Institute, St George's,
University of London, London, UK
e-mail: achild@sgul.ac.uk

© Springer-Verlag London 2016

A.H. Child (ed.), *Diagnosis and Management of Marfan Syndrome*,
DOI 10.1007/978-1-4471-5442-6_17

Medical Management

Early recognition and prompt medical management of allergic rhinitis or sinusitis may prevent secondary infections. Antibiotics for infection must be used earlier in the sinusitis, otitis or tonsillitis attack, and for longer than for a normal child or adult.

Surgical Management

Grommets for "glue ear" may help resolve the problem of recurrent otitis media. However, early removal of tonsils and/or adenoids is recommended, as surgical experience shows that these structures are surprisingly large and can actually contribute, through obstruction, to chronic otitis and sleep apnoea [5].

Surgical correction of deviated septum can be very helpful in management of nasal obstruction, mouth breathing and sleep apnoea. Cautery for recurrent nosebleeds may be necessary.

Bacterial Endocarditis Prophylaxis

The prevention of bacterial endocarditis is all-important because of the high risk of incidence of heart valve involvement. High risk patients are those who have had cardiac surgery or a previous attack of bacterial endocarditis. Therefore antibiotic prophylaxis is mandatory for any invasive procedure involving bleeding. Guidelines for antibiotic prophylaxis are periodically updated in the British National Formulary. The possibility of a bleeding tendency, probably due to vascular fragility, has been noted in some affected individuals, and this should be taken into consideration when planning surgery.

General Anaesthesia

Patients with Marfan syndrome are recognised to have a slightly increased morbidity and mortality risk associated with general anaesthesia. Factors contributing to this are cardiovascular abnormalities and arrhythmia, impaired respiratory function, scoliosis, the potential to develop endocarditis, and a tendency to spontaneous pneumothorax especially in adolescence. Rarely, difficulty with intubation has been reported, due to limited neck extension, high palate and narrow trachea [6]. Preoperative assessment should include a through medical examination with a chest x-ray, electrocardiogram and echocardiogram looking for valvular insufficiency and aortic root dilatation in the sinuses of Valsalva. Any treatment must be carried out in conjunction with the patient's cardiologist.

Conclusion

In summary, the patient's doctor and ENT specialist must be aware of all the problems associated with treating a patient who has Marfan syndrome. Prompt management of ENT infections in childhood, together with surgical removal of tonsils and adenoids, where indicated, and correction of deviated septum or inadequate sinus drainage, will preserve health and hearing.

The classical marfanoid appearance of the face, mouth and ears can be recognised by a physician or surgeon, and could be the first vital step towards a diagnosis of the underlying condition. If the diagnosis is suspected, the patient should be referred for echocardiography and genetic counselling through the family practitioner.

References

1. Pyeritz R. The Marfan syndrome. In: Royce PM, Steinmann B, editors. Connective tissue and its heritable disorders. London: Wiley Liss; 1993. p. 427–68.
2. Crosher R, Holmes A. Marfan syndrome: dental problems and management. Dent Update. 1988;15(3):120–2.
3. Cistulli PA, Sullivan CE. Sleep-disordered breathing in Marfan's sundrome. Am Rev Respir Dis. 1993;147:645–8.
4. Cistulli PA, Sullivan CE. Influence of maxillary morphology on nasal airways resistance in Marfan syndrome. Acta Otolaryngol. 2000;120:401–13.
5. Rybczynski M, Koschyk D, Karmeier A, et al. Frequency of sleep apnea in adults with the Marfan syndrome. Am J Cardiol. 2010;105(12):1836–41. Erratum in: Am J Cardiol. 2010;106(5):755.
6. Verghese C. Anaesthesia in the Marfan syndrome. Anaesthesia. 1984;33:917–22.

18 Gastrointestinal Symptoms in Patients with Marfan Syndrome

Benedict Scoones and Anne H. Child

Introduction

According to the Ghent criteria, two of three main body systems must be affected for the diagnosis of MFS: the heart and blood vessels, the eyes and the skeleton. Other body systems are also affected to a lesser extent. It has been suggested that the gastrointestinal system is one. St George's, University of London has a database of 3,500 patients with MFS. Assessment of many of these patients in clinic has led to the hypothesis that an increased number of patients with MFS have gastrointestinal disturbances constituting irritable bowel syndrome (IBS). This anecdotal evidence strongly suggests a prevalence of IBS in MFS of 20 %, compared to a population incidence of 10.5 % (6.6 % for men and 14 % for women) [1, 2].

There are no previous reports in the literature of IBS being a feature of MFS. Reports of gastrointestinal problems in MFS are limited and generally restricted to abnormal gastrointestinal anatomy. They include one of diverticulosis coli in a 38-year old woman [3], diagnosed post mortem. Death occurred following surgery for a thoracic aortic aneurysm, which confirmed the diagnosis of MFS. In the letter, however, there is no report of gastrointestinal symptoms, if any, in this woman prior to death. More recent reports include one of multiple gastrointestinal problems in a 36 year old woman including diaphragmatic hernia, inguinal hernia, diverticulosis coli and a Zenker's diverticulum [4]. Both inguinal and diaphragmatic hernias are known to be problems associated with MFS.

B. Scoones, BSc, MBBS
Norfolk and Norwich University Hospital, Norwich, UK
e-mail: benscoones@doctors.org.uk

A.H. Child, MD, FRCP (✉)
Cardiovascular and Cell Sciences Research Institute,
St George's, University of London, London, UK
e-mail: achild@sgul.ac.uk

© Springer-Verlag London 2016

A.H. Child (ed.), *Diagnosis and Management of Marfan Syndrome*,
DOI 10.1007/978-1-4471-5442-6_18

In 2013, Thakur et al. reported a 25 year old Marfan syndrome female who presented with acute abdominal pain for 1 day [5]. Contrasted-enhanced computed tomography revealed that the port of herniation was the lax, dilated oesophageal hiatus, and at exploratory laparotomy, herniation into the chest, of stomach, part of ascending and transverse colon, splenic flexure and hernia omentum was revealed. The hernial contents were returned to the abdominal cavity after assessing the viability. The hiatus was approximated and fundoplication successfully achieved, with uneventful recovery. Arena et al. [6] reported a rare case of neonatal intrathoracic gastric volvulus in MFS.

Another report [7] is of a 15 year old boy with features suggestive but not diagnostic of MFS because there was only involvement of the skeletal system and there was not a FBN1 mutation reported, nor affected family members. The gastrointestinal presentation although of interest, consisting of an absent suspensory ligament of the liver and a massively dilated liver, cannot be said to be related to MFS which is not definitively diagnosed. Despite requests [4, 7] for further research into gastrointestinal problems in MFS we believe this present report to be the first such piece of research.

Although mention of gastrointestinal symptoms in MFS is very limited there is more widespread reporting of gastrointestinal problems in Ehlers-Danlos Syndrome (EDS) which overlaps clinically with MFS. The basis for Ehlers-Danlos Syndrome is collagen deficiency. In the gut this presents problems in two forms: tissue extensibility and tissue fragility specifically in EDS type IV. The problems can include diverticula throughout the GI system, visceroptosis, gastric atony, megaoesophagus and megacolon. Constipation is thought to be caused by flaccidity of the large bowel, and reflux and IBS are complications seen in the classical form of EDS. Hernias are common and can recur after correction; diverticulae can lead to perforation and bleeding. The relevance of the occurrence of these problems in patients with EDS is that it is known that collagen and fibrillin usually occur together in connective tissue and deficiencies in one or the other can lead to similar problems.

Patients and Methods

Marfan Syndrome Patients

Patients with MFS were recruited from our clinical database. All patients involved had a clinical diagnosis of classical MFS; half of the patients had been screened for fibrillin-1 mutations [8]. Two hundred and seventeen questionnaires were sent out to patients currently attending a specialist MFS clinic at St George's Hospital.

Hospital Outpatient Controls

Hospital controls were recruited from outpatients attending a hypertension clinic at St George's Hospital. This is because the drug therapy for MFS patients before and after aortic root replacement is broadly similar to treatment for hypertensive patients.

Approximately half of all MFS patients take a beta-blocker of some kind and over a quarter take warfarin postoperatively. It was felt that it was important to control for some of the drugs used in the treatment of MFS as the effect that these may have on the gastrointestinal system could be noticeable. Hospital outpatients were matched by sex and age (±7 years). All patients completed the questionnaire themselves whilst waiting for their clinic appointment.

Community Controls

Community controls were selected from the patient list of a general practice sited close to St George's Hospital. We stratified the list into 5-year age groups from 20 to 80 years for both males and females. We then extracted 20 names from each of the 24 sex-age groups by taking the fourth name from each group. A questionnaire was sent, with a covering letter from the general practitioner, and a stamped addressed envelope. No financial or other inducements were given. Patients who did not return their questionnaires were sent a reminder after 6 weeks. Those whose addresses were incorrect, or who had moved, were replaced by additional names from the same age-sex group. We then selected one community control for each MFS patient, matched for sex and age (±10 years) and ethnicity [9]. For each patient, the first suitable control on the returned questionnaire list was used.

Questionnaire Design and Validation

After reviewing methods of evaluating bowel disease [10, 11], our questionnaire was designed. A locally validated version of the Rome II criteria was used [12]. Additional questions on stool frequency, use of laxative and drug treatment were added. MFS patients and the hypertensive patients were also asked to fill out a hospital anxiety and depression score [13], as these can influence the perception of pain [14].

Gastrointestinal symptoms were classified according to the following categories [12]:

1. Oesophageal disorders (globus, rumination syndrome, chest pain of presumed oesophageal origin, heartburn, dysphagia).
2. Gastroduodenal disorders (dyspepsia, aerophagia, vomiting).
3. Bowel disorders (irritable bowel syndrome, abdominal bloating, constipation, diarrhoea and unspecified bowel disorder).
4. Abdominal pain syndrome or unspecified.
5. Biliary disorders (gallbladder or sphincter of Oddi dysfunction).
6. Anorectal disorders (functional incontinence and functional anorectal pain).

Statistical Analyses

Statistical analyses were performed using the Statistical Package for the Social Sciences (SPSS) software version 10.1. The Fisher's exact test and chi-square test were used for comparing categorical variables. As multiple comparisons were made, a probability value of 0.01 was taken to denote statistical significance.

Ethical Considerations

The study protocol was approved by the Wandsworth Research Ethics Committee, and informed written consent was obtained from all patients and control subjects.

Results

Questionnaire Validation and Community Controls

Seventy-three patients took part in the validation studies. Out of 54 questions, the kappa score was greater than 4.0 in every case, and above 7.0 for 45 questions. For the community controls, 400 questionnaires were sent. One hundred and ninety-four were completed and returned, giving a response rate of 49 %.

Hospital Outpatient Controls

43 hypertensive patients were recruited from outpatient clinics. There were 26 females and 17 males, with age range from 22 to 80 years. There were more MFS patients than hypertensive patients; because of this each hypertensive patient was age-sex matched with 2 MFS patients.

MFS Patients

118 MFS patients responded to the questionnaire; these included 56 men and 62 women, ranging in age from 18 to 82 years (Table 18.1). Of the 118 patients all had a clinical diagnosis of MFS according to the Ghent Criteria. 58 of the 118 (49 %) had had a genetic test for mutations in the FBN1 gene. Of these 58, 37 (64 %) had a putative mutation identified in their FBN1 gene using SSCP method. Of the other 21, 17 had no putative mutation found, and 4 had variants identified that were considered to be less common polymorphisms.

Table 18.1 Showing all results

	Marfan patients	Outpatient controls	Community controls
M:F	56:62 (118)	17:26 (43)	56:62 (118)
Globus	8 (7 %)	0	2 (2 %)
Rumination syndrome	0	1 (2 %)	2 (2 %)
Chest pain, presumed oesophageal	7 (6 %)	0	1 (1 %)
Functional heartburn	24 (20 %)	5 (12 %)	20 (17 %)
Functional dysphagia	5 (4 %)	0	3 (3 %)
Functional dyspepsia	5 (4 %)	0	4 (3 %)
Ulcer type dyspepsia	3 (3 %)	0	1 (1 %)
Dysmotility type dyspepsia	2 (2 %)	0	3 (3 %)
Aerophagia	9 (8 %)	2 (5 %)	10 (9 %)
Functional vomiting	0	0	1 (1 %)
Abdominal pain	**47 (40 %)**	**6 (13 %)**[a]	**18 (15 %)**[a]
IBS	**31 (26 %)**	6 (13 %)	**12 (10 %)**[a]
Diarrhoea predominate IBS	9 (8 %)	2 (5 %)	2 (2 %)
Constipation predominate IBS	12 (10 %)	0	3 (3 %)
Functional abdominal bloating	19 (16 %)	3 (7 %)	17 (14 %)
Functional diarrhoea	6 (5 %)	2 (5 %)	6 (5 %)
Functional constipation	22 (19 %)	2 (5 %)	17 (14 %)
Unspecified bowel disorder	29 (25 %)	8 (19 %)	30 (25 %)
Incontinence: soiling	14 (12 %)	0	4 (3 %)
Gross incontinence	5 (4 %)	0	3 (3 %)
Levator ani syndrome	3 (3 %)	2 (5 %)	1 (1 %)
Proctalgia fugax	4 (3 %)	0	12 (10 %)
Pelvic floor dyssynergia	2 (2 %)	1 (2 %)	4 (3 %)
Laxative use	21 (18 %)	3 (7 %)	NA

[a]$p<0.01$

Shows the results for all questions, comparing the patients with MFS to the community controls and the outpatient control group

Oesophageal Disorders in Patients with MFS

MFS patients did not report globus, rumination syndrome, heartburn or dysphagia more often then community controls or the outpatients. MFS patients did however, report more functional chest pain then the community controls 7:1 ($p<0.05$); this result was not found with the outpatient group.

Gastroduodenal Disorders in MFS Patients

There were no significant differences between the MFS patients and the two control groups all reporting similar levels of dyspepsisa, ulcer type dyspepsia, dysmotility dyspepsia, aerophagia and functional vomiting.

Bowel Disorders in MFS Patients

MFS patients suffered more abdominal discomfort and IBS then the community control group. Abdominal discomfort was reported by 47 of the 118 MFS patients (40 %), but only 18/194 (10 %) of the community controls ($p < 0.0001$). When compared to the outpatient group this result was not quite so significant ($p < 0.005$). 31 of the MFS patients reported symptoms of IBS compared to 12 of the community control group ($p < 0.005$). The levels of IBS in the outpatient control group were not significantly lower than the MFS group (6/43:31/118). When looking at the two subsets of IBS, diarrhoea predominating or constipation predominating, the MFS patients suffered from both more than the community control group. IBS (diarrhoea predominating) affected 9 MFS patients but only 2 of the community controls ($p < 0.05$), IBS (constipation predominating) affected 12 MFS patients and just 3 of the community controls ($p < 0.05$). The outpatient control group did report significantly lower rates of IBS (constipation predominating) ($p < 0.05$) and functional constipation ($p < 0.05$) then the MFS group. There were however, no significant differences with respect to diarrhoea. There were no major differences with regards to bloating, diarrhoea, constipation or unspecified functional bowel disorders between the community controls and the MFS group.

Anorectal Disorders in MFS Patients

MFS patients did report higher rates of incontinence (soiling) than both the outpatient control group ($p < 0.05$) and the community control group ($p < 0.05$). The rates of gross incontinence, levator ani syndrome and pelvic floor dyssynergia were not significantly different.

Differences between Male and Female MFS Patients

The only difference found was that women with MFS had higher rates of abdominal bloating ($p < 0.05$) and constipation ($p < 0.005$) than men with MFS (Table 18.2).

Effect of Anxiety

Of the MFS patients 16 of the 118 (14 %) had anxiety according to the criteria used [9]. Of the outpatients only 34 of the 43 filled out the form sufficiently to assess

Table 18.2 Comparing men and women with Marfan syndrome

	MFS men (56)	MFS women (62)
Globus	5 (9 %)	3 (5 %)
Rumination syndrome	0	0
Chest pain, presumed oesophageal	2 (4 %)	5 (8 %)
Functional heartburn	8 (14 %)	16 (26 %)
Functional dysphagia	3 (5 %)	2 (3 %)
Functional dyspepsia	1 (2 %)	4 (6 %)
Ulcer type dyspepsia	0	3 (5 %)
Dysmotility type dyspepsia	1 (2 %)	1 (2 %)
Aerophagia	4 (7 %)	5 (8 %)
Functional vomiting	0	0
Abdominal pain	18 (32 %)	29 (47 %)
IBS	13 (23 %)	18 (29 %)
Diarrhoea predominate IBS	6 (10 %)	3 (5 %)
Constipation predominate IBS	4 (7 %)	8 (13 %)
Functional abdominal bloating	4 (7 %)	15 (24 %)
Functional diarrhoea	4 (7 %)	2 (3 %)
Functional constipation	**4 (7 %)**	**18 (29 %)**[a]
Unspecified bowel disorder	13 (23 %)	16 (26 %)
Incontinence: soiling	8 (14 %)	6 (10 %)
Gross incontinence	2 (4 %)	3 (5 %)
Levator ani syndrome	1 (2 %)	2 (3 %)
Proctalgia fugax	2 (4 %)	2 (3 %)
Pelvic floor dyssynergia	0	2 (3 %)
Laxative use	6 (11 %)	15 (24 %)

[a]$p<0.01$

anxiety and of these 6 were found to be anxious (18 %); thus there was no significant difference in the numbers of anxious patients between the two groups. In the MFS group there were no significant differences between anxious and non-anxious patients. In the outpatient group diarrhoea was more common in anxious patients ($p<0.05$) (Tables 18.3 and 18.4).

Effect of Depression

Of the MFS patients 9 of the 118 (8 %) were depressed according to the criteria; only 34 of the outpatient controls filled out the depression questionnaire fully and of these none were depressed. Comparing the depressed MFS patients to the non-depressed MFS patients, more of the depressed patients reported heartburn ($p<0.05$), more reported abdominal pain ($p<0.05$), more IBS ($p<0.01$), more IBS

Table 18.3 Comparing anxious Marfan syndrome patients with anxious outpatients

	Anxious Marfans (16)	Anxious outpatients (6)
M:F	6:10	1:5
Globus	2 (13 %)	0
Rumination syndrome	0	0
Chest pain, presumed oesophageal	1 (6 %)	0
Functional heartburn	6 (38 %)	0
Functional dysphagia	1 (6 %)	0
Functional dyspepsia	0	0
Ulcer type dyspepsia	0	0
Dysmotility type dyspepsia	0	0
Aerophagia	1 (6 %)	0
Functional vomiting	0	0
Abdominal pain	10 (63 %)	0
IBS	6 (38 %)	0
Diarrhoea predominate IBS	0	0
Constipation predominate IBS	2 (13 %)	0
Functional abdominal bloating	3 (19 %)	0
Functional diarrhoea	1 (6 %)	2 (33 %)
Functional constipation	2 (13 %)	0
Unspecified bowel disorder	6 (38 %)	0
Incontinence: soiling	4 (25 %)	0
Gross incontinence	0	0
Levator ani syndrome	1 (6 %)	0
Proctalgia fugax	1 (6 %)	0
Pelvic floor dyssynergia	1 (6 %)	0
Laxative use	5 (31 %)	0

(constipation predominating) ($p<0.05$), more levator ani syndrome ($p<0.05$) and greater use of laxatives ($p<0.01$) (Table 18.5).

Effect of Calcium Channel Blockers

Of the MFS patients 12 of the 118 (10 %) were taking a calcium channel blocker at the time of the survey; 8 of the 43 (19 %) outpatient hypertensive control group were taking a calcium channel blocker. There were no differences between those patients taking calcium channel blockers and those not taking calcium channel blockers in either the MFS patient group or the outpatient group (Table 18.6).

Table 18.4 Comparing non-anxious MFS patients with non-anxious outpatients

	Non-anxious MFS patients	Non-anxious outpatients
M:F	50:52	13:15
Globus	6 (6 %)	0
Rumination syndrome	0	1 (4 %)
Chest pain, presumed oesophageal	6 (6 %)	0
Functional heartburn	18 (18 %)	3 (11 %)
Functional dysphagia	4 (4 %)	0
Functional dyspepsia	5 (5 %)	0
Ulcer type dyspepsia	3 (3 %)	0
Dysmotility type dyspepsia	2 (2 %)	0
Aerophagia	8 (8 %)	2 (7 %)
Functional vomiting	0	0
Abdominal pain	**37 (36 %)**	**3 (11 %)**[a]
IBS	25 (25 %)	3 (11 %)
Diarrhoea predominate IBS	9 (9 %)	2 (7 %)
Constipation predominate IBS	10 (10 %)	0
Functional abdominal bloating	16 (16 %)	3 (11 %)
Functional diarrhoea	5 (5 %)	0
Functional constipation	20 (20 %)	1 (4 %)
Unspecified bowel disorder	23 (23 %)	8 (29 %)
Incontinence: soiling	10 (10 %)	0
Gross incontinence	5 (5 %)	0
Levator ani syndrome	2 (2 %)	2 (7 %)
Proctalgia fugax	3 (3 %)	0
Pelvic floor dyssynergia	1 (1 %)	0
Laxative use	16 (16 %)	2 (7 %)

[a] $p < 0.01$

Discussion

The findings presented in this study represent the first scientific study to be found in the literature of gastrointestinal symptoms in Marfan syndrome. Therefore there are no previous studies with which to compare these results. To validate the results, further research with other populations of Marfan syndrome patients should be performed. The first point to note is that compared to community controls patients with Marfan syndrome suffer from both more abdominal pain and more IBS. Compared to outpatient controls, the patients with Marfan syndrome suffer from more abdominal pain, but the rates of IBS are not significantly higher. Abdominal pain is of course not always due to gastrointestinal pathology. Specifically with respect to Marfan

Table 18.5 Comparing non-depressed MFS patients and non-depressed outpatients

	Non-depressed Marfans	Non-depressed outpatients
M:F	51:58	14:20
Globus	6 (6 %)	0
Rumination syndrome	0	1 (3 %)
Chest pain, presumed oesophageal	7 (6 %)	0
Functional heartburn	22 (20 %)	3 (9 %)
Functional dysphagia	3 (3 %)	0
Functional dyspepsia	5 (5 %)	0
Ulcer type dyspepsia	3 (3 %)	0
Dysmotility type dyspepsia	2 (2 %)	0
Aerophagia	8 (7 %)	2 (6 %)
Functional vomiting	0	0
Abdominal pain	**40 (37 %)**	**3 (9 %)**[a]
IBS	25 (23 %)	3 (9 %)
Diarrhoea predominate IBS	9 (8 %)	2 (6 %)
Constipation predominate IBS	9 (8 %)	0
Functional abdominal bloating	18 (17 %)	3 (9 %)
Functional diarrhoea	6 (6 %)	2 (6 %)
Functional constipation	20 (18 %)	1 (3 %)
Unspecified bowel disorder	28 (26 %)	8 (24 %)
Incontinence: soiling	11 (10 %)	0
Gross incontinence	5 (5 %)	0
Levator ani syndrome	1 (1 %)	2 (6 %)
Proctalgia fugax	4 (4 %)	0
Pelvic floor dyssynergia	2 (2 %)	0
Laxative use	16 (15 %)	2 (6 %)

[a] $p<0.01$

syndrome, aortic dissection can cause abdominal pain, but this would be an acute severe event that is unlikely to have been reported in response to this questionnaire.

Summary

A significant proportion of patients with Marfan syndrome have gastrointestinal disturbances constituting irritable bowel syndrome (IBS).

In a St George's Hospital project, 118 Marfan syndrome patients (56 men and 62 women) aged 18–88 years were asked to fill out a bowel questionnaire. The results were compared with two control groups. Hospital patients participating also filled out anxiety and depression questionnaires as these can influence the perception of pain.

MFS patients suffered more abdominal discomfort and IBS than control groups. 40 % of the MFS group as compared to 15 % of the control group reported symptoms, consisting of both types of IBS, namely diarrhea predominant or constipation

Table 18.6 Comparing MFS patients not taking calcium channel blockers with outpatient controls not taking calcium channel blockers

	Marfans not on calcium channel blockers	Outpatients not on calcium channel blockers
M:F	50:56	15:20
Globus	7 (7 %)	0
Rumination syndrome	0	1 (3 %)
Chest pain, presumed oesophageal	6 (6 %)	0
Functional heartburn	21 (20 %)	3 (9 %)
Functional dysphagia	5 (5 %)	0
Functional dyspepsia	5 (5 %)	0
Ulcer type dyspepsia	3 (3 %)	0
Dysmotility type dyspepsia	2 (2 %)	0
Aerophagia	8 (8 %)	1 (3 %)
Functional vomiting	0	0
Abdominal pain	**42 (40 %)**	**5 (14 %)**[a]
IBS	27 (25 %)	5 (14 %)
Diarrhoea predominate IBS	9 (8 %)	2 (6 %)
Constipation predominate IBS	10 (9 %)	0
Functional abdominal Bloating	16 (15 %)	2 (6 %)
Functional diarrhoea	6 (6 %)	2 (6 %)
Functional constipation	20 (19 %)	1 (3 %)
Unspecified bowel disorder	26 (25 %)	5 (14 %)
Incontinence: soiling	11 (10 %)	0
Gross incontinence	5 (5 %)	0
Levator ani syndrome	2 (2 %)	2 (6 %)
Proctalgia fugax	2 (2 %)	0
Pelvic floor dyssynergia	2 (2 %)	0
Laxative use	17 (16 %)	1 (3 %)

[a]$p<0.01$

predominant. Women with MFS had higher rates of bloating and constipation than men. There was no significant difference in bowel complaints between anxious and non anxious patients. However, depressed patients reported more symptoms. Medication for Marfan syndrome, for example antihypertensives including beta-blockers, did not make any difference to bowel symptoms.

Management

There is no blood test for IBS, however blood tests can rule out more serious conditions such as coeliac disease. The cause of IBS is unknown, but overactivity of the gut, emotional stress, and intolerance to certain foods may play a part. Specific dietary advice and medical management should be sought through the general practitioner, and may include referrals to hospital dietician and gastroenterologist.

Careful attention to diet, avoiding foods such as wheat, dairy products, coffee and alcohol may be helpful, as well as eliminating stress and taking regular exercise [15–17].

Acknowledgments We are grateful to all patients and physicians who participated in this study, undertaken as a special project by St George's Hospital Medical School student, Benedict Scoones, with supervision by Dr JY Kang, Consultant Gastroenterologist, St George's Hospital, and Dr Anne Child, Reader in Cardiovascular Genetics, St George's, University of London.

References

1. Wilson S, Roberts L, Roalfe A, Bridge P, Singh S. Prevalence of irritable bowel syndrome: a community survey. Br J Gen Pract. 2004;54:490–1.
2. Jones R, Lydeard S. Irritable bowel syndrome in the general population. BMJ. 1992;304(6819):87–90.
3. Suster SM, Ronnen M, Bubis JJ. Diverticulosis coli in association with Marfan syndrome. Arch Intern Med. 1984;144:203.
4. Eliasher R, Sichel JY, Biron A, Dano I. Multiple gastrointestinal complications in Marfan syndrome. Postgrad Med J. 1998;74:495–508.
5. Thakur S, Jhobta A, Sharma B, Chauhan A, Thakur CS. Unusual presentation of adult Marfan syndrome as a complex diaphragmatic hiatus hernia. Asian J Surg. 2014;xx:1–4.
6. Arena F, Impellizzeri P, Antonuccio P, Montalto S, Racchiusa S, Romeo C. Neonatal intrathoracic gastric volvulus in Marfan syndrome. Minerva Pediatr. 2009;61(5):565–7.
7. Atta HM, Schaffner D, Pilzer E. The association of absent suspensory ligaments of the liver and Marfan syndrome. J Pediztr Surg. 1999;34:1575–7.
8. Comeglio P, Johnson P, Arno G, Brice G, Evans A, Aragon-Martin J, da Silva FP, Kiotsekoglou A, Child A. The importance of mutation detection in Marfan syndrome and Marfan-related disorders: report of 193 FBN1 mutations. Hum Mutat. 2007;28(9):928–50.
9. Kang JY. Systematic review: the influence of geography and ethnicity in irritable bowel syndrome. Aliment Pharmacol Ther. 2005;21(6):663–76.
10. Svedlund J, Sjodin I. Dotevall G GSRS – a clinical rating scale for gastrointestinal symptoms in patients with irritable bowel syndrome and peptic ulcer disease. Dig Dis Sci. 1988;33(2):129–34.
11. Talley NJ, Phillips SF, Melton 3rd J, Wiltgen C, Zinsmeister AR. A patient questionnaire to identify bowel disease. Ann Intern Med. 1989;111(8):671–4.
12. Drossman DA, Corazziari E, Talley N, Grant W, Whitehead W, editors. Rome II: the functional gastrointestinal disorders. 2nd ed. McLean, VA: Degnon Associates; 2000.
13. Zigmond AS, Snaith RP. The hospital anxiety and depression scale. Acta Psychiatr Scand. 1983;67(6):361–70.
14. Henningsen P, Zimmermann T, Sattel H. Medically unexplained physical symptoms, anxiety, and depression: a meta-analytic review. Psychosom Med. 2003;65:528–33.
15. Irritable Bowel Syndrome, NICE Clinical Guidelines CG61 (2008) (Updated 2015). Irritable bowel syndrome in adults: diagnosis and management. www.nice.org.uk/guidance/cg61.
16. Jones R. Treatment of irritable bowel syndrome in primary care. Br Med J. 2008;337:A2213.
17. IBS Treatment Options, International Foundation for Functional Gastrointestinal Disorders (IFFGD). www.aboutibs.org. Sept 2014.

The Neurosurgical Manifestations of Marfan Syndrome

19

Timothy L. Jones and Marios C. Papadopoulos

Background

Antoine-Bernard Marfan first described the skeletal manifestations of Marfan's syndrome (MFS) in 1896. Since then, a variety of associated clinical manifestations have been identified and numerous diagnostic criterions for MFS proposed. Following the identification of *FBN1* as a causal gene for MFS, more stringent diagnostic criteria were put forth, referred to as the 'Ghent nosology' [1]. This employed a set of 'major' and 'minor' manifestations of MFS in numerous tissues. It has been criticised as difficult to use in children, that it includes non-specific physical manifestations and has poorly validated diagnostic thresholds. To address these issues a 'revised Ghent nosology' was proposed [2] based on clinical characteristics of large published patient cohorts and expert opinion. These systems include systemic features relevant to neurosurgical practice, most notably the identification of dural ectasia (DE). This chapter focuses on the diagnosis and management of this condition and discusses some of the other possible spinal and cerebro-vascular sequelae of MFS relevant to neurosurgical practice.

Dural Ectasia (DE)

Definition and Pathophysiology

Dural ectasia has been defined as: "enlargement of the neural canal anywhere along the spinal column, but nearly always in the lower lumbar and sacral regions; thinning of the cortex of the pedicles and laminae of the vertebrae; widening of the

T.L. Jones, PhD, FRCS(SN) (✉) • M.C. Papadopoulos, MD, FRCS(SN)
Academic Neurosurgery Unit, St George's University of London,
Room 1.122 Jenner Wing, London SW17 0RE, UK
e-mail: timothy.jones@stgeorges.nhs.uk

© Springer-Verlag London 2016

A.H. Child (ed.), *Diagnosis and Management of Marfan Syndrome*,
DOI 10.1007/978-1-4471-5442-6_19

neural foramina; or an anterior meningocele." A more recent definition of DE is widening of the dural sac or spinal nerve root sleeves, usually associated with bony erosions of the posterior vertebral body [3]. In MFS, it is typically identified in the lumbosacral spine and associated with the thinning of adjacent osseous structures. DE is one of the 'major' criteria in the Ghent nosology and has an incidence ranging from 63 to 92 % in Ghent positive patients [4, 5].

DE is considered a sign of potential MFS however is not specific to the syndrome. DE has been observed in scoliosis, neurofibromatosis [6], ankylosing spondylitis [7, 8] and Ehlers-Danlos syndrome [9] as well as following trauma. It has been suggested that DE may be more a sign of inherited connective tissue disorders than MFS alone, as DE has been found in persons with mutations in *TGFBR1* and *TGFBR2* genes, some of these individuals fulfilling the Ghent criteria, and some not [10–12]. It is proposed that defective fibrillin results in abnormally weak connective tissues causing incompetence of the dural sac. This theory is supported by the fact that the ectasia mostly occurs in the caudal portions of the spinal column, where the cerebrospinal fluid pressure is highest with the patient in the upright position [4, 13]. Animal studies of dural ectasia have shown increased levels of TGF-b in the dura [14] correlating with the current understanding of MFS as a fibrillin-1 deficiency resulting in an increased expression of TGF-b [15].

Clinical Presentation

In the majority of cases, DE is asymptomatic and may only be identified incidentally on imaging studies or as part of clinical surveillance. The range of commonest reported symptoms in patients with radiologically confirmed DE, based on previous studies, are summarised in Table 19.1.

The prevalence of moderate to severe back pain in patients with MFS is common [17], reportedly in as many as 53 % of patients in the largest series [18] however DE may be present without any significant back pain [16]. The amount of pain may correlate with the intradural volume (i.e. severity of ectasia). Interestingly, this is not the case in MFS patients with associated spinal dysraphism. This may be because the enlarged bony canal in dysraphia allows more room for the DE to expand without eroding vertebral structures [16]. The pathophysiology of DE pain is not fully understood. Theories include: direct pressure on the periosteum, erosion

Table 19.1 Frequency of symptoms in MFS patients with radiologically confirmed dural ectasia [16]

Symptom	Incidence (previous studies)	%
Back pain	20/63	31.7
Headache	5/16	31.3
Radiculopathic leg pain	8/30	26.7
Neurologic deficit	3/36	8.33
Gait abnormality	1/19	5.3
Abdominal pain	1/20	5.0
Sphincter disturbance	3/20	15.0

of structural lumbosacral elements, nerve root traction and sacral bone thinning resulting in microfractures [17, 19–22]. Symptoms associated with anterior meningoceles associated with MFS include abdominal discomfort, constipation and incontinence and are discussed later in this chapter [16, 22–24].

Headache is reported in approximately 30 % of MFS patients with DE. In the majority of cases, patients report an improvement when they are in the supine position. A direct association between the volume of ectasia and presence of headache has not been found; however, there may be an association between headache and persistent CSF leak from DE, which is considered later in the context of intracranial hypotension.

It is rare to identify neurological deficits in patients with MFS-associated DE [4, 22]. However neurological deficits have been observed in DE associated with ankylosing spondylitis [25, 26]. There are also reports of radiculopathic dysfunction (pain and weakness) due to DE and scoliosis associated with MFS in adults [27]. Less common presentations of DE in MFS include sepsis [28], where enteric flora (e.g. E.coli) may enter into the central nervous system via recto-thecal fistulas and vertebral/meningeal anomalies.

Natural History

The natural history of dural ectasia in MFS is relatively unknown [14, 29]. In one study, dural ectasia was noted in 40 % of children with MFS at a median age of 12.6 years [30]. A 10 year follow up study of patients with MFS-associated DE, (age range 40–60 years old), did not identify any significant change in imaging features, supporting the concept that dural ectasia size peaks during adolescence or early adulthood and then plateaus [5]. The same study did not identify a significant increase in Oswestry Disability Index (ODI) scores, dural volume or any progression of any associated spondylolisthesis [5].

Diagnosis

A number of methods of how to best assess DE in MFS have been reported using conventional radiographs, CT, and MR imaging [9, 29, 31, 32], yet no gold standard for DE diagnosis has emerged. A number of radiologic features of DE have been defined (Figs. 19.1 and 19.2), including:

- Anterior sacral meningocele: herniation of a dural sac via a defect in the anterior sacral surface [33] or through a widened foramen.
- Lateral herniation of the dura along the nerve root sleeves [29] (widened root sleeve throughout the neuroforamen).
- Dural sac ratios (DSR) >0.48 at L5 and >0.57 at S1. DSR is the ratio between the dural sac diameter (DSD) measured on the midline sagittal image and the vertebral body diameter (VBD) at the same level [32].

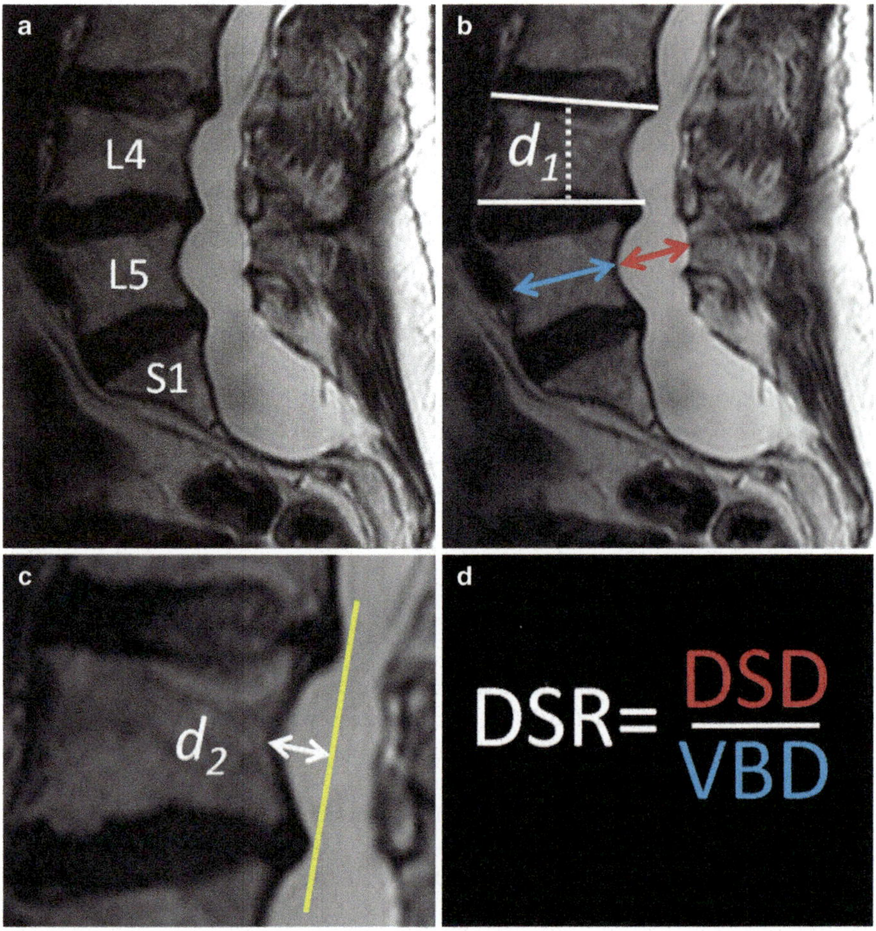

Fig. 19.1 Quantitative radiological assessment of DE. (**a**) Sagittal T2-weighted MRI acquired from a patient with DE, centred on L4, L5 and S1. (**b**) *White lines* drawn through the plane of the superior and inferior endplates of the vertebral body of L4. The perpendicular distance between them (d_1) is a measurement of the vertebral body height and the mid-point of this line ($d_1/2$) is nominated at the level at which to measure corresponding axial metrics such as dural sac diameter (DSD, *red arrow*) and vertebral body diameter (VBD) and to assess for scalloping. Dural sac ratio can be determined at each level using equation D. (**c**) Assessment of scalloping. Posterior vertebral margin drawn for L4 (*yellow line*). The distance in mm (d_2) between this line and the posterior margin of the vertebral body through the plane of the mid-point of the body is measured. A value of d_2 greater than 2 mm suggests scalloping

- Scalloping of the vertebra (posterior vertebral margin halfway between the superior and inferior endplates was greater than 2 mm anterior to a line drawn from the upper to lower posterior margin of the vertebral body [34].
- Perineural or Tarlov cysts (cystic dilation containing spinal fluid along the nerve root) [35].

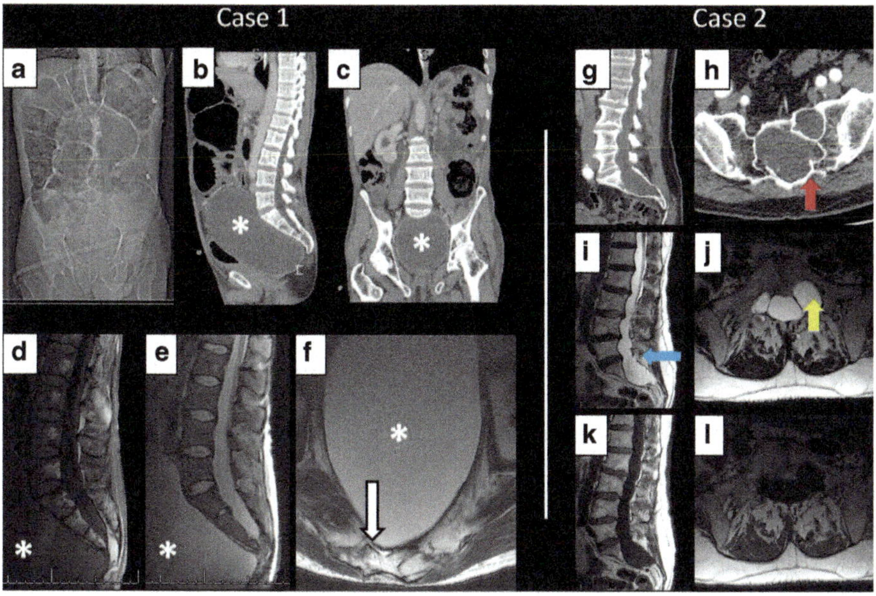

Fig. 19.2 Case 1. A 45 year old 'Marfanoid' man presents with a painful, distended abdomen. Plain radiographs (**a**) confirm acute large bowel obstruction. He proceeded to CT scanning (**b** sagittal reconstructed & **c** coronal reconstructed) which identifies a large cystic mass within the pelvis, thinned sacral bone and a possible defect in the anterior sacrum. This is further characterised by MRI (**d** sagittal T1-weighted, **e** sagittal T2-weighted, **f** axial T2-weighted through the level S3) which confirms a diagnosis of anterior meningocele (*), filling via an antero-lateral ectactic defect at S3 (*white arrow* on **f**). He was managed conservatively and went on to make a full recovery. Case 2. A 36 year old Ghent positive MFS patient presents to clinic with chronic back pain with no radiculopathy, neurological deficit or reported headaches. Sagittal reconstructed CT (**g**) and axial images (**h**) identify a widened lumbosacral canal (S1 > L5), thinning of the sacral laminae (*red arrow*) and enlarged sacral foraminae. Subsequent MR imaging (**i** sagittal T2-weighted, **j** axial T2-weighted, **k** sagittal T1-weighted, **l** axial T1-weighted) confirms the diagnosis of dural ectasia (*blue arrow*) with nerve root enlargement (*yellow arrow*) with early signs of lateral meningocele. As a result the body of the sacrum is severely thinned due to remodelling around the expanded theca. Some disc and facet degeneration is also observed as well as 'scalloping' of the posterior vertebral bodies at other levels. She was successfully treated with oral analgesia and a course of physiotherapy

CT and conventional radiographs are best suited to identify the osseous changes associated with DE. MRI allows direct visualisation of soft tissues of the spine [16, 17, 29]. Sagittal images best identify the antero-posterior (AP) spinal canal and vertebral body diameters, whereas additional information may be obtained from axial and coronal images. The latter are of particular importance to characterise lateral or anterior meningoceles. It has been proposed that quantitative signs of DE (e.g. DSR & DSD) have major advantages over qualitative assessments (e.g. presence of Tarlov cysts and vertebral scalloping) as definitive diagnostic 'cut-off' values can be applied and tested more uniformly than qualitative signs [32, 36].

The role of vertebral body scalloping as a diagnostic marker of DE is controversial. Habermann et al. found no differences in scalloping between patients with MFS and controls [36]. Ahn et al. [29] found scalloping at S1 a useful minor criterion for DE however another study found significantly higher scalloping at S1 level in Ghent-positive patients than in others [34].

Lundby et al. [34] investigated imaging criteria to characterise DE in patients with MFS. They studied 105 subjects divided into three groups: (i) those already fulfilling the Ghent criteria for MFS, independent of a diagnosis of DE (group 1, n = 73), (ii) those fulfilling the Ghent criteria dependent on a diagnosis of DE (group 2, n = 14) and (iii) those suspected of having MFS, but not fulfilling the criteria (group 3, n = 18). 91 % of all Ghent-positive patients (group 1) had DE on the basis of lateral or anterior meningoceles, the latter were only found in Ghent-positive patients. Lateral meningoceles were present in 37 % of group 1 patients and 14 % in group 2 patients. The sensitivity of this finding in diagnosing MFS was 37 % and the specificity, 100 %. Herniation of the nerve root sleeve was frequently present in Ghent-positive patients. They were most commonly found at levels S1 and S2. A larger DSD at S1 than L4 was found in a high proportion of Ghent-positive patients and could be assessed with high inter-observer agreement, agreeing with previous studies [29, 36].

Oosterhof et al. [32] reported that DSR could be used to identify MFS with 95 % sensitivity and 98 % specificity. Their method has been discussed and tested in later studies, but similar results have not been reproduced [37, 38]. Weigang et al. [39] detected DE in 94 % of patients with MFS and in 44 % without MFS when they followed the methods and cut-off values of Oosterhof et al. [32]. Habermann et al. [36] found a difference in DSR between patients with MFS and controls at L5 and S1 only. At S1, they calculated a diagnostic sensitivity of this metric of only 56 % and a specificity of 65 %. Lundby et al's study applied the DSR cut-off values from Oosterhof et al. to a group of normal controls and found DE 'diagnostic' levels in 12 % at S1 and 19 % at L5, suggesting that these cut-off values are too low. In practice, the radiological diagnosis of DE is formed by a qualitative appreciation of a range of imaging features and the variation of opinion on the clinical utility of spinal measurements, mean these techniques are suited more to the stratification of disease in clinical trials at this stage.

Spondylolisthesis is found in 6 % of patients with Marfan syndrome [18], usually as a high-grade slip. It is not known if dural ectasia leads to the progression or development of spondylolisthesis/spondylolysis over time [18]. It has been postulated that this slip may be due to the underlying connective tissue disorder affecting ligament and disc properties [5].

Management of DE

Several previous reports present posterior laminectomy as a technique to relieve back pain secondary to dural ectasia [21, 40, 41]. Owing to the risk of peri- and post-operative cerebrospinal fluid (CSF) leak plus the lack of long-term data on spinal stability, DE, in the majority of cases, should be managed non-operatively. This may especially the case in DE associated with MFS owing to potential anaesthetic risks associated with the cardiovascular features of the syndrome. Dural ectasia results in erosion of the osseous structures of the lumbosacral spine [42, 43]. Mean pedicle widths and lamina thickness in the lumbosacral spine are significantly less than in normal controls [42]. The combination of thin pedicles, thin laminae, and weak dural connective tissue in MFS can make operative fixation of the Marfan spine perilous with a conservative estimate of dural tear rate of 8 % and a 8 % rate of adjacent segment lamina fracture reported [44].

Surgery for anterior sacral meningocele (Fig. 19.2, case 1) is not indicated for stable and asymptomatic lesions [45]. The presence of escalating pelvic discomfort, neurologic deficits, altered bowel habit and urinary frequency may lead the surgeon to consider operating. The two classical approaches are either posteriorly via sacral laminectomy or anteriorly via an open transperitoneal approach. A more recent case series proposed employing a laparoscopic transperitoneal drainage of the cyst [46]. We propose that the management of these lesions is complex and that surgery is reserved for selected cases requiring allied general and neurological surgical input.

Intracranial Hypotension

Spontaneous intracranial hypotension (SIH) is an important cause of new-onset headache, which are typically orthostatic in character and relieved by recumbency. SIH may be caused by a spinal cerebrospinal fluid (CSF) leak, the exact cause of which usually remains unknown however a combination of an underlying weakness of the spinal meninges and a trivial precipitating event is generally suspected. The underlying pathological substrate may range from small dural rents and tears to complex fragile meningeal diverticula or absence of the dura normally enveloping the spinal nerve roots.

Auditory and visual vestibular symptoms often accompany SIH [47]. Intracranial subdural haematoma with accompanying signs and symptoms of meningeal irritation is a recognised complication. The presumed aetiology of haematoma is rupture of the bridging veins between the cortical surface of the brain and the dura when the brain descends as CSF volume decreases. These changes are mirrored radiologically on MRI scan as a ‘sinking brain’, with herniation of the cerebellar tonsils through the foramen magnum. There is often accompanying enhancement of the dura evident on gadolinium-enhanced T1-weighted MR images. The mechanism of pain production in SIH is unclear [47]. It has been hypothesised that it is not low CSF pressure, rather displacement of pain sensitive structures in the cranial vault that cause headache when the patient is upright.

Retrospective studies suggest connective tissue disorders are present in 16–36 % of patients presenting with spontaneous spinal CSF leaks [48–50]. In some cases a heritable connective-tissue disorder is suspected on the basis of physical examination alone, e.g., isolated joint hyper-mobility in up to two-thirds of patients with SIH [51]. Isolated skeletal features of MFS (i.e. absence of the major ocular or cardiovascular manifestations) are found in 10–20 % of patients with SIH [48, 51]. These patients do not typically harbour mutations in *FBN1* gene [52], however, abnormalities of fibrillin-1 containing microfibrils have been demonstrated in these patients. Studies have failed to show a direct relationship between SIH and MFS using clinical examination techniques (e.g. joint hypemorbility scores) [53, 54] or gene studies alone [52]. A small study of 18 patients with spontaneous intracranial hypotension found that seven (38 %) did have subtle signs of connective tissue disorders with three of the patients having some of the minor skeletal features of MFS [51].

Conservative management of SIH may include bed rest, hydration, analgesia, a high-salt diet and caffeine in the first instance [55]. Refractory cases may require epidural venous blood patching [56] and a period of flat bed rest, even in the context of SIH and intracranial subdural collections [57]. A report exists of Chiari malformation secondary to the CSF leak in MFS [58]. In this case, primary surgical decompression of the foramen magnum did not relieve the patient's symptoms however a subsequent recovery was noted following blood patching. In most cases of MFS associated SIH, the suspected site of CSF leak is lumbo-sacral ectatic dura however there exists a report of a leak via a CSF fistula located in the clivus [59], presumably caused by a failure in bone development. This patient was successfully treated by trans-sphenoidal approach to perform a graft repair covering the fistulous defect.

Other Spinal Manifestations of MFS

Atlanto-Axial Subluxation

There is an increased prevalence of focal kyphosis in the cervical spine and atlanto-axial translation (on flexion and extension) reported in patients with MFS [60]. The Marfan population also has an increased rate of basilar impression, possibly explained by an associated general increase in odontoid height when compared to age-matched controls. In light of these features, it is possible that MFS patients are at increased risk of cervical spine injuries, particularly when muscle tone is attenuated by muscle relaxants peri-operatively. Several authors recommend that MFS patients avoid sports at risk of high-impact loading of the cervical spine. However, the rarity of actual neurologic injuries in MFS means that pre-operative radiographs for all patients with MFS undergoing general anaesthesia is not necessary or recommended. Our experience (Fig. 19.3) and those of small case series however have reported incidence of rotational atlanto-axial subluxation following minor trauma and neck manipulation during intubation for general anaesthesia [61]. This may be due to ligamentous laxity coupled with dysmorphic cervical spine anatomy. Of particular concern, the combination of atlanto-axial hypermobility and increased odontoid height may predispose MFS to life-threatening cervicomedullary compression. The typical cause of sudden death in MFS is cardiac arrhythmias, especially in the presence of ventricular dilation [62], there exists however reports of sudden death in patients with MFS with a normal cardiovascular system on post mortem examination however abnormal anterior axis height and cervical stenosis suggesting cervical subluxation as the likely cause [63].

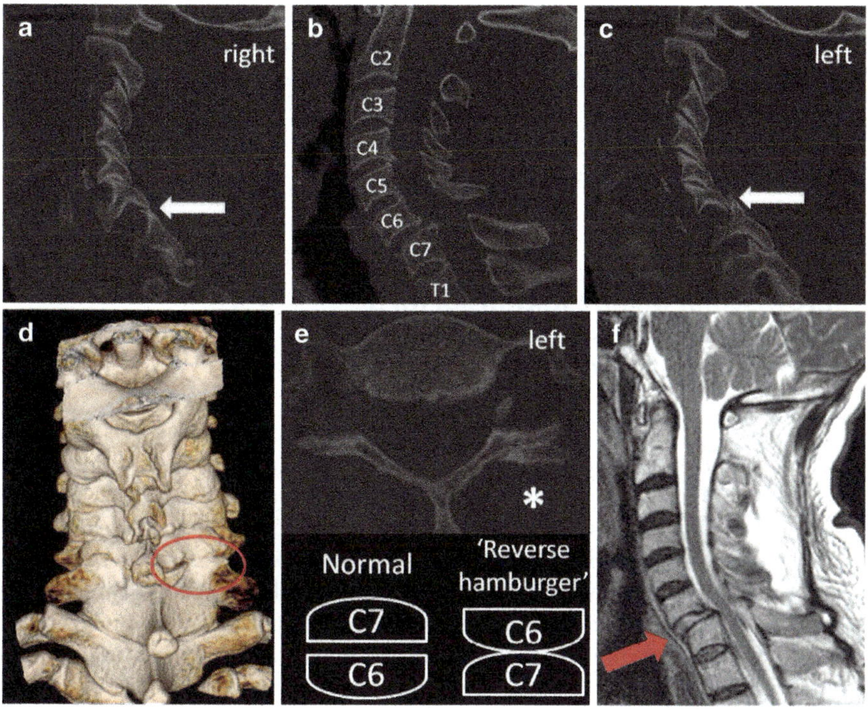

Fig. 19.3 Twenty-nine year old male with known Ghent positive MFS, who was admitted with neck following a trivial fall. No neurological deficit noted on examination. Cervical spine CT reconstructions in the sagittal plane through *right facet complexes* (**a**), *midline* (**b**) and *left facet complexes* (**c**). 3D reconstruction (**d**) showing the bilateral 'jumped' facet joints at C6/C7 (*white arrows*, *red circle* on 3D-reconstruction) which is also shown on the axial CT slice through the C6/C7 facet joint (**e**) revealing the classic 'reverse hamburger sign' in the left sided C6/7 facet (* on **e**), NB not seen on the same CT slice on the right due to angulation of the acquisition). Sagittal T2-weighted MRI shows the step deformity at C6/7 (*red arrow*), kinking of the spinal cord however no cord compression due to ruptured C6/7 intervertebral disc prior to treatment. He was successfully treated with open (operative) reduction and underwent anterior cervical discectomy and plating followed by the posterior stabilisation using lateral mass screw fixation

Spinal Scoliosis

Scoliosis, defined as curvature of the spine in the coronal plane of more than 10°, is seen in slightly more a half of individuals with MFS and can be mild to severe as well as atypically progressive [18, 64]. Close monitoring using a 'forward-bending test' at yearly intervals and management with physiotherapy is preferred to invasive and high risk surgical stabilisation of the spine [65]. Application of a spinal brace is less successful if the curves are greater than 35–40° but may have some role in prevention for smaller curves. A spinal curvature of less than 30° is associated with a good long-term prognosis with dramatic progression often seen with curvatures greater than 50°. This progression can occur well into adulthood.

Thoracic kyphosis is also common in MFS and can be postural or a result of bony over-growth and ligamentous laxity [66]. Postural education and joint stabilisation with core strengthening may be of benefit but have unproven long-term outcomes. Spinal deformities can lead to chronic back pain and, in some cases, restrictive lung disease. As with DE, the surgical management of scoliosis in these patients is complex and should be performed only by those with experience in treating patients with MFS [67].

Neurovascular Manifestations of MFS

Neurovascular Compression

The genetic defect in MFS codes for fibrillin, a glycoprotein which is a major structural component of elastic tissues within artery walls [68]. Patients with MFS may demonstrate tortuous and elongated intracranial vessels causing dissection of the internal carotid [69] or vertebral artery [70] or to intracranial giant aneurysms [71, 72]. Although these tortuous vessels can theoretically cause neurovascular compression syndromes, only two cases of hemifacial spasm [71, 73] and one case of trigeminal neuralgia [74] have been reported so far. In these case reports, digital subtraction angiography or MR angiography showed tortuous and ectatic vertebral arteries causing the neurovascular compression and all were successfully treated with microvascular decompression (MVD). MVD may in these cases be easier as patients tend to be younger and the vessels less atherosclerotic.

Cerebrovascular Ischaemia

Cerebrovascular complications of MFS are rare, with an incidence of only 3.5 % in one retrospective study of 513 patients, the majority of which were a cardio-embolic ischemic stroke [75]. Reports of cervico-cephalic extension of aortic dissection associated with MFS with consequent cerebral ischemic symptoms and of extracranial arterial dissection exist in the literature [76]. Cystic medial necrosis and fibromuscular dysplasia has been identified in extracranial arterial vessels in MFS, but neither finding is considered specific for dissection [77]. Pathological analysis of intracranial arteries of three patients with MFS identified a range of findings; from normal arterial segments to combinations of intimal proliferation, medial degeneration, and fragmentation of the internal elastic lamina [78]. The physiologic stressors of hypertension, extreme physical exertion, and migraine noted before development of acute neurologic signs and symptoms may contribute to the dissection of intracranial vessels. The best approach to treat dissection remains unclear, especially in children. Recent guidelines that address both stroke and anticoagulation therapy do not recommend the use of anticoagulation for the treatment of intracranial arterial dissection [79, 80].

Intracranial Aneurysms

Intracranial aneurysms have historically been reported as a feature of MFS [78, 81]. Case series [82, 83] however have not identified an increased prevalence of intracranial aneurysm or rate of rupture in MFS and they are in fact likely to be of similar prevalence to that seen in the general population. The differential diagnosis for MFS includes multiple hereditary disorders of connective tissue (HDCT). HDCTs associated with intracranial aneurysm include pseudoxanthoma elasticum, Loeys-Dietz syndrome and Ehlers-Danlos syndrome. There was no observed increase in the prevalence of symptomatic or asymptomatic intracranial aneurysm in MFS patients compared to the general population in two large case series using post-mortem and neurosurgery audit data [82, 84, 85]. It has been proposed that the previously reported association between MFS and intracranial aneurysms came from a series of combined single-patient reports of patients. A significant proportion these patients did not, in fact, fulfil the diagnostic nosology for MFS at that time [82]. Furthermore, the autopsy series from the Mayo Clinic [78] may suffer from a sampling bias (i.e. due to its volume of neurovascular throughput). In selected cases of headache, presumed to secondary to cerebral aneurysm, alternative diagnoses such as temporo-mandibular joint dysfunction may be found [86], which affects up to 52 % of patients with MFS [87].

Migraine

The aetiology of migraine is multi-factorial, due to a combination of genetic and environmental factors. Migraine with aura has been associated with cardiac shunts, non-shunting congenital heart defects, congenital abnormalities of the aorta, pulmonary arteriovenous malformation and connective tissue disorders such as Ehlers–Danlos and MFS [88]. A questionnaire study of 457 MFS patients [89] and a multicentre study of 123 MFS patients [88] found that the lifetime prevalence of migraine with aura (but not migraine without aura), is increased in patients with MFS. This association is driven by a history of aortic root surgery and was not influenced by the presence or absence of dural ectasia [88] as previously proposed [90]. It has been postulated that the increased extracellular matrix degeneration observed in the systemic blood vessels of MFS patients results in an endothelial cell reaction, secreting vasoactive mediators (e.g. vasodilator nitric oxide and vasoconstrictor endothelin-1). Several studies have found increased levels of these mediators to be present in patients with migraine. Another possibility is the presence of micro-emboli in the affected aortic root, which can act as a trigger for spreading cortical depression. There exists one case report of a 38 year old man known to have MFS presenting with headache and neck pain and a ventral epidural mass which was found to be an engorged and thrombosed epidural venous plexus [91]. The authors postulate that MFS may have predisposed the patient to engorged veins due to a disorder of the venous connective tissue however appreciate that it may be sequelae of CSF leak resulting in a reduced CSF volume.

Conclusion

The influence of the genetic abnormality causing MFS is characterised by its multi-system involvement and variability in phenotypic expression. Whereas patients with MFS may frequently present to cardiothoracic surgeons, they are a rare entity in general neurosurgical practice and even more rarely require surgery. Despite this, the range of symptoms and signs described in the preceding sections represent the bulk of our practice. It is paramount therefore that a possible diagnosis of MFS is not overlooked, enabling referral to the relevant specialty and appreciation of the increased surgical risks associated with treating this condition.

References

1. De Paepe A, Devereux RB, Dietz HC, Hennekam RC, Pyeritz RE. Revised diagnostic criteria for the Marfan syndrome. Am J Med Genet [Internet]. 1996 [cited 2014 Feb 15];62(4):417–26. Available from: http://www.ncbi.nlm.nih.gov/pubmed/8723076.
2. Loeys BL, Dietz HC, Braverman AC, Callewaert BL, De Backer J, Devereux RB, et al. The revised Ghent nosology for the Marfan syndrome. J Med Genet [Internet]. 2010 [cited 2014 Jan 29];47(7):476–85. Available from: http://www.ncbi.nlm.nih.gov/pubmed/20591885.
3. Avivi E, Arzi H, Paz L, Caspi I, Chechik A. Skeletal manifestations of Marfan syndrome. Isr Med Assoc J [Internet]. 2008 [cited 2014 Feb 13];10(3):186–8. Available from: http://www.ncbi.nlm.nih.gov/pubmed/18494229.
4. Pyeritz RE, Fishman EK, Bernhardt BA, Siegelman SS. Dural ectasia is a common feature of the Marfan syndrome. Am J Hum Genet [Internet]. 1988 [cited 2014 Feb 12];43(5):726–32. Available from: http://www.pubmedcentral.nih.gov/articlerender.fcgi?artid=1715546&tool=pmcentrez&rendertype=abstract.
5. Mesfin A, Ahn NU, Carrino JA, Sponseller PD. Ten-year clinical and imaging follow-up of dural ectasia in adults with Marfan syndrome. Spine J [Internet]. Elsevier Inc; 2013 [cited 2014 Feb 11];13(1):62–7. Available from: http://www.ncbi.nlm.nih.gov/pubmed/23218825.
6. Gajeski BL, Kettner NW, Awwad EE, Boesch RJ. Neurofibromatosis type I: clinical and imaging features of Von Recklinghausen's disease. J Manipulative Physiol Ther [Internet]. 2003 [cited 2014 Jan 24];26(2):116–27. Available from: http://www.ncbi.nlm.nih.gov/pubmed/12584510.
7. Lan HH-C, Chen D-Y, Chen CC-C, Lan J-L, Hsieh C-W. Combination of transverse myelitis and arachnoiditis in cauda equina syndrome of long-standing ankylosing spondylitis: MRI features and its role in clinical management. Clin Rheumatol [Internet]. 2007 [cited 2014 Feb 13];26(11):1963–7. Available from: http://www.ncbi.nlm.nih.gov/pubmed/17332972.
8. Ahn NU, Ahn UM, Nallamshetty L, Springer BD, Buchowski JM, Funches L, et al. Cauda equina syndrome in ankylosing spondylitis (the CES-AS syndrome): meta-analysis of outcomes after medical and surgical treatments. J Spinal Disord [Internet]. 2001 [cited 2014 Feb 13];14(5):427–33. Available from: http://www.ncbi.nlm.nih.gov/pubmed/11586143.
9. Villeirs GM, Van Tongerloo AJ, Verstraete KL, Kunnen MF, De Paepe AM. Widening of the spinal canal and dural ectasia in Marfan's syndrome: assessment by CT. Neuroradiology [Internet]. 1999 [cited 2014 Feb 13];41(11):850–4. Available from: http://www.ncbi.nlm.nih.gov/pubmed/10602862.
10. Adès LC, Haan EA, Colley AF, Richard RI. Characterisation of four novel fibrillin-1 (FBN1) mutations in Marfan syndrome. J Med Genet [Internet]. 1996 [cited 2014 Feb 13];33(8):665–71. Available from: http://www.pubmedcentral.nih.gov/articlerender.fcgi?artid=1050701&tool=pmcentrez&rendertype=abstract.
11. Loeys BL, Chen J, Neptune ER, Judge DP, Podowski M, Holm T, et al. A syndrome of altered cardiovascular, craniofacial, neurocognitive and skeletal development caused by mutations in TGFBR1 or TGFBR2. Nat Genet [Internet]. 2005 [cited 2014 Jan 20];37(3):275–81. Available from: http://www.ncbi.nlm.nih.gov/pubmed/15731757.

12. Loeys BL, Schwarze U, Holm T, Callewaert BL, Thomas GH, Pannu H, et al. Aneurysm syndromes caused by mutations in the TGF-β receptor. N Engl J Med [Internet]. 2006 [cited 2014 Feb 7];355(8):788–98. Available from: http://www.ncbi.nlm.nih.gov/pubmed/16928994.
13. Fishman EK, Zinreich SJ, Kumar AJ, Rosenbaum AE, Siegelman SS. Sacral abnormalities in Marfan syndrome. J Comput Assist Tomogr [Internet]. 1983 [cited 2014 Feb 12];7(5):851–6. Available from: http://www.ncbi.nlm.nih.gov/pubmed/6224826.
14. Jones KB, Sponseller PD, Erkula G, Sakai L, Ramirez F, Dietz HC, et al. Symposium on the musculoskeletal aspects of Marfan syndrome: meeting report and state of the science. J Orthop Res [Internet]. 2007 [cited 2014 Feb 12];25(3):413–22. Available from: http://www.ncbi.nlm.nih.gov/pubmed/17143900.
15. Dietz HC, Cutting GR, Pyeritz RE, Maslen CL, Sakai LY, Corson GM, et al. Marfan syndrome caused by a recurrent de novo missense mutation in the fibrillin gene. Nature [Internet]. 1991 [cited 2014 Feb 12];352(6333):337–9. Available from: http://www.ncbi.nlm.nih.gov/pubmed/1852208.
16. Ahn NU, Sponseller PD, Ahn UM, Nallamshetty L, Kuszyk BS, Zinreich SJ. Dural ectasia is associated with back pain in Marfan syndrome. Spine (Phila Pa 1976) [Internet]. 2000;25(12):1562–8. Available from: http://www.ncbi.nlm.nih.gov/pubmed/10851107.
17. Foran JR, Pyeritz RE, Dietz HC, Sponseller PD. Characterization of the symptoms associated with dural ectasia in the Marfan patient. Am J Med Genet A [Internet]. 2005 [cited 2014 Feb 12];134A(1):58–65. Available from: http://www.ncbi.nlm.nih.gov/pubmed/15690402.
18. Sponseller PD, Hobbs W, Riley LH, Pyeritz RE. The thoracolumbar spine in Marfan syndrome. J Bone Joint Surg Am [Internet]. 1995 [cited 2014 Feb 12];77(6):867–76. Available from: http://www.ncbi.nlm.nih.gov/pubmed/7782359.
19. Duncan RW, Esses S. Marfan syndrome with back pain secondary to pedicular attenuation. A case report. Spine (Phila Pa 1976) [Internet]. 1995 May 15 [cited 2014 Feb 12];20(10):1197–8. Available from: http://www.ncbi.nlm.nih.gov/pubmed/7638665.
20. Nallamshetty L, Ahn NU, Ahn UM, Nallamshetty HS, Rose PS, Buchowski JM, et al. Dural ectasia and back pain: review of the literature and case report. J Spinal Disord Tech [Internet]. 2002 [cited 2014 Feb 12];15(4):326–9. Available from: http://www.ncbi.nlm.nih.gov/pubmed/12177551.
21. Smith MD. Large sacral dural defect in Marfan syndrome. A case report. J Bone Joint Surg Am [Internet]. 1993 [cited 2014 Feb 12];75(7):1067–70. Available from: http://www.ncbi.nlm.nih.gov/pubmed/8335666.
22. Stern WE. Dural ectasia and the Marfan syndrome. J Neurosurg [Internet]. 1988 [cited 2014 Feb 12];69(2):221–7. Available from: http://www.ncbi.nlm.nih.gov/pubmed/3392569.
23. Raftopoulos C, Pierard GE, Rétif C, Braude P, Brotchi J. Endoscopic cure of a giant sacral meningocele associated with Marfan's syndrome: case report. Neurosurgery [Internet]. 1992 [cited 2014 Feb 12];30(5):765–8. Available from: http://www.ncbi.nlm.nih.gov/pubmed/1584392.
24. Strand RD, Eisenberg HM. Anterior sacral meningocele in association with Marfan's syndrome. Radiology [Internet]. 1971 [cited 2014 Feb 12];99(3):653–4. Available from: http://www.ncbi.nlm.nih.gov/pubmed/5578713.
25. Sparling MJ, Bartleson JD, McLeod RA, Cohen MD, Ginsburg WW. Magnetic resonance imaging of arachnoid diverticula associated with cauda equina syndrome in ankylosing spondylitis. J Rheumatol [Internet]. 1989 [cited 2014 Feb 12];16(10):1335–7. Available from: http://www.ncbi.nlm.nih.gov/pubmed/2509695.
26. Abelló R, Rovira M, Sanz MP, Gili J, Capdevila A, Escalada J, et al. MRI and CT of ankylosing spondylitis with vertebral scalloping. Neuroradiology [Internet]. 1988 [cited 2014 Feb 12];30(3):272–5. Available from: http://www.ncbi.nlm.nih.gov/pubmed/3405419.
27. Voermans NC, Dijk KGJ van, Bos MM, Geus-Oei L-F de, Verrips A, Lindert EJ van. Postural headache in marfan syndrome associated with spinal cysts and liquor hypotension. Neuropediatrics [Internet]. 2009 [cited 2014 Feb 15];40(4):201–4. Available from: http://www.ncbi.nlm.nih.gov/pubmed/20135580.
28. Kangath RV, Midturi J. An unusual case of E coli meningitis in a patient with Marfan's syndrome. BMJ Case Rep [Internet]. 2013 [cited 2014 Feb 11];2013:1–2. Available from: http://www.ncbi.nlm.nih.gov/pubmed/23462652.

29. Ahn NU, Sponseller PD, Ahn UM, Nallamshetty L, Rose PS, Buchowski JM, et al. Dural ectasia in the Marfan syndrome: MR and CT findings and criteria. Genet Med [Internet]. 2000 [cited 2014 Feb 12];2(3):173–9. Available from: http://www.ncbi.nlm.nih.gov/pubmed/11256662.
30. Knirsch W, Kurtz C, Häffner N, Binz G, Heim P, Winkler P, et al. Dural ectasia in children with Marfan syndrome: a prospective, multicenter, patient-control study. Am J Med Genet A [Internet]. 2006 [cited 2014 Feb 12];140(7):775–81. Available from: http://www.ncbi.nlm.nih.gov/pubmed/16523504.
31. Ahn NU, Nallamshetty L, Ahn UM, Buchowski JM, Rose PS, Garrett ES, et al. Dural ectasia and conventional radiography in the Marfan lumbosacral spine. Skeletal Radiol [Internet]. 2001 [cited 2014 Feb 13];30(6):338–45. Available from: http://www.ncbi.nlm.nih.gov/pubmed/11465775.
32. Oosterhof T, Groenink M, Hulsmans FJ, Mulder BJ, van der Wall EE, Smit R, et al. Quantitative assessment of dural ectasia as a marker for Marfan syndrome. Radiology [Internet]. 2001;220(2):514–8. Available from: http://www.ncbi.nlm.nih.gov/pubmed/11477262.
33. Oren M, Lorber B, Lee SH, Truex RC, Gennaro AR. Anterior sacral meningocele: report of five cases and review of the literature. Dis Colon Rectum [Internet]. 1977 [cited 2014 Feb 15];20(6):492–505. Available from: http://www.ncbi.nlm.nih.gov/pubmed/143361.
34. Lundby R, Rand-Hendriksen S, Hald JK, Lilleås FG, Pripp a H, Skaar S, et al. Dural ectasia in Marfan syndrome: a case control study. AJNR Am J Neuroradiol [Internet]. 2009 [cited 2014 Feb 11];30(8):1534–40. Available from: http://www.ncbi.nlm.nih.gov/pubmed/19461064.
35. Acosta FL, Quinones-Hinojosa A, Schmidt MH, Weinstein PR. Diagnosis and management of sacral Tarlov cysts. Case report and review of the literature. Neurosurg Focus [Internet]. 2003 [cited 2014 Feb 15];15(2):E15. Available from: http://www.ncbi.nlm.nih.gov/pubmed/15350046.
36. Habermann CR, Weiss F, Schoder V, Cramer MC, Kemper J, Wittkugel O, et al. Radiology MR evaluation of dural ectasia in Marfan syndrome: reassessment of the established criteria in children adolescents, and young adults. Radiology. 2005;234(2):535–41.
37. Rose PS, Levy HP, Ahn NU, Sponseller PD, Magyari T, Davis J, et al. A comparison of the Berlin and Ghent nosologies and the influence of dural ectasia in the diagnosis of Marfan syndrome. Genet Med [Internet]. 2000 [cited 2014 Feb 15];2(5):278–82. Available from: http://www.ncbi.nlm.nih.gov/pubmed/11399208.
38. Fattori R, Nienaber CA, Descovich B, Ambrosetto P, Reggiani LB, Pepe G, et al. Importance of dural ectasia in phenotypic assessment of Marfan's syndrome. Lancet [Internet]. 1999 [cited 2014 Feb 12];354(9182):910–3. Available from: http://www.ncbi.nlm.nih.gov/pubmed/10489951.
39. Weigang E, Ghanem N, Chang X-C, Richter H, Frydrychowicz A, Szabó G, et al. Evaluation of three different measurement methods for dural ectasia in Marfan syndrome. Clin Radiol [Internet]. 2006 [cited 2014 Feb 15];61(11):971–8. Available from: http://www.ncbi.nlm.nih.gov/pubmed/17018311.
40. Weir B. Leptomeningeal cysts in congenital ectopia lentis. Case report. J Neurosurg [Internet]. 1973 [cited 2014 Feb 12];38(5):650–4. Available from: http://www.ncbi.nlm.nih.gov/pubmed/4711641.
41. Cilluffo JM, Gomez MR, Reese DF, Onofrio BM, Miller RH. Idiopathic ("congenital") spinal arachnoid diverticula. Clin Diagn Surg Results. Mayo Clin Proc [Internet]. 1981 [cited 2014 Feb 12];56(2):93–101. Available from: http://www.ncbi.nlm.nih.gov/pubmed/6780735.
42. Sponseller PD, Ahn NU, Ahn UM, Nallamshetty L, Rose PS, Kuszyk BS, et al. Osseous anatomy of the lumbosacral spine in Marfan syndrome. Spine (Phila Pa 1976) [Internet]. 2000 [cited 2014 Feb 12];25(21):2797–802. Available from: http://www.ncbi.nlm.nih.gov/pubmed/11064525.
43. Jones KB, Myers L, Judge DP, Kirby PA, Dietz HC, Sponseller PD. Toward an understanding of dural ectasia: a light microscopy study in a murine model of Marfan syndrome. Spine (Phila Pa 1976) [Internet]. 2005 [cited 2014 Feb 12];30(3):291–3. Available from: http://www.ncbi.nlm.nih.gov/pubmed/15682009.

44. Jones KB, Erkula G, Sponseller PD, Dormans JP. Spine deformity correction in Marfan syndrome. Spine (Phila Pa 1976) [Internet]. 2002 [cited 2014 Feb 12];27(18):2003–12. Available from: http://www.ncbi.nlm.nih.gov/pubmed/12634560.
45. Anderson FM, Burke BL. Anterior sacral meningocele. A presentation of three cases. JAMA [Internet]. 1977 [cited 2014 Feb 16];237(1):39–42. Available from: http://www.ncbi.nlm.nih.gov/pubmed/576128.
46. Trapp C, Farage L, Clatterbuck RE, Romero FR, Rais-Bahrami S, Long DM, et al. Laparoscopic treatment of anterior sacral meningocele. Surg Neurol [Internet]. 2007 [cited 2014 Feb 15];68(4):443–8; discussion 448. Available from: http://www.ncbi.nlm.nih.gov/pubmed/17905071.
47. Milledge JT, Ades LC, Cooper MG, Jaumees A, Onikul E. Severe spontaneous intracranial hypotension and Marfan syndrome in an adolescent. J Paediatr Child Health [Internet]. 2005 [cited 2014 Feb 13];41(1–2):68–71. Available from: http://www.ncbi.nlm.nih.gov/pubmed/15670230.
48. Schrijver I, Schievink WI, Godfrey M, Meyer FB, Francke U. Spontaneous spinal cerebrospinal fluid leaks and minor skeletal features of Marfan syndrome: a microfibrillopathy. J Neurosurg [Internet]. 2002 [cited 2014 Feb 15];96(3):483–9. Available from: http://www.ncbi.nlm.nih.gov/pubmed/11883832.
49. Schievink WI, Meyer FB, Atkinson JL, Mokri B. Spontaneous spinal cerebrospinal fluid leaks and intracranial hypotension. J Neurosurg [Internet]. 1996 [cited 2014 Feb 15];84(4):598–605. Available from: http://www.ncbi.nlm.nih.gov/pubmed/8613851.
50. Mokri B, Maher CO, Sencakova D. Spontaneous CSF leaks: underlying disorder of connective tissue. Neurology [Internet]. 2002 [cited 2014 Feb 15];58(5):814–6. Available from: http://www.ncbi.nlm.nih.gov/pubmed/11889250.
51. Schievink WI, Gordon OK, Tourje J. Connective tissue disorders with spontaneous spinal cerebrospinal fluid leaks and intracranial hypotension: a prospective study. Neurosurgery [Internet]. 2004 [cited 2014 Feb 5];54(1):65–70; discussion 70–1. Available from: http://www.ncbi.nlm.nih.gov/pubmed/14683542.
52. Schievink WI, Gordon OK, Hyland JC, Ala-Kokko L. Absence of TGFBR2 mutations in patients with spontaneous spinal CSF leaks and intracranial hypotension. J Headache Pain [Internet]. 2008 [cited 2014 Feb 15];9(2):99–102. Available from: http://www.pubmedcentral.nih.gov/articlerender.fcgi?artid=3476180&tool=pmcentrez&rendertype=abstract.
53. Liu F-C, Fuh J-L, Wang Y-F, Wang S-J. Connective tissue disorders in patients with spontaneous intracranial hypotension. Cephalalgia [Internet]. 2011 [cited 2014 Feb 5];31(6):691–5. Available from: http://www.ncbi.nlm.nih.gov/pubmed/21220378.
54. Hall WA, Martin A, Liu H, Truwit CL. Improving diagnostic yield in brain biopsy: coupling spectroscopic targeting with real-time needle placement. J Magn Reson Imaging. 2001;13(1):12–5.
55. Rosser T, Finkel J, Vezina G, Majd M. Postural headache in a child with Marfan syndrome: case report and review of the literature. J Child Neurol [Internet]. 2005 [cited 2014 Feb 13];20(2):153–5. Available from: http://www.ncbi.nlm.nih.gov/pubmed/15794185.
56. Albayram S, Baş A, Ozer H, Dikici S, Gulertan SY, Yuksel A. Spontaneous intracranial hypotension syndrome in a patient with marfan syndrome and autosomal dominant polycystic kidney disease. Headache [Internet]. 2008 [cited 2014 Feb 15];48(4):632–6. Available from: http://www.ncbi.nlm.nih.gov/pubmed/18194297.
57. Cheuret E, Edouard T, Mejdoubi M, Acar P, Pienkowski C, Cances C, et al. Intracranial hypotension in a girl with Marfan syndrome: case report and review of the literature. Childs Nerv Syst [Internet]. 2008 [cited 2014 Feb 15];24(4):509–13. Available from: http://www.ncbi.nlm.nih.gov/pubmed/17906865.
58. Puget S, Kondageski C, Wray A, Boddaert N, Roujeau T, Di Rocco F, et al. Chiari-like tonsillar herniation associated with intracranial hypotension in Marfan syndrome. Case report. J Neurosurg [Internet]. 2007 [cited 2014 Feb 15];106(1 Suppl):48–52. Available from: http://www.ncbi.nlm.nih.gov/pubmed/17233313.
59. Ramos A, García-Uría J, Ley L, Saucedo G. Transclival cerebrospinal fluid fistula in a patient with Marfan's syndrome. Acta Neurochir (Wien) [Internet]. 2007 [cited 2014 Feb 15];

149(7):723–5; discussion 725. Available from: http://www.ncbi.nlm.nih.gov/pubmed/17558456.
60. Hobbs WR, Sponseller PD, Weiss AP, Pyeritz RE. The cervical spine in Marfan syndrome. Spine (Phila Pa 1976) [Internet]. 1997 [cited 2014 Feb 13];22(9):983–9. Available from: http://www.ncbi.nlm.nih.gov/pubmed/9152448.
61. Herzka A, Sponseller PD, Pyeritz RE. Atlantoaxial rotatory subluxation in patients with Marfan syndrome. A report of three cases. Spine (Phila Pa 1976) [Internet]. 2000 [cited 2014 Feb 13];25(4):524–6. Available from: http://www.ncbi.nlm.nih.gov/pubmed/10707402.
62. Yetman AT, Bornemeier RA, McCrindle BW. Long-term outcome in patients with Marfan syndrome: is aortic dissection the only cause of sudden death? J Am Coll Cardiol [Internet]. 2003 [cited 2014 Feb 13];41(2):329–32. Available from: http://www.ncbi.nlm.nih.gov/pubmed/12535830.
63. MacKenzie JM, Rankin R. Sudden death due to atlantoaxial subluxation in marfan syndrome. Am J Forensic Med Pathol [Internet]. 2003 [cited 2014 Feb 13];24(4):369–70. Available from: http://www.ncbi.nlm.nih.gov/pubmed/14634478.
64. Glard Y, Launay F, Edgard-Rosa G, Collignon P, Jouve J-L, Bollini G. Scoliotic curve patterns in patients with Marfan syndrome. J Child Orthop [Internet]. 2008 [cited 2014 Feb 13];2(3):211–6. Available from: http://www.pubmedcentral.nih.gov/articlerender.fcgi?artid=2656803&tool=pmcentrez&rendertype=abstract.
65. Di Silvestre M, Greggi T, Giacomini S, Cioni A, Bakaloudis G, Lolli F, et al. Surgical treatment for scoliosis in Marfan syndrome. Spine (Phila Pa 1976) [Internet]. 2005 [cited 2014 Feb 13];30(20):E597–604. Available from: http://www.ncbi.nlm.nih.gov/pubmed/16227876.
66. Demetracopoulos CA, Sponseller PD. Spinal deformities in Marfan syndrome. Orthop Clin North Am [Internet]. 2007 [cited 2014 Feb 13];38(4):563–72, vii. Available from: http://www.ncbi.nlm.nih.gov/pubmed/17945136.
67. Shirley ED, Sponseller PD. Marfan syndrome. J Am Acad Orthop Surg [Internet]. 2009 [cited 2014 Feb 13];17(9):572–81. Available from: http://www.ncbi.nlm.nih.gov/pubmed/19726741.
68. Collod-Béroud G, Boileau C. Marfan syndrome in the third Millennium. Eur J Hum Genet [Internet]. 2002 [cited 2014 Feb 7];10(11):673–81. Available from: http://www.pubmedcentral.nih.gov/articlerender.fcgi?artid=2695985&tool=pmcentrez&rendertype=abstract.
69. Maski KP, Sengupta S, Silvera M, Rivkin MJ. Intracranial artery dissection in an adolescent with Marfan syndrome. Pediatr Neurol [Internet]. 2011 [cited 2014 Feb 13];45(1):39–41. Available from: http://www.ncbi.nlm.nih.gov/pubmed/21723458.
70. Kondo M, Itoh S, Nagano K, Namba M, Imai T, Onishi S. A 10-year-old boy with Marfan syndrome exhibiting cerebrovascular abnormalities. Brain Dev [Internet]. 2001 [cited 2014 Feb 13];23(4):251–4. Available from: http://www.ncbi.nlm.nih.gov/pubmed/11377006.
71. Nagatani T, Inao S, Yoshida J. Hemifacial spasm associated with Marfan's syndrome: a case report. Neurosurg Rev [Internet]. 1998 [cited 2014 Feb 13];21(2–3):152–4. Available from: http://www.ncbi.nlm.nih.gov/pubmed/9795950.
72. Hainsworth PJ, Mendelow AD. Giant intracranial aneurysm associated with Marfan's syndrome: a case report. J Neurol Neurosurg Psychiatry [Internet]. 1991 [cited 2014 Feb 13];54(5):471–2. Available from: http://www.pubmedcentral.nih.gov/articlerender.fcgi?artid=488560&tool=pmcentrez&rendertype=abstract.
73. Braca J, Hornyak M, Murali R. Hemifacial spasm in a patient with Marfan syndrome and Chiari I malformation. Case report. J Neurosurg [Internet]. 2005 [cited 2014 Feb 13];103(3):552–4. Available from: http://www.ncbi.nlm.nih.gov/pubmed/16235689.
74. Sakakura K, Akutsu H, Yamamoto T, Masuda Y, Ishikawa E, Matsumura A. Trigeminal neuralgia in a patient with Marfan syndrome: case report. Neurol Med Chir (Tokyo) [Internet]. 2013 [cited 2014 Feb 11];1–5. Available from: http://jlc.jst.go.jp/DN/JST.JSTAGE/nmc/cr.2013-0072?lang=en&from=CrossRef&type=abstract.
75. Wityk RJ, Zanferrari C, Oppenheimer S. Neurovascular complications of marfan syndrome: a retrospective, hospital-based study. Stroke [Internet]. 2002 [cited 2014 Feb 13];33(3):680–4. Available from: http://www.ncbi.nlm.nih.gov/pubmed/11872887.

76. Youl BD, Coutellier A, Dubois B, Leger JM, Bousser MG. Three cases of spontaneous extracranial vertebral artery dissection. Stroke [Internet]. 1990 [cited 2014 Feb 13];21(4):618–25. Available from: http://www.ncbi.nlm.nih.gov/pubmed/2326844.
77. Schievink WI, Björnsson J, Piepgras DG. Coexistence of fibromuscular dysplasia and cystic medial necrosis in a patient with Marfan's syndrome and bilateral carotid artery dissections. Stroke [Internet]. 1994 [cited 2014 Feb 13];25(12):2492–6. Available from: http://www.ncbi.nlm.nih.gov/pubmed/7974595.
78. Schievink WI, Parisi JE, Piepgras DG, Michels VV. Intracranial aneurysms in Marfan's syndrome: an autopsy study. Neurosurgery [Internet]. 1997 [cited 2014 Feb 13];41(4):866–70; discussion 871. Available from: http://www.ncbi.nlm.nih.gov/pubmed/9316048.
79. Monagle P, Chalmers E, Chan A, DeVeber G, Kirkham F, Massicotte P, et al. Antithrombotic therapy in neonates and children: American College of Chest Physicians Evidence-Based Clinical Practice Guidelines (8th ed). Chest [Internet]. 2008 [cited 2014 Jan 21];133(6 Suppl):887S–968S. Available from: http://www.ncbi.nlm.nih.gov/pubmed/18574281.
80. Roach ES, Golomb MR, Adams R, Biller J, Daniels S, Deveber G, et al. Management of stroke in infants and children: a scientific statement from a Special Writing Group of the American Heart Association Stroke Council and the Council on Cardiovascular Disease in the Young. Stroke [Internet]. 2008 [cited 2014 Jan 23];39(9):2644–91. Available from: http://www.ncbi.nlm.nih.gov/pubmed/18635845.
81. Finney LH, Roberts TS, Anderson RE. Giant intracranial aneurysm associated with Marfan's syndrome. Case report. J Neurosurg [Internet]. 1976 [cited 2014 Feb 13];45(3):342–7. Available from: http://www.ncbi.nlm.nih.gov/pubmed/948022.
82. Conway JE, Hutchins GM, Tamargo RJ. Marfan syndrome is not associated with intracranial aneurysms. Stroke [Internet]. 1999 [cited 2014 Feb 11];30(8):1632–6. Available from: http://stroke.ahajournals.org/cgi/doi/10.1161/01.STR.30.8.1632.
83. Van den Berg JS, Limburg M, Hennekam RC. Is Marfan syndrome associated with symptomatic intracranial aneurysms? Stroke [Internet]. 1996 [cited 2014 Feb 13];27(1):10–2. Available from: http://www.ncbi.nlm.nih.gov/pubmed/8553383.
84. Brooke BS, Habashi JP, Judge DP, Patel N, Loeys B, Dietz HC. Angiotensin II blockade and aortic-root dilation in Marfan's syndrome. N Engl J Med [Internet]. 2008 [cited 2014 Jan 31];358(26):2787–95. Available from: http://www.pubmedcentral.nih.gov/articlerender.fcgi?artid=2692965&tool=pmcentrez&rendertype=abstract.
85. Wityk RJ, Zanferrari C, Oppenheimer S. Neurovascular complications of Marfan syndrome: a retrospective, hospital-based study. Stroke [Internet]. 2002 [cited 2014 Feb 13];33(3):680–4. Available from: http://stroke.ahajournals.org/cgi/doi/10.1161/hs0302.103816.
86. Vandersteen AM, Kenny J, Khan NL, Male A. Marfan syndrome presenting with headache and coincidental ophthalmic artery aneurysm. BMJ Case Rep [Internet]. 2013 [cited 2014 Feb 11];2013:2012–3. Available from: http://www.ncbi.nlm.nih.gov/pubmed/23505274.
87. Bauss O, Sadat-Khonsari R, Fenske C, Engelke W, Schwestka-Polly R. Temporomandibular joint dysfunction in Marfan syndrome. Oral Surg Oral Med Oral Pathol Oral Radiol Endod [Internet]. 2004 [cited 2014 Feb 13];97(5):592–8. Available from: http://www.ncbi.nlm.nih.gov/pubmed/15153871.
88. Koppen H, Vis JC, Gooiker DJ, Knudsen S, Bouma BJ, Tijssen JG, et al. Aortic root pathology in Marfan syndrome increases the risk of migraine with aura. Cephalalgia [Internet]. 2012 [cited 2014 Feb 15];32(6):467–72. Available from: http://www.ncbi.nlm.nih.gov/pubmed/22492422.
89. Vis JC, Timmermans J, Post MC, Budts W, Schepens MA, Thijs V, et al. Increased prevalence of migraine in Marfan syndrome. Int J Cardiol [Internet]. 2009 [cited 2014 Feb 15];136(3):330–4. Available from: http://www.ncbi.nlm.nih.gov/pubmed/18678417.
90. Knudsen S, Russell MB. Increased risk of migraine in Marfan's syndrome? Acta Neurol Scand [Internet]. 2006 [cited 2014 Feb 15];114(4):281–6. Available from: http://www.ncbi.nlm.nih.gov/pubmed/16942549.
91. Chun JY, Dillon WP, Berger MS. Case report symptomatic enlarged cervical anterior epidural venous plexus in a patient with Marfan syndrome. AJNR Am J Neuroradiol. 2002; 23(2):622–4.

Genitourinary Tract in Women with Marfan Syndrome

20

Corrine Jabs and Anne H. Child

Pelvic organ prolapse and urinary stress incontinence in women are multifactorial in etiology. The etiologic factors associated with these two conditions are thought to have considerable overlap. Stress incontinence is associated with hypermobility of the bladder neck as well as intrinsic sphincter weakness with most patients having overlap of these two components. Hypermobility of the bladder neck can be elicited on physical examination with the presence of cystourethrocele.

The denervation of the pelvic floor and physical trauma which occurs with childbirth is thought to contribute to these conditions but individual predisposition also has a considerable effect. The strength and resilience of the connective tissue of the pelvis is thought to have a major influence on the occurrence of pelvic organ prolapse and stress incontinence.

A constitutional predisposition to stress incontinence and pelvic organ prolapse has been sought by studying joint hypermobility and collagen. Joint hypermobility has been associated with pelvic organ prolapse [1, 2]. Ehlers-Danlos syndrome, a connective tissue disorder involving collagen, has been studied in association with gynecologic disorders and while incontinence was a frequent complaint, joint hypermobility was not correlated with pelvic floor prolapse [3, 4]. Weaker collagen cross linking [5], reduced overall collagen production [6, 7] and changes in the ratios of collagen types [8] have all been studied in relation to stress incontinence or prolapse and suggest an etiologic role for reduced overall fascial strength as a predisposing factor for stress incontinence and prolapse.

C. Jabs, MD, FRCS-C
Department of Obstetrics and Gynecology,
Regina Qu'Appelle Health Region,
Regina, Saskatchewan, Canada
e-mail: corrinejabs@hotmail.com

A.H. Child, MD, FRCP (✉)
Cardiovascular and Cell Sciences Research Institute,
St George's, University of London, London, UK
e-mail: achild@sgul.ac.uk

© Springer-Verlag London 2016

A.H. Child (ed.), *Diagnosis and Management of Marfan Syndrome*,
DOI 10.1007/978-1-4471-5442-6_20

Collagen and fibrillin are essential components of connective tissue. Marfan syndrome is an autosomal dominant hereditary condition which results from mutations in the FBN1 gene which encodes fibrillin-1 on chromosome 15q21.1. Fibrillin-1 is an extracellular matrix component found in non-collagenous microfibrils in virtually every tissue. Microfibrils contribute to the formation of elastic fibers as well as serving an anchoring function in non-elastic tissue.

Marfan syndrome was first described more than 100 years ago [9] and remains a clinical diagnosis which can be confirmed by demonstrating a mutation in the FBN1 gene. Two of the three main systems (ocular, cardiovascular, skeletal) must be affected to make the diagnosis [10]. If a first degree relative is classically affected, involvement of one system is sufficient to make the diagnosis. Marfan syndrome affects approximately 1 in 5000 population world-wide and 25 % of cases are a result of a new mutation [11]. There are many overlapping syndromes affecting these systems which are related to defects in specific domains of the fibrillin gene or other mutations affecting microfibrils.

Medline literature search for Marfan syndrome, fibrillin, prolapse and incontinence did not reveal any studies of these urogynecological disorders in women with Marfan syndrome despite the frequent mention of connective tissue disorders as etiologic features of pelvic organ prolapse and stress incontinence. One study on pelvic organ prolapse in women less than 35 years of age found an increased number of women with neurological, autoimmune and congenital diseases but included no cases of Marfan syndrome or Ehlers-Danlos syndrome. The association of medical diseases with prolapse may also have been related to the treatment of these disorders (e.g. corticosteroids) or to the university hospital setting predisposing to an increased number of referrals of young women with underlying medical conditions [12].

A postal survey was undertaken with 240 questionnaires sent to addresses obtained from the Marfan Association in the United Kingdom. Surveys were sent to both men and women and asked questions eliciting presence of diseases involving the renal, urinary and reproductive systems (unpublished data, Anne Child). Responses were received from 42 females who had a mean age of 41 years (range 14–63). Eleven women were age 50 years or above. There were 14 positive responses to the question regarding stress incontinence. This corresponds to a 33 % crude prevalence rate of stress incontinence in this group. Due to the embarrassing nature of urinary incontinence, we suspect the prevalence rate of the postal survey to be an underestimate of the true rate of incontinence.

An observational study by Jabs showed a prevalence of pelvic organ prolapse and stress incontinence in a population of women with Marfan syndrome. The association between pelvic organ prolapse, stress incontinence and joint hypermobility in women with Marfan syndrome was also studied and found not to be correlated.

The study involved recruitment of female subjects from the clinical genetics practice of Anne Child. Female patients, 18 years of age or older, who could be contacted were invited to participate. Seventy-five names of adult female patients with Marfan syndrome were obtained from the records of Dr. Child. Four patients were deceased and 12 patients were unable to be contacted by any means leaving 59 patients available for recruitment. Of the 25 women who agreed to participate,

Table 20.1 Effect of parity

	Nulliparous	Parous
Stress/mixed incontinence (18)	7	11
Prolapse (9)	3	6
Total study group (25)	10	15

14 patients underwent interview, questionnaire and examination. An additional 11 were interviewed by telephone and completed the questionnaire. Information collected included: age, obstetrical history, gynecological history, medical complications associated with Marfan syndrome, medical conditions unrelated to Marfan syndrome, and medications. Symptoms of urinary incontinence, pelvic organ prolapse and bowel dysfunction were elicited. A standardized urinary symptom questionnaire was used to document bladder function, type of incontinence and effects on quality of life [13]. Physical examination determined joint hypermobility using the method described by Beighton [14] which allocates a score of 0–9 with a score of 4 or more indicating hypermobility. Pelvic examination was carried out with pelvic organ prolapse staging recorded according to the International Continence Society guidelines in the left lateral position at maximum Valsalva maneuver.

Of the 25 women with Marfan syndrome recruited to the study, the mean age was 43 years (range 22–59 years). Ten women were postmenopausal of whom eight were using hormone replacement therapy. Ten women were nulliparous. Four women had undergone abdominal hysterectomy, 1 had undergone vaginal hysterectomy. A history of urinary incontinence was elicited in 22/25 (88 %) of patients, of whom 13/25 (52 %) considered the problem significant. Five had undergone surgical treatment for stress incontinence and 1 had medical treatment of urge incontinence. Of the women with a history of incontinence, 18/25 (72 %) had a history of stress incontinence (pure or mixed) and 10/25 (40 %) felt that stress incontinence interfered with their life. Twenty-four percent of women had undergone treatment for stress incontinence. Women with stress incontinence were older than women without stress incontinence (47.6 vs. 31 years, $p=0.004$). Seven of the 18 women with stress incontinence were nulliparous (Table 20.1). Parity was not associated with stress incontinence in this population.

Nine women had Stage II prolapse on examination, one patient had undergone Manchester repair on history and one additional patient had symptomatic prolapse but was not available for examination and had not undergone treatment therefore 11/25 (44 %) of the total group had history or evidence of prolapse. Six women (24 %) had undergone surgical treatment of prolapse. The average age of women with prolapse on examination was similar to women without prolapse (47.2 vs. 42.6 years, $p=0.3$). Nine (64 %) of the women examined had Stage II prolapse (descent to −1, 0 or +1 cm from the hymenal ring). Seven women had anterior wall prolapse, all of whom had stress incontinence and two were symptomatic with a genital bulging sensation. Three had Stage II posterior wall descent, two of which complained of incomplete evacuation and the third had fecal soiling. Three of the 9 women with prolapse were nulliparous and parity was not associated with the finding of prolapse (Table 20.1).

Table 20.2 Examination – hypermobility and prolapse

N = 14	Prolapse	No prolapse
Hypermobility	5	3
No hypermobility	4	2

Three of the 6 women with Stage II anterior descent (cystocele/cystourethrocele) had undergone previous anterior repair for prolapse or stress incontinence and now had recurrent prolapse. One of the 2 women with Stage II posterior wall descent (rectocele) had previously undergone a vaginal prolapse repair. The patient with anterior and posterior prolapse had previously undergone anterior and posterior repair. Of note is that of the 5 women with previous surgical repair of prolapse, all now had findings of recurrent Stage II prolapse.

Eight of the 14 women examined had evidence of joint hypermobility with a score of 4 or more out of 9. Of the 9 women with Stage II prolapse, 5 occurred in the hypermobile group and 4 occurred in the group without hypermobility (Table 20.2). Eleven of the 14 women examined complained of stress incontinence of whom 6 were in the hypermobile group while 5 were not. Prolapse and stress incontinence were not significantly associated with hypermobility.

The etiology of pelvic organ prolapse and stress incontinence is not yet fully understood. Individual variation has a significant impact as patients presumed to be at high risk are commonly seen with no stress incontinence and no evidence of prolapse, while nulliparous women at low risk are sometimes found to have these conditions. This is presumed to be due to variation in pelvic floor muscle and connective tissue. Marfan syndrome affects strength and elasticity of connective tissue. An abstract by Carley and Schaffer at the American Urogynecologic Society Meeting 1998 presented interview data on 12 women with Marfan syndrome and found a rate of urinary incontinence of 42 % and pelvic organ prolapse of 33 %. There is no other published article defining the incidence of these disorders in women with Marfan syndrome.

The prevalence of incontinence in women in the general population is not easily ascertained as the methodologic problems in epidemiologic studies include the sample population chosen, the definition of stress incontinence used and the under-reporting of embarrassing conditions. There is also variation between studies which estimate the prevalence of "any incontinence" versus "severe incontinence." This has led to a wide range of estimates for incontinence in the literature from 5 to 51 % [15]. A prevalence of approximately 30 % may be a clinically useful figure with approximately 5 % considered to have "severe" incontinence. In females, stress incontinence accounts for nearly 50 % of symptomatic women with approximately 30 % complaining of mixed symptoms and 20 % complaining of isolated urge incontinence [16]. In the study by Jabs, 88 % of women with Marfan syndrome had experienced urinary incontinence, 72 % had experienced episodes of stress incontinence, 52 % considered stress incontinence a problem and 24 % had undergone previous treatment for stress incontinence. These rates are considerably higher than those quoted for the general population despite the wide range of prevalence found in the literature.

The prevalence of pelvic organ prolapse in the general population is even less well defined than that of urinary incontinence. One study estimates the lifetime risk of a woman undergoing at least one operation for treatment for prolapse and stress incontinence to be 11.1 % [17]. A study of the prevalence of prolapse in women 20–59 years of age found a prevalence of 30.8 % for any degree of prolapse and 2 % of prolapse that reached the introitus [18]. Age, parity, pelvic floor muscle strength and maximum birth weight were independently associated with prolapse [18]. In one population with Marfan syndrome, 24 % had undergone surgical treatment for prolapse. Of the 14 women examined, 9 (64 %) had Stage II pelvic organ prolapse of whom 5 were recurrent and 3 occurred in nulliparous women.

The high risk of recurrence following operation for prolapse repair in the Marfan population is discouraging. Patients need to be counseled that their risk of recurrence is higher than the general population. Consideration should be given to a trial of conservative therapy for prolapse such vaginal pessary. Anterior repair was used to correct prolapse and stress incontinence in 4 women in this study group. Anterior repair has been shown to be a less effective treatment for stress incontinence in the general population [19, 20] and it should also be avoided in this population with high risk of recurrence. A colposuspension using the strong attachment point of the iliopectineal ligament and permanent suture or a vaginal tape may prove more successful for treatment of stress incontinence.

It appears that there is a higher prevalence of pelvic organ prolapse and stress incontinence in women affected by Marfan syndrome. This agrees with the assumed association of connective tissue disease and these conditions. As prolapse and stress incontinence are multifactorial in origin, it is difficult to determine what, if any, preventive techniques are effective for this high-risk group. Certainly these patients should be counseled to minimize additional theoretical risk factors for these conditions such as constipation, straining at stool, chronic cough, heavy lifting and increased body weight. Pelvic floor exercises with or without the assistance of a physiotherapist, are risk-free and should be encouraged. Elective cesarean delivery cannot be recommended as prophylaxis against prolapse since these patients are at higher surgical risk and prolapse has also been shown to occur in nulliparous women.

Patients with Marfan syndrome are known to have delayed wound healing due to abnormal fibrillin production. The vasculature of Marfan syndrome patients is also fragile which can lead to increased blood loss and hematoma formation [21]. They should be considered at higher risk for incisional hernia and dehiscence. Meticulous surgical technique is required with attention to hemostasis and consideration should be given to using suture material with prolonged delayed absorption (Maxon or PDS) or non-absorbable suture where possible. Suture and staple removal should also be delayed compared with patients with normal wound healing. Antibiotic prophylaxis is required for bacterial endocarditis prevention.

The care of Marfan syndrome patients may be co-ordinated through their family physician but often they are seen more regularly by specialists for complications of Marfan syndrome.

Specialists such as cardiologists, geneticists, ophthalmologists or orthopedic surgeons may be involved depending on the individual patient's health status. Effective treatment for cardiovascular complications of Marfan syndrome has increased the life expectancy for these patients [22]. As a result, Marfan syndrome patients will more commonly experience diseases that increase in prevalence with age, such as incontinence and pelvic organ prolapse. Physicians caring for these patients should be aware of the diverse manifestations of this disease and request input from a gynecologist or urogynecologist when appropriate.

References

1. Al-Rawi ZS, Al Rawa ZT. Joint hypermobility in women with genital prolapse. Lancet. 1982;1(8287):1439–41.
2. Norton PA, Baker JE, Sharp HC, Warenski JC. Genitourinary prolapse and joint hypermobility in women. Obstet Gynecol. 1995;85:225–8.
3. McIntosh LJ, Mallett VT, Frahm JK, Richardson DA, Evans MI. Gynecologic disorders in women with Ehlers-Danlos syndrome. J Soc Gynecol Investig. 1995;2(3):559–64.
4. McIntosh LJ, Stanitski DF, Mallett VT, Frahm JD, Richardson DA, Evans MI. Ehlers-Danlos syndrome: relationship between joint hypermobility, urinary incontinence and pelvic floor prolapse. Gynecol Obstet Invest. 1996;41(2):135–9.
5. Sayer TR, Dixon JS, Hosker GL, Warrell DW. A study of paraurethral connective tissue in women with stress incontinence of urine. Neurourol Urodynam. 1990;9:319–20.
6. Falconer C, Ekman G, Malmstrom A, Ulmsten U. Decreased collagen synthesis in stress incontinent women. Obstet Gynecol. 1994;84:583–6.
7. Jackson SR, Avery NC, Tarilton JF, Eckford SK, Abrams P, Bailey AJ. Changes in metabolism of collagen in genitourinary prolapse. Lancet. 1996;347:1658–61.
8. Keane DP, Sims TJ, Abrams P, Bailey AJ. Analysis of collagen status in premenopausal nulliparous women with genuine stress incontinence. Br J Obstet Gynaecol. 1997;104:994–8.
9. Marfan MA. Un cas de deformation congenitale des quatre membres, plus prononcee aux extremities, caracterisee par l'allongement des os avec un certain degre d'eminicissement. Bull Mem Soc Med Hos Paris. 1896;13:220–6.
10. Beighton P, de Paepe A, Danks K, Finidori G, Gedde-Dahl T, Goodman R, et al. International nosology of heritable disorders of connective tissue. Am J Med Genet. 1988;53:46–54.
11. Dietz HC, Pyeritz RE. Mutations in human gene for fibrillin-1 (FBN-1) in Marfan syndrome and related disorders. Hum Mol Genet. 1995;4:1799–809.
12. Strohbehn K, Jakary JA, Delancey JOL. Pelvic organ prolapse in young women. Obstet Gynecol. 1997;90:33–6.
13. Jackson S, Donavan J, Brookes S, Eckford S, Swithinbank L, Abrams P. The Bristol female lower urinary tract symptoms questionnaire: development and psychometric testing. Br J Urol. 1996;77:805–12.
14. Beighton PH, Solomon L, Soskolne CL. Articular mobility in an African population. Ann Rheum Dis. 1973;32:413–8.
15. Hempel C, Wienhold D, Denker N, Eggersmann C, Thuroff JW. Definition of overactive bladder and epidemiology of urinary incontinence. Urology. 1997;50(Suppl 6A):4–14.
16. Bump RC, Mattiasson A, Bo K, Brubaker LP, DeLancey JOL, Klarskov P, et al. The standardization of terminology of female pelvic organ prolapse and pelvic floor dysfunction. Am J Obstet Gynecol. 1996;175:10–7.
17. Olsen AL, Smith VJ, Bergstrom JO, Colling JC, Clark AL. Epidemiology of surgically managed pelvic organ prolapse and urinary incontinence. Obstet Gynecol. 1997;89:501–6.
18. Samuelsson EC, Victor FTA, Tibblin G, Svardsudd KF. Signs of genital prolapse in a Swedish population of women 20 to 59 years of age and possible related factors. Am J Obstet Gynecol. 1999;180:299–305.
19. Black NA, Downs SH. The effectiveness of surgery for stress incontinence in women: a systematic review. Br J Urol. 1996;78:497–510.

20. Leach GE, Dmochowski RR, Appell RA, Blaivas JG, Hadley HR, Luber KM, et al. Female stress urinary incontinence clinical guidelines panel summary report on surgical management of female stress urinary incontinence. J Urol. 1997;158:875–80.
21. McLaren M, Bridges AB, Gray JR, Tamei H, Belch JJF. Endothelial cell and platelet function in Marfan syndrome. Endothelium. 1993;1:203–7.
22. Silverman DI, Burton KJ, Gray J, Bosner MS, Kouchoukos NT, Roman MJ, Boxer M, Devereux RB, Tsipouras P. Life expectancy in the Marfan syndrome. Am J Cardiol. 1995;75(2):157–60.

Pregnancy Management in Marfan Syndrome

21

Fiona Walker and Anne H. Child

Introduction

Cardiac disease is the leading cause of maternal mortality in the developed world [1]. In women with MFS and a significantly dilated aorta (over 4.0 cm) [2] the risk of aortic dissection rises to at least 10 % and increases further with an increasing aortic diameter [2, 3].

Preconception Counselling

All women with MFS should have preconception counselling to discuss MFS inheritance risk: the risk of an affected foetus is 50 %. The actual prediction of severity of the disease is based on the male and female phenotypes within the proband's family. The proband's mutation should be sought through DNA analysis of the FBN-1 gene, all 65 exons plus MLPA, in the 6 months prior to planned conception. This can be used for chorionic villus biopsy at 11 weeks' gestation, pre-implantation genetic diagnosis [5, 6], or postnatal diagnosis, according to the couple's wishes. (see Chap. 23).

F. Walker, BM(Hons), FRCP, FESC (✉)
Barts Heart Centre, St Bartholomew's Hospital,
West Smithfield, London EC1A 7BE, UK
e-mail: fiona.walker@bartshealth.nhs.uk

A.H. Child, MD, FRCP
Cardiovascular and Cell Sciences Research Institute,
St George's, University of London, London, UK
e-mail: achild@sgul.ac.uk

© Springer-Verlag London 2016

A.H. Child (ed.), *Diagnosis and Management of Marfan Syndrome*,
DOI 10.1007/978-1-4471-5442-6_21

Maternal cardiovascular risk; the cardiologist should review current and past serial echo data (if available) and also take a detailed family history. Specific echocardiographic considerations include aortic dimensions, aortic valve function, mitral valve anatomy and function, and myocardial function. A cardiac MRI should be undertaken to assess the whole of the distal aorta. With regards the family history the details of aortic dissection (AOD) in any family members including intra-operative or post-mortem findings is helpful in knowing if AOD occurred in the context of normal aortic dimensions or aortic enlargement. If AOD occurred with normal aortic size the threshold for undertaking elective root replacement pre-pregnancy is 40 mm, otherwise elective root replacement should be considered at 45 mm. All women should be advised of the symptoms of AOD and told to have a low threshold for seeking urgent medical attention if such symptoms occur. It is better that an A&E attendance is unnecessary and the diagnosis is indigestion rather than missing the early symptoms of AOD.

Obstetric risk; The miscarriage rate for the normal population is 10–20 % prior to 20 weeks gestation. In MFS this rate is higher but the main cause of foetal mortality and morbidity relates to prematurity and premature rupture of membranes (~5 %). Other complications include increased joint pain and joint dislocation, and respiratory complications due to kyphoscoliosis. Symphysis pubis dysfunction is particularly painful and can be debilitating.

Advice with regards contraception should also be provided, [4] both prior to planned pregnancy, and postpartum.

Pregnancy Management

All women with MFS embarking on pregnancy should be referred to a tertiary centre, with a multi-disciplinary team (MDT) in place for pregnancy care. Such joint expert care reduces maternal and foetal risks [10–12].

Drug Therapy

Beta-blockers, have been shown to reduce aortic growth in pregnancy and are therefore the preferred treatment option. Women should switch from ACE inhibitors (ACEI) or Angiotensin receptor blockers (e. g Losartan) to beta-blockers pre-pregnancy where possible, but should also be advised of their potential associated foetal effects including growth retardation [7], and bradycardia in the newborn [8]. Although tiny amounts of beta-blockers are secreted in breast milk, breastfeeding is not contraindicated and the benefits of treatment outweigh the small foetal risks. ACEI and ARBs are contraindicated in pregnancy due to a risk of foetal renal abnormalities and an increased risk of intra-uterine death but they can re-instated post-partum and are safe in breast-feeding [9].

Echo Surveillance

Echocardiography to assess the aortic dimensions should be undertaken each trimester but more frequently if the aorta is between 40 and 45 mm. Surveillance should continue post-partum for up to 6 months as the peak risk for aortic dissection is in the last trimester and postpartum period. If aortic dimensions increase during pregnancy the degree and accuracy of this increase in size must be validated by blinded measurements and repeat CMRI. The recommendation to interrupt a pregnancy early is a significant decision with important consequences, therefore changes in dimension must be genuine and pathological and the decision made by the MDT.

Delivery Planning

Each delivery plan must be individualized taking into account the patients echo/CMRI findings and family history. For patients with no FHX of AOD and normal aortic dimensions, a vaginal delivery with epidural anaesthesia is entirely appropriate. Epidural is preferable to general anaesthesia, as intubation may lead to marked fluctuations in blood pressure [13]. Intubation may be difficult due to high palate, limited neck extension, jaw dislocation and floppy larynx [14]. Note, if regional anaesthesia is planned, that the anaesthetist should be made aware of the presence of dural ectasia as the local anaesthetic dosing regime can be affected [15]. Dural ectasia is present in 65 % of MFS patients and can be determined prior to pregnancy by MRI [16, 17]. The optimal mode of delivery for other patients with perhaps a positive FHX of AOD or aorta size of 40–45 mm is less clear. Usually a vaginal delivery with epidural anaesthesia and instrumental assistance to shorten the second stage, along with tight blood pressure control is appropriate, but an elective caesarean section is equally appropriate and also safe. The risk of postpartum haemorrhage is increased in MFS.

Aortic Dissection and Pregnancy

Acute aortic dissection in pregnancy is a catastrophic complication with a high maternal and foetal mortality. Maternal health is the priority and any intervention should focus on preserving maternal health and well-being. Treatment should follow current guidelines for acute AOD [18]. There are many case reports regarding vascular complications requiring surgery during pregnancy [19–21]. Of 11 pregnant patients (4 had Marfan syndrome) undergoing aortic surgery, Yates et al. [22] reported no maternal deaths, 8 healthy babies born at term and 3 pregnancies resulting in intra-uterine demise within one week of surgery. With appropriate maternal and foetal monitoring, attention to cardiopulmonary bypass, pulsatile perfusion, near-normothermia, and avoidance of vasoconstrictors any risks may be minimised (see Chap. 9).

The risk of AOD persists for up to 6 months post-partum irrespective of mode of delivery [23, 24], therefore ongoing surveillance and vigilance for symptoms suggestive of AOD is essential. Breastfeeding prolongs the risk period, however most mothers still prefer to breastfeed.

Further Pregnancy

Any subsequent pregnancy should be deferred for 12 months after stopping breastfeeding and new baseline investigations including TTE and CMRI undertaken to inform pre-conception risk discussions [25].

Conclusions

Pregnancy in MFS women is associated with significant maternal, foetal and neonatal risks. At best there is a background AOD risk of ~1 % which has an associated mortality of up to 30 %. In light of this, all women with MFS who wish to embark on pregnancy should be offered expert pre-pregnancy counselling and specialist multidisciplinary care in a tertiary hospital setting, and made aware of the symptoms of aortic dissection and the need for urgent medical attention should these occur.

References

1. Emmanuel Y, Thorne SA. Heart disease in pregnancy. Best Pract Res Clin Obstet Gynaecol. 2015;29(5):579–97.
2. Lipscombe KJ, et al. Outcome of pregnancy in women with Marfan syndrome. Br J Obstet Gynaecol. 1997;104:201–6.
3. Rossiter J, et al. A prospective longitudinal evaluation of pregnancy in the Marfan syndrome. Am J Obstet Gynecol. 1995;183:1599–606.
4. Royal College of Obstetricians and Gynaecologists: Cardiac Disease and Pregnancy. Good Practice Guideline: No 13. 22 June 2011. https://www.rcog.org.uk/en/guidelines-research-services/guidelines/good-practice-13/.
5. Vlahos NF, Triantafyllidou O, Vitoratos N, Grigoriadis C, Creatsas G. Preimplantation genetic diagnosis in Marfan syndrome. Case Rep Obstet Gynaecol. 2013;2013:542961.
6. Loeys B, et al. Strategies for prenatal and preimplantation genetic diagnosis in Marfan syndrome (MFS). Prenat Diagn. 2002;22:22–8.
7. Ersboll AS, Hedegaard M, Sondergaard L, Ersboll M, Johansen M. Treatment with oral beta-blockers during pregnancy complicated by maternal heart disease increases the risk of fetal growth restriction. BJOG. 2014;121(5):618–26.
8. Regitz-Zagrosek V, Blomstrom Lundqvist C, Borghi C, et al. SC Guidelines in the management of cardiovascular diseases during pregnancy: the Task Force on the Management of Cardiovascular Diseases during Pregnancy of the European Society of Cardiology (ESC). Eur Heart J. 2011;32(24):3147–97.
9. Daikha-Dahmane F, Levy-Beff E, Jugie M, Lenclen R. Foetal kidney maldevelopment in maternal use of antiotensin II type I receptor antagonists. Pediatr Nephrol. 2006;21(5):729–32.
10. Curry RA, Gelson E, Swan L, Dob D, Babu-Narayan SV, Gatzoulis MA, Steer PJ, Johnson MR. Marfan syndrome and pregnancy: maternal and neonatal outcomes. BJOG. 2014;121(5):610–7.

11. Omnes S, Jondeau G, Deaint D, Dumont A, Yzabeck C, Guglielminotti J, Luton D, Azria E. Pregnancy outcomes among women with Marfan syndrome. Int J Gynaecol Obstet. 2013;122(3):219–23.
12. Cox DA, Ginde S, Kuhlmann RS, Earing MG. Management of the pregnant woman with Marfan syndrome complicated by ascending aorta dilation. Arch Gynecol Obstet. 2014;290(4):797–802.
13. Allyn J, Guglielminotti J, Omnes S, Guezouli L, Egan M, Jondeau G, Longrois D, Montravers P. Marfan's syndrome during pregnancy: anesthetic management of delivery in 16 consecutive patients. Anesth Analg. 2013;116(2):392–8.
14. Verghese C. Anaesthesia in the Marfan syndrome. Anaesthesia. 1984;33:917–22.
15. Lacassie HJ, et al. Dural ectasia: a likely cause of inadequate spinal anaesthesia in two parturients with Marfan's syndrome. Br J Anaesth. 2005;94(4):500–4.
16. Heck A, Clayton R, Robinson C. Dural ectasia in Marfan syndrome. Int J Obstet Anesth. 2014;23(3):287–8.
17. McNeilly G, Nicholl A, Broadway J, Rao S. Dural ectasia in Marfan's syndrome: magnetic resonance imaging appearances and anaesthetic experience of three deliveries. Int J Obstet Anesth. 2013;22(4):337–9.
18. Hiratzka LF, Bakris GL, Beckman JA, et al. ACCF/AHA/AATS/ACR/ASA/SCA/SCAI/SIR/STS/SVM guidelines for the diagnosis and management of aortic disease. Circulation. 2010;121:e266–369.
19. Sato A, Ishida M, Ishibashi K, Shirasawa H, Akahira S, Miura H, Sato M, Kumagai J, Terada Y. A case of acute aortic dissection in a woman with Marfan syndrome at 29 weeks' gestation. J Obstet Gynaecol. 2014;34(4):358.
20. Master M, Day G. Acute aortic dissection in pregnancy in a woman with undiagnosed Marfan syndrome. Case Rep Obstet Gynaecol. 2012;2012:490169.
21. Tang GH, Malekan R, Lansman SL, Spielvogel D. Aortic valve-sparing reimplantation and mitral repair in a pregnant, second trimester Marfan patient: surgical decision. Ann Thorac Surg. 2013;95(2):701–3.
22. Yates MT, Soppa G, Smelt J, Fletcher N, van Besouw JP, Thilaganathan B, Jahangiri M. Perioperative management and outcomes of aortic surgery during pregnancy. J Thorac Cardiovasc Surg. 2015;149(2):607–10.
23. Yuan SM. Postpartum aortic dissection. Taiwan J Obstet Gynecol. 2013;52(3):318–22.
24. Sato S, Nishida M, Furukawa Y, Nasu K, Narahara H. Acute aortic dissection after caesarean section in a patient with Marfan syndrome. J Obstet Gynaecol. 2014;34(4):354.
25. Zamlynski J, Olejek A, Gajewska-Kucharek A, Horzelska E, Carson MP, Rykaczewska-Czerwinska M, Chudek J, Bodzek P. Three pregnancies in a Marfan syndrome patient after a mitral and tricuspid valve surgery. Ginekol Pol. 2013;84(4):314–7.

Marfan Syndrome (MFS): Inherited Microfibrillar Disorder Caused by Mutations in the Fibrillin-1 Gene

22

Jose Antonio Aragon-Martin and Anne H. Child

There have been several studies suggesting that *FBN1* gene was responsible for the Marfan syndrome (MFS) phenotype [1–4] before announcing the localisation of the gene on chromosome 15q21.1 in 1991 [3, 5, 6]. Subsequently, many research laboratories started to screen *FBN1* in their MFS patients. Many mutations have been mapped to this gene due to this increase in genetic screening and international collaborations confirming *FBN1* as the gene responsible for Marfan syndrome [7–15]. This has been the final proof to confirm that the *FBN1* gene is the cause of MFS.

MFS displays an autosomal dominant [16] inheritance pattern. Although infrequent, there have been recessive [17–21] and compound-heterozygote [22, 23] cases with mutations in the *FBN1* gene where the phenotype tends to be more severe than the autosomal dominant form. Most of the *FBN1* mutations occur at the germline, either by spontaneous mutation (*de Novo* mutation) [12] or inherited (familial mutation) [7]. Though very rare, there have been cases of mosaicism by either germline [8] or somatic mutations [9, 10]. The syndrome has been reported with an estimated incidence of 1 in 3000–5000 [24–26] live births, Gray has reported an incidence of 1 in 9800 [27] live births; and approximately 25 % [25, 27] of cases arising as the result of spontaneous mutations.

J.A. Aragon-Martin, PhD (✉)
Sonalee Laboratory, Cardiovascular and Cell Sciences Research Institute,
St George's, University of London, London, UK
e-mail: jaragon@sgul.ac.uk

A.H. Child, MD, FRCP
Cardiovascular and Cell Sciences Research Institute, St George's, University of London,
London, UK
e-mail: achild@sgul.ac.uk

© Springer-Verlag London 2016

A.H. Child (ed.), *Diagnosis and Management of Marfan Syndrome*,
DOI 10.1007/978-1-4471-5442-6_22

In 1995 it was reported that life expectancy for patients with MFS had increased about 25 % [28] since 1972. One of the reasons was the addition of one year of life expectancy per every year of research in the field, but the main reason was due to the increased frequency of diagnosis helped by mutation screening [29].

FBN1 gene codes for fibrillin-1 protein, which is composed of 47 (~75 % of the protein) repeated EGF-like (epidermal growth factor-like) domains; 43 of them have calcium-binding properties [30] (cbEGF-like - calcium binding EGF-like). Between the EGF-like domains there are 7 (~11 % of the protein) TGFBP (transforming growth factor-β binding protein-like) domains, defined as 8-cysteine domains (Fig. 22.1).

MFS occurs when a causative mutation appears in the nucleotide sequence of the *FBN1* gene disrupting the normal assembly of the protein [32]. This extracellular matrix protein is produced as profibrillin-1 (~350 kD), which is transformed to fibrillin-1 (~320 kD) in a calcium-dependent process [33, 34]. Fibrillin-1 is a cysteine-rich glycoprotein that is a major structural component of the 10–12 nm calcium-binding extracellular microfibrils [1]. A better understanding of the role of fibrillin-1 is being obtained due to the mapping of novel and recurrent causative mutations and by the study of their effect on protein structure and expression.

A region of interest is between exons 24–32 (neonatal region). Causative mutations in this region tend to create severe phenotypes [35–37] and patients generally die in the first years of life of cardiopulmonary failure [32].

Another region to be noticed is between exons 23–29. Causative mutations in this region tend to create phenotypes with no ocular anomalies. The UMD (universal mutation database) shows that half of causative mutations in these patients are located in this region [8].

FBN1 is a relatively large and highly fragmented gene. It consists of 65 coding exons (Exons 1–66 – Exon 1 is a non-coding exon) contained in ~237 kb of genomic DNA [31, 38, 39]. About 3000 mutations associated with *FBN1* gene have been reported in the UMD to date [40]. The majority of the mutations occur throughout the gene in exons 2 through 66. Each mutation is unique to a specific family (rare exceptions occur) implying that spontaneous de novo mutations are common. A great number of mutations are base changes that result in amino acid substitutions (non-synonymous variants) within the EGF-like domains of fibrillin-1 [41]. These

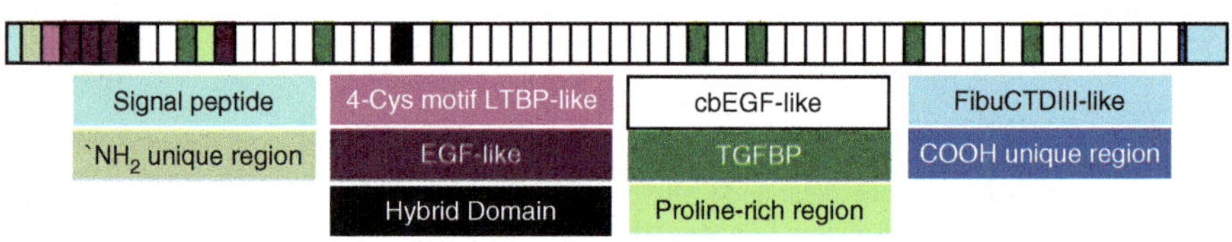

Fig. 22.1 Drawing of the 62 different domains of profibrillin-1 protein. Each domain is made of a black box and the box is coloured depending on the type of domain. The location of the signal peptide cleavage, the 2 tetrabasic Furin/PACE cleavage site, the N-terminus and C-terminus cleavage, the cell attachment signal location and the 15 N-glycosilation sites has been omitted to focus on a clear understanding of the domains. *EGF* epidermal growth factor, *TGFBP* transforming growth factor-β binding protein-like, *cbEGF* calcium binding EGF (Modified from Pereira et al. [31])

variants are expected to alter calcium binding or disulphide bond formation, which mediate protein interactions in the extracellular matrix [42, 43].

There are 43 calcium binding epidermal growth factor-like (cbEGF-like) domains in fibrillin-1. The amino acid sequence in these 43 domains differs between 2–7 amino acids but the core amino acids are highly conserved. Calcium binds to a highly conserved region in the cb-EGF-like domain made of the following amino acid sequence [D]–[x_1]–[D/N]–[E]–[C_1]–[x_{4-6}]–[C_2]–[x_{3-6}]–[C_3]–[x_1]–[N/D]. The example in Fig. 22.2 is from cb-EGF-like number 35 with its conserved sequence [D]–[x_1]–[D]–[E]–[C_1]–[x_6]–[C_2]–[x_6]–[C_3]–[x_1]–[N] (Fig. 22.2).

Non-synonymous causative mutations in the conserved calcium-binding region have been found in Marfan patients [7, 40, 45–47]. This is probably due to the inability of the conserved region to bind calcium ions and as a consequence the protein might breakdown at the domain affected by the mutation. Proteolysis of fibrilin-1 can occur but it has been studied that calcium ions in the cb-EGF-like domains have a protective effect [48–52].

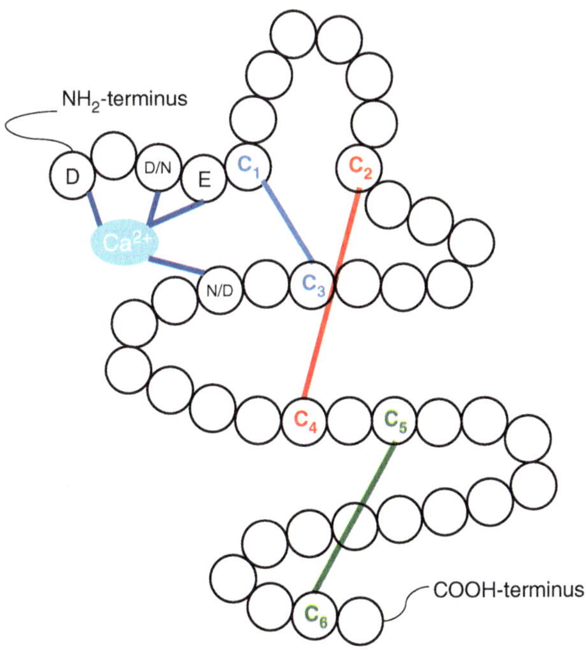

Fig. 22.2 This picture represents cbEGF-like domain number 35 in fibrillin-1, from the amino terminus (NH2-terminus) to the carboxyl terminus (COOH-terminus). *Black circles* represent amino acids. Black circles C1-C3 (*light blue*), C2-C4 (*red*), C5-C6 (*green*) reveal the position of cysteine residues. Cysteine residues are attached by disulphide bonds, which are represented by *dotted colour lines*. Calcium (Ca2+) is represented as oval shape and attached (*solid blue lines*) to a highly conserved amino acid sequence ([D]–[x1]–[D/ N]–[E]–[C1]–[x4-6]–[C2]–[x3-6]–[C3]–[x1]–[N/D]) found in cb-EGF-like domains. x = amino acids not conserved. x4–6 = 4–6 amino acids (Modified from Micheal et al. [44])

Cysteine changes are very important because cysteine tends to create disulphide bonds with another cysteine. Other non-synonymous causative mutations are found in Marfan patients where one of the 6 cysteines found in the cbEGF-like domain has been changed to an amino acid that might disrupt the normal assembly of the disulphide bonds, therefore, destabilising the domain [7, 53, 54]. There are Marfan patients where a normal amino acid in the protein sequence has been changed to a new cysteine, which might disrupt the natural assembly of the disulphide bonds [7, 40].

Other types of DNA mutations can affect the normal splicing of the FBN1 transcript either by inserting [55] or skipping [7, 40] exons. There is a large and complex molecular machine behind the normal splicing called spliceosome. Proteins involved in the spliceosome need to recognise and bind to consensus sequences in pre-mRNA molecules to splice their introns. Several studies in Marfan patients have found causative mutations in the sequence of FBN1 pre-mRNA molecules that disrupt the involvement of the spliceosome [7, 40, 55, 56].

There are cases where the transcription of fibrillin-1 message is prematurely terminated or part of the *FBN1* gene is deleted; if there is no degradation of the mRNA it will produce truncated fibrillin-1 polypeptides disrupting the normal function of fibrillin-1 protein [7, 40, 57, 58]. On the other hand, if there is degradation of the mRNA the Marfan patient will develop FBN1 haploinsufficiency; this happens when one of the alleles for *FBN1* gene is not expressed as protein due to an anomaly, leaving one copy of the good gene to do the entire job but it is not sufficient to stop the development of Marfan phenotype. One study suggests that patients with haploinsufficiency respond better to drug treatment [59].

It is understandable to think that the importance of knowing the type of causative mutation will tell us more about the Marfan phenotype. This is something that scientists are working hard on, at present, to get an explanation. There have been several genotype-phenotype association studies in Marfan syndrome but none of them with a conclusive answer [60–62].

Diagnosis of MFS relies on clinical criteria and mutation screening helps to find the genetic cause. Scientists have been investigating to improve mutation sensitive techniques to get a clear idea of the molecular genetic cause in MFS. Heteroduplex (~78 %) [63] and SSCP (~75 %) [7] techniques had a low mutation rate in *FBN1* screening. An improvement in sensitivity came with dHPLC analysis technique (~91 %) [7] but when it comes to sensitivity there is nothing like the gold standard, Sanger sequencing (~98 %), which all the other techniques have to use to validate their variants.

Mutation screening by Sanger sequencing technique (Fig. 22.3) is very powerful but even this technique has sensitivity issues. It cannot detect large deletions or duplications in the DNA sequence and to solve this problem MLPA technique has come to the rescue. The combination of MLPA with Sanger sequencing has improved the mutation screening technique to ~99 % accuracy. One of the reasons it is not 100 % is because these techniques do not normally cover promoter or whole intron regions when screening for mutations. It is known that variations can occur

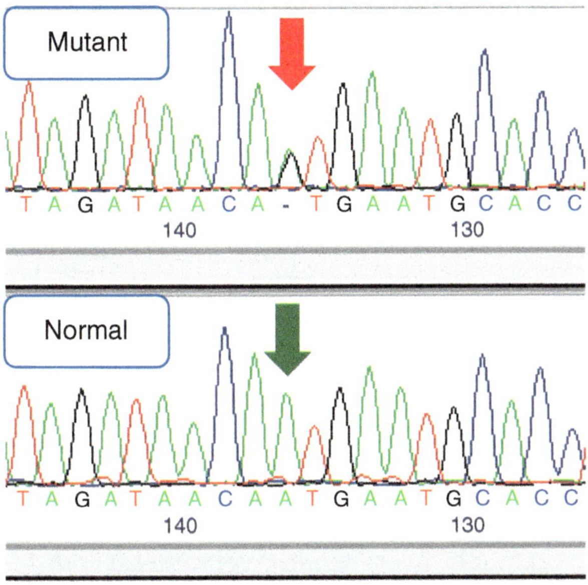

Fig. 22.3 This picture represents the visual result of using Sanger sequencing technique. It was visualised with Gap4 program. The *red arrow* points to the location of a mutant nucleotide and the *green arrow* to the normal variant. This FBN1 causative mutation is found in Exon 61. It alters the nucleotide sequence at a codon (AAT>AGT), where its amino acid affects the calcium binding consensus sequence in the domain cbEGF-like number 40. This causative mutation is called c.7577A>G (nucleotide sequence) and p.N2526S (amino acid sequence) based on HGVS nomenclature and NM_000138 transcript

deep within an intron and some of them can be causative mutations [55] but the majority of causative mutations occur within the coding region of a gene. It would be astronomically expensive to screen whole introns of *FBN1* gene by Sanger sequencing.

The world has been working very hard since 2004 to solve this monetary problem. The latest techniques that scientists trust for mutation screening are called whole genome/exome sequencing, which are part of next generation sequencing (NGS). The difference between them is that whole exome sequencing will only screen the coding regions of all the genes in a genome; on the other hand, whole genome sequencing will screen the whole genome of a patient (including promoter and intron regions). Major drawback points of these techniques are random low coverage of regions in the genome, accuracy when sequencing repetitive regions with one nucleotide and the reliability of the programs used to find variants [64]. Although the programs are very convenient and fast, increasing the coverage or even the usage of visual interfaces like IGV (Fig. 22.4) to screen manually the sequences will help to increase NGS reliability [64]. A minor drawback is that every single variant that needs to be studied has to be confirmed by the "gold standard": Sanger sequencing.

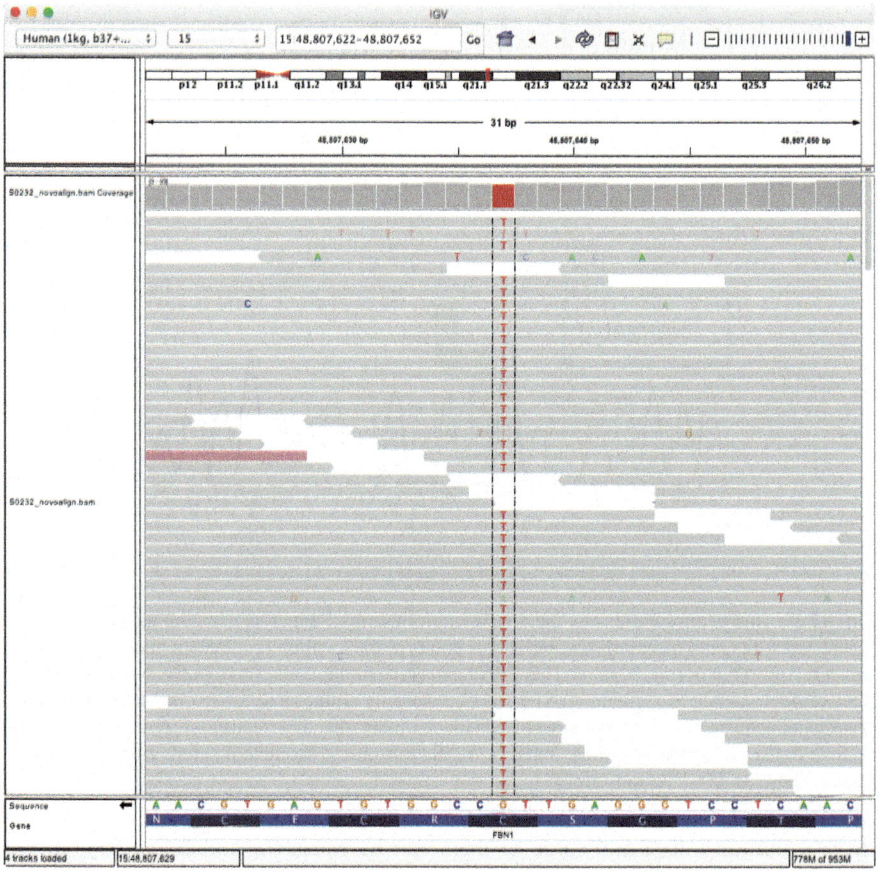

Fig. 22.4 Picture taken from IGV program to visualize exome sequencing data. Fragments with nucleotide sequence identical to the reference genome are coloured *grey* and nucleotides that are different will be shown in colours (*blue = C*; *black = G*; *green = A*; *red = T*). The reference genome sequence is located at the *bottom* of the picture. The location of the two *black dotted lines* is centred in a particular nucleotide. This variant was found in exon 11 of the FBN1 gene with the names c.1415G>A & p.C472Y (based on HGVS nomenclature and NM_000138 transcript). The nucleotide and the coverage region are coloured to facilitate the location of important variants in the genome. Some other possibly important nucleotides in the vicinity are shown in lighter colour but the program analysing the data could be calling the wrong nucleotide

Advance on these last two techniques is going even further. In the past years there has been a growing interest with a company called Oxford Nanopore Technologies. The previous NGS platforms are going to be renamed 2nd Generation Sequencing (2GenSeq) since the technique from this last company is going to be called 3rd Generation Sequencing (3GenSeq). The previous platforms must use fragmented DNA, while Oxford Nanopore is using whole DNA molecules to pass through a very tiny pore where each nucleotide gives a different electric charge (Fig. 22.5). If it

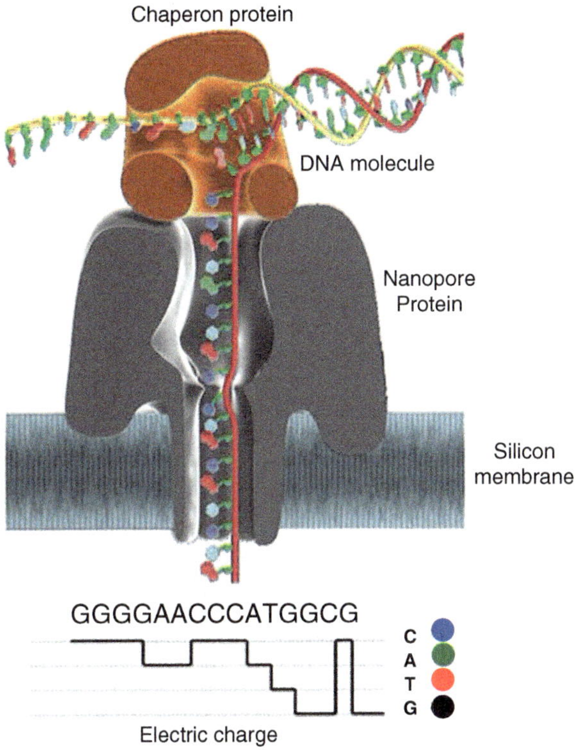

Fig. 22.5 Top picture: translocation of a DNA molecule through a nanopore. *Grey* figure is the nanopore. *Orange* figure is a DNA chaperon. *Bottom picture*: electric charge when different nucleotides pass through the nanopore (*blue* for *C*, *green* for *A*, *red* for *T* and *black* for *G*) with its nucleotide sequence (Modified from Schneider and Dekker 2012 and Bayley 2006 [65, 66])

really works one day, this will definitely solve the reliability of the nucleotide sequences. At the moment there is a major challenge with the fast speed of DNA molecules when they pass through the pores [67].

The importance of 2nd & 3rd Generation Sequencing comes from the current understanding that other genes could influence the mild or severe phenotype of Marfan syndrome patients. These other genes are called modifiers and therefore variations in these genes will modify the severity of a Marfan phenotype. It is well known that Marfan syndrome is clinically variable between families and between members of the same family, making the research into the genotype-phenotype association very difficult. This is why the arrival of NGS platforms is critical. NGS techniques provide data that not only will screen the whole *FBN1* gene but also will allow the study of other genes that can be classified as modifiers. This will help to better understand the genotype-phenotype association in Marfan syndrome patients.

One last point to consider here is the incidence of many overlapping syndromes when it comes to diagnosing a patient with Marfan syndrome where patients with similar features are not linked to the *FBN1* gene [68]. Also, other connective tissue disorders may be linked to the *FBN1* gene. There are many connective tissue disorders that are similar to the phenotype encountered in Marfan syndrome like Loeys-Dietz syndrome (LDS) or Ehlers-Danlos syndrome (EDS type IV), which do not have mutations in the *FBN1* gene. On the other hand, depending on the location of the causative mutation within the *FBN1* gene, different clinical phenotypes, apart from Marfan syndrome may appear, and some of them are: Mitral valve, Aorta, Skeleton, and Skin syndrome (MASS), Thoracic Aortic Aneurysm and Dissection (TAAD) or familial Ectopia Lentis (EL) [35, 41].

Because other connective tissue disorders are very similar clinically to Marfan syndrome, when researching it is imperative to focus on these overlapping conditions, their different phenotypes and the genes they are associated with. It is understood that some TAAD genes are involved in the same pathway as the Marfan syndrome gene (*FBN1*) and these other genes could be modifier genes that researchers are looking for to clarify the understanding of the genotype-phenotype relationship in Marfan syndrome.

We are coming from a long way and we are still going places.

References

1. Sakai LY, Keene DR, Engvall E. Fibrillin, a new 350-kD glycoprotein, is a component of extracellular microfibrils. J Cell Biol. 1986;103(6 Pt 1):2499–509.
2. Hollister DW, Godfrey M, Sakai LY, Pyeritz RE. Immunohistologic abnormalities of the microfibrillar-fiber system in the Marfan syndrome. N Engl J Med. 1990;323(3):152–9.
3. Dietz HC, Pyeritz RE, Hall BD, Cadle RG, Hamosh A, Schwartz J, Meyers DA, Francomano CA. The Marfan syndrome locus: confirmation of assignment to chromosome 15 and identification of tightly linked markers at 15q15-q21.3. Genomics. 1991;9(2):355–61.
4. Kainulainen K, Pulkkinen L, Savolainen A, Kaitila I, Peltonen L. Location on chromosome 15 of the gene defect causing Marfan syndrome. N Engl J Med. 1990;323(14):935–9.
5. Magenis RE, Maslen CL, Smith L, Allen L, Sakai LY. Localization of the fibrillin (FBN) gene to chromosome 15, band q21.1. Genomics. 1991;11(2):346–51.
6. Lee B, Godfrey M, Vitale E, Hori H, Mattei MG, Sarfarazi M, Tsipouras P, Ramirez F, Hollister DW. Linkage of Marfan syndrome and a phenotypically related disorder to two different fibrillin genes. Nature. 1991;352(6333):330–4.
7. Comeglio P, Johnson P, Arno G, Brice G, Evans A, Aragon-Martin J, da Silva FP, Kiotsekoglou A, Child A. The importance of mutation detection in Marfan syndrome and Marfan-related disorders: report of 193 FBN1 mutations. Hum Mutat. 2007;28(9):928–50.
8. Collod-Béroud G, Lackmy-Port-Lys M, Jondeau G, Mathieu M, Maingourd Y, Coulon M, Guillotel M, Junien C, Boileau C. Demonstration of the recurrence of Marfan-like skeletal and cardiovascular manifestations due to germline mosaicism for an FBN1 mutation. Am J Hum Genet. 1999;65(3):917–21.
9. Blyth M, Foulds N, Turner C, Bunyan D. Severe Marfan syndrome due to FBN1 exon deletions. Am J Med Genet A. 2008;146A(10):1320–4.
10. Montgomery RA, Geraghty MT, Bull E, Gelb BD, Johnson M, McIntosh I, Francomano CA, Dietz HC. Multiple molecular mechanisms underlying subdiagnostic variants of Marfan syndrome. Am J Hum Genet. 1998;63(6):1703–11.
11. Hayward C, Porteous ME, Brock DJ. Mutation screening of all 65 exons of the fibrillin-1 gene in 60 patients with Marfan syndrome: report of 12 novel mutations. Hum Mutat. 1997;10(4):280–9.
12. Hayward C, Keston M, Brock DJ, Dietz HC. Fibrillin (FBN1) mutations in Marfan syndrome. Hum Mutat. 1992;1(1):79.
13. Dietz HC, Cutting GR, Pyeritz RE, Maslen CL, Sakai LY, Corson GM, Puffenberger EG, Hamosh A, Nanthakumar EJ, Curristin SM. Marfan syndrome caused by a recurrent de novo missense mutation in the fibrillin gene. Nature. 1991;352(6333):337–9.

14. Dietz HC, McIntosh I, Sakai LY, Corson GM, Chalberg SC, Pyeritz RE, Francomano CA. Four novel FBN1 mutations: significance for mutant transcript level and EGF-like domain calcium binding in the pathogenesis of Marfan syndrome. Genomics. 1993;17(2):468–75.
15. Tynan K, Comeau K, Pearson M, Wilgenbus P, Levitt D, Gasner C, Berg MA, Miller DC, Francke U. Mutation screening of complete fibrillin-1 coding sequence: report of five new mutations, including two in 8-cysteine domains. Hum Mol Genet. 1993;2(11):1813–21.
16. McKUSICK VA. The cardiovascular aspects of Marfan's syndrome: a heritable disorder of connective tissue. Circulation. 1955;11(3):321–42.
17. de Vries BB, Pals G, Odink R, Hamel BC. Homozygosity for a FBN1 missense mutation: clinical and molecular evidence for recessive Marfan syndrome. Eur J Hum Genet. 2007;15(9):930–5.
18. Hogue J, Lee C, Jelin A, Strecker MN, Cox VA, Slavotinek AM. Homozygosity for a FBN1 missense mutation causes a severe Marfan syndrome phenotype. Clin Genet. 2013;84(4):392–3.
19. Capotorti L, de Benedetti Gaddini R, Rizzo P. Contribution to the study of the heredity of Marfan's syndrome: description of a family tree of 4 generations with marriage between consanguineous parents. Acta Genet Med Gemellol (Roma). 1959;8:455–82.
20. Chemke J, Nisani R, Feigl A, Garty R, Cooper M, Bårash Y, Duksin D. Homozygosity for autosomal dominant Marfan syndrome. J Med Genet. 1984;21(3):173–7.
21. Schollin J, Bjarke B, Gustavson KH. Probable homozygotic form of the Marfan syndrome in a newborn child. Acta Paediatr Scand. 1988;77(3):452–6.
22. Karttunen L, Raghunath M, Lönnqvist L, Peltonen L. A compound-heterozygous Marfan patient: two defective fibrillin alleles result in a lethal phenotype. Am J Hum Genet. 1994;55(6):1083–91.
23. Van Dijk FS, Hamel BC, Hilhorst-Hofstee Y, Mulder BJ, Timmermans J, Pals G, Cobben JM. Compound-heterozygous Marfan syndrome. Eur J Med Genet. 2009;52(1):1–5.
24. Keane MG, Pyeritz RE. Medical management of Marfan syndrome. Circulation. 2008;117(21):2802–13.
25. Judge DP, Dietz HC. Marfan's syndrome. Lancet. 2005;366(9501):1965–76.
26. Chiu HH, Wu MH, Chen HC, Kao FY, Huang SK. Epidemiological profile of Marfan syndrome in a general population: a national database study. Mayo Clin Proc. 2014;89(1):34–42.
27. Dean JC. Management of Marfan syndrome. Heart. 2002;88(1):97–103.
28. Silverman DI, Burton KJ, Gray J, Bosner MS, Kouchoukos NT, Roman MJ, Boxer M, Devereux RB, Tsipouras P. Life expectancy in the Marfan syndrome. Am J Cardiol. 1995;75(2):157–60.
29. Pyeritz RE. Marfan syndrome: 30 years of research equals 30 years of additional life expectancy. Heart. 2009;95(3):173–5.
30. Corson GM, Chalberg SC, Dietz HC, Charbonneau NL, Sakai LY. Fibrillin binds calcium and is coded by cDNAs that reveal a multidomain structure and alternatively spliced exons at the 5' end. Genomics. 1993;17(2):476–84.
31. Pereira L, D'Alessio M, Ramirez F, Lynch JR, Sykes B, Pangilinan T, Bonadio J. Genomic organization of the sequence coding for fibrillin, the defective gene product in Marfan syndrome. Hum Mol Genet. 1993;2(7):961–8.
32. Summers KM, Nataatmadja M, Xu D, West MJ, McGill JJ, Whight C, Colley A, Adès LC. Histopathology and fibrillin-1 distribution in severe early onset Marfan syndrome. Am J Med Genet A. 2005;139(1):2–8.
33. Milewicz DM, Pyeritz RE, Crawford ES, Byers PH. Marfan syndrome: defective synthesis, secretion, and extracellular matrix formation of fibrillin by cultured dermal fibroblasts. J Clin Invest. 1992;89(1):79–86.
34. Raghunath M, Kielty CM, Steinmann B. Truncated profibrillin of a Marfan patient is of apparent similar size as fibrillin: intracellular retention leads to over-N-glycosylation. J Mol Biol. 1995;248(5):901–9.
35. Kainulainen K, Karttunen L, Puhakka L, Sakai L, Peltonen L. Mutations in the fibrillin gene responsible for dominant ectopia lentis and neonatal Marfan syndrome. Nat Genet. 1994;6(1):64–9.

36. Milewicz DM, Duvic M. Severe neonatal Marfan syndrome resulting from a de novo 3-bp insertion into the fibrillin gene on chromosome 15. Am J Hum Genet. 1994;54(3):447–53.
37. Putnam EA, Cho M, Zinn AB, Towbin JA, Byers PH, Milewicz DM. Delineation of the Marfan phenotype associated with mutations in exons 23–32 of the FBN1 gene. Am J Med Genet. 1996;62(3):233–42.
38. Sakai LY, Keene DR. Fibrillin: monomers and microfibrils. Methods Enzymol. 1994; 245:29–52.
39. Biery NJ, Eldadah ZA, Moore CS, Stetten G, Spencer F, Dietz HC. Revised genomic organization of FBN1 and significance for regulated gene expression. Genomics. 1999;56(1):70–7.
40. Collod-Béroud G, Le Bourdelles S, Ades L, Ala-Kokko L, Booms P, Boxer M, Child A, Comeglio P, De Paepe A, Hyland JC. and others. Update of the UMD-FBN1 mutation database and creation of an FBN1 polymorphism database. Hum Mutat. 2003;22(3):199–208.
41. Dietz HC, Saraiva JM, Pyeritz RE, Cutting GR, Francomano CA. Clustering of fibrillin (FBN1) missense mutations in Marfan syndrome patients at cysteine residues in EGF-like domains. Hum Mutat. 1992;1(5):366–74.
42. Smallridge RS, Whiteman P, Doering K, Handford PA, Downing AK. EGF-like domain calcium affinity modulated by N-terminal domain linkage in human fibrillin-1. J Mol Biol. 1999;286(3):661–8.
43. Kielty CM, Rantamäki T, Child AH, Shuttleworth CA, Peltonen L. Cysteine-to-arginine point mutation in a 'hybrid' eight-cysteine domain of FBN1: consequences for fibrillin aggregation and microfibril assembly. J Cell Sci. 1995;108(Pt 3):1317–23.
44. Micheal S, Khan MI, Akhtar F, Weiss MM, Islam F, Ali M, Qamar R, Maugeri A, den Hollander AI. Identification of a novel FBN1 gene mutation in a large Pakistani family with Marfan syndrome. Mol Vis. 2012;18:1918–26.
45. Collod-Béroud G, Béroud C, Ades L, Black C, Boxer M, Brock DJ, Holman KJ, de Paepe A, Francke U, Grau U. Marfan Database (third edition): new mutations and new routines for the software. Nucleic Acids Res. 1998;26(1):229–33.
46. Liu WO, Oefner PJ, Qian C, Odom RS, Francke U. Denaturing HPLC-identified novel FBN1 mutations, polymorphisms, and sequence variants in Marfan syndrome and related connective tissue disorders. Genet Test. 1997;1(4):237–42.
47. Lönnqvist L, Child A, Kainulainen K, Davidson R, Puhakka L, Peltonen L. A novel mutation of the fibrillin gene causing ectopia lentis. Genomics. 1994;19(3):573–6.
48. Reinhardt DP, Mechling DE, Boswell BA, Keene DR, Sakai LY, Bächinger HP. Calcium determines the shape of fibrillin. J Biol Chem. 1997;272(11):7368–73.
49. Reinhardt DP, Ono RN, Sakai LY. Calcium stabilizes fibrillin-1 against proteolytic degradation. J Biol Chem. 1997;272(2):1231–6.
50. Reinhardt DP, Ono RN, Notbohm H, Müller PK, Bächinger HP, Sakai LY. Mutations in calcium-binding epidermal growth factor modules render fibrillin-1 susceptible to proteolysis. A potential disease-causing mechanism in Marfan syndrome. J Biol Chem. 2000;275(16):12339–45.
51. Ashworth JL, Murphy G, Rock MJ, Sherratt MJ, Shapiro SD, Shuttleworth CA, Kielty CM. Fibrillin degradation by matrix metalloproteinases: implications for connective tissue remodelling. Biochem J. 1999;340(Pt 1):171–81.
52. McGettrick AJ, Knott V, Willis A, Handford PA. Molecular effects of calcium binding mutations in Marfan syndrome depend on domain context. Hum Mol Genet. 2000;9(13):1987–94.
53. Loeys B, Nuytinck L, Van Acker P, Walraedt S, Bonduelle M, Sermon K, Hamel B, Sanchez A, Messiaen L, De Paepe A. Strategies for prenatal and preimplantation genetic diagnosis in Marfan syndrome (MFS). Prenat Diagn. 2002;22(1):22–8.
54. Schrijver I, Liu W, Brenn T, Furthmayr H, Francke U. Cysteine substitutions in epidermal growth factor-like domains of fibrillin-1: distinct effects on biochemical and clinical phenotypes. Am J Hum Genet. 1999;65(4):1007–20.
55. Gillis E, Kempers M, Salemink S, Timmermans J, Cheriex EC, Bekkers SC, Fransen E, De Die-Smulders CE, Loeys BL, Van Laer L. An FBN1 deep intronic mutation in a familial case of Marfan syndrome: an explanation for genetically unsolved cases? Hum Mutat. 2014;35(5):571–4.

56. Dietz HC, Valle D, Francomano CA, Kendzior RJ, Pyeritz RE, Cutting GR. The skipping of constitutive exons in vivo induced by nonsense mutations. Science. 1993;259(5095):680–3.
57. Kainulainen K, Sakai LY, Child A, Pope FM, Puhakka L, Ryhänen L, Palotie A, Kaitila I, Peltonen L. Two mutations in Marfan syndrome resulting in truncated fibrillin polypeptides. Proc Natl Acad Sci U S A. 1992;89(13):5917–21.
58. Körkkö J, Kaitila I, Lönnqvist L, Peltonen L, Ala-Kokko L. Sensitivity of conformation sensitive gel electrophoresis in detecting mutations in Marfan syndrome and related conditions. J Med Genet. 2002;39(1):34–41.
59. Franken R, den Hartog A, Radonic T, Micha D, Maugeri A, van Dijk FS, Meijers-Heijboer HE, Timmermans J, Scholte AJ, van den Berg MP. Beneficial Outcome of Losartan Therapy Depends on Type of FBN1 Mutation in Marfan Syndrome. Circ Cardiovasc Genet. 2015;8(2):383–8.
60. Franken R, Heesterbeek T, de Waard V, Zwinderman A, Pals G, Mulder B, Groenink M. Diagnosis and genetics of Marfan syndrome. Expert Opinion Orphan Drugs. 2014;2(10):1049–62.
61. Attias D, Stheneur C, Roy C, Collod-Béroud G, Detaint D, Faivre L, Delrue MA, Cohen L, Francannet C, Béroud C. and others. Comparison of clinical presentations and outcomes between patients with TGFBR2 and FBN1 mutations in Marfan syndrome and related disorders. Circulation. 2009;120(25):2541–9.
62. Hilhorst-Hofstee Y, Hamel BC, Verheij JB, Rijlaarsdam ME, Mancini GM, Cobben JM, Giroth C, Ruivenkamp CA, Hansson KB, Timmermans J. and others. The clinical spectrum of complete FBN1 allele deletions. Eur J Hum Genet. 2011;19(3):247–52.
63. Nijbroek G, Sood S, McIntosh I, Francomano CA, Bull E, Pereira L, Ramirez F, Pyeritz RE, Dietz HC. Fifteen novel FBN1 mutations causing Marfan syndrome detected by heteroduplex analysis of genomic amplicons. Am J Hum Genet. 1995;57(1):8–21.
64. McInerney-Leo AM, Marshall MS, Gardiner B, Coucke PJ, Van Laer L, Loeys BL, Summers KM, Symoens S, West JA, West MJ. Whole exome sequencing is an efficient, sensitive and specific method of mutation detection in osteogenesis imperfecta and Marfan syndrome. Bonekey Rep. 2013;2:456.
65. Bayley H. Sequencing single molecules of DNA. Curr Opin Chem Biol. 2006;10(6):628–37.
66. Schneider GF, Dekker C. DNA sequencing with nanopores. Nat Biotechnol. 2012;30(4):326–8.
67. Wang Y, Yang Q, Wang Z. The evolution of nanopore sequencing. Front Genet. 2014;5:449.
68. Boileau C, Jondeau G, Babron MC, Coulon M, Alexandre JA, Sakai L, Melki J, Delorme G, Dubourg O, Bonaïti-Pellié C. Autosomal dominant Marfan-like connective-tissue disorder with aortic dilation and skeletal anomalies not linked to the fibrillin genes. Am J Hum Genet. 1993;53(1):46–54.

Reproductive Decisions

23

Karen Sage

Reproductive Options for Marfan Syndrome

The majority of individuals diagnosed with Marfan syndrome have a mutation in the fibrillin 1 (FBN1) gene located on chromosome 15. This genetic change will have either been inherited (75 % chance) from one of the parents or the mutation will have arisen as result of a new or "*de novo*" change (25 %). Discussions with health care professionals trained in genetics, a genetic counsellor or clinical geneticist specialising in cardiac conditions would be recommended so that individuals can fully understand their options prior to planning a family.

Reproductive Risk

When a parent has Marfan syndrome, each pregnancy and child has a 50 % chance of inheriting the mutation; the pattern of inheritance is described as autosomal dominant. If both parents have Marfan syndrome there is a 75 % chance that the child will be affected. However, a child inheriting an altered FBN1 gene copy from each parent would be severely affected and the pregnancy will often not proceed to term, or the child will have serious complications after birth resulting in neonatal death.

The following discussion on reproductive options considers the situation where the risk of having a child with Marfan syndrome is 50 % with one parent affected and the gene mutation is known.

K. Sage, BSc, MSc, GC
Department of Preimplantation Genetic Diagnosis,
The Bridge Centre, London Fertility Clinic, London, UK
e-mail: k.sage@thebridgecentre.co.uk

© Springer-Verlag London 2016

A.H. Child (ed.), *Diagnosis and Management of Marfan Syndrome*,
DOI 10.1007/978-1-4471-5442-6_23

Reproductive Options

There are several reproductive options available to couples with Marfan syndrome who wish to minimise the risk of passing on the condition to their children.

- **Prenatal Diagnosis (PND)**
- **Pre-implantation Genetic Diagnosis (PGD)**
- **Natural Conception**
- **Gamete (egg or sperm) Donation**
- **Adoption**

Prenatal Diagnosis

Prenatal Diagnosis is available during a pregnancy to diagnose and confirm whether the foetus has inherited the genetic mutation from the parent. There are two routinely used procedures for prenatal diagnosis currently available [1]:

1. **Chorionic villus sampling (CVS)**.
2. **Amniocentesis**.

Chorionic Villus Sampling

Chorionic villus sampling (CVS) is routinely performed between 10 and 12 weeks of gestation under ultrasound guidance and can be performed trans-abdominally or trans-cervically (Figs. 23.1 and 23.2).

The chorion is the outermost layer of the foetal membranes and the sampling is carefully carried out to ensure that the amniotic cavity is not penetrated. Using ultrasonography guidance, a needle attached to a syringe is inserted through the abdomen for the trans-abdominal procedure, the most commonly used method. If performing the procedure trans-cervically, a tube or forceps are inserted through the cervix to reach the chorion. The sample is collected and dissected to separate foetal material from maternal cells. The chorionic villi can be used for DNA extraction and for rapid molecular analysis using the techniques described below.

Polymerase Chain Reaction (PCR)

There is only a very small amount of DNA present in the villi sample. In order to accurately detect the specific mutation being investigated, more copies of the small section of DNA are required. PCR is highly selective and it allows copies of the section of DNA required for the test targeting the mutation site. PCR can only amplify a small length of DNA (typically up to 1–2 thousand bases) known as an amplicon. Since most genes are larger than this, several PCR reactions will be needed to copy a whole gene.

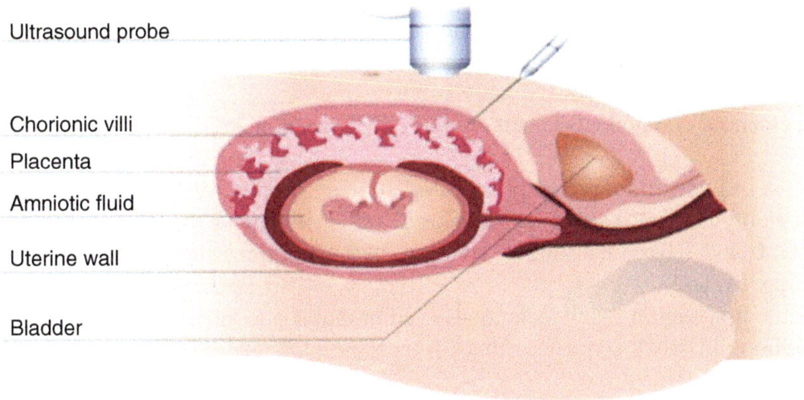

Fig. 23.1 Transabdominal chorionic villus sampling (CVS)

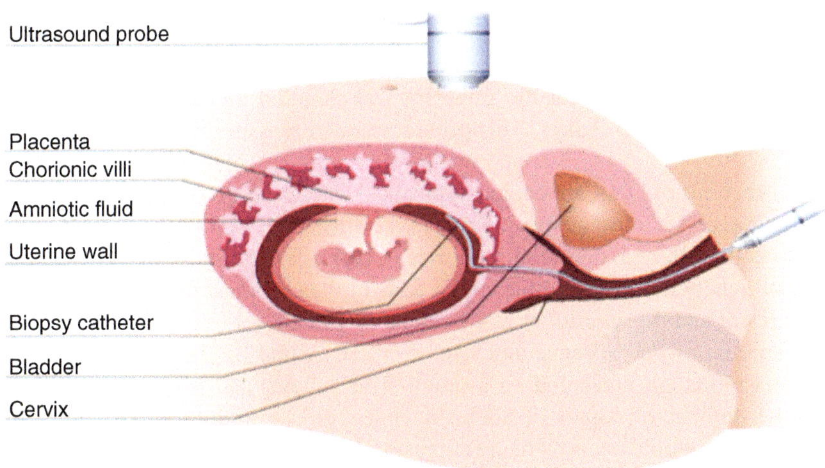

Fig. 23.2 Transcervical chorionic villus sampling

How PCR Works

Before a particular DNA sequence can be PCR-amplified it is necessary to design two short single-stranded DNA fragments called "primers". The primers will match and bind specifically to sequences flanking the section of DNA which is to be amplified. The primers are chemically synthesised by specialist diagnostic companies. The samples are placed on an automated machine that undergoes a series of amplification cycles of programmed temperature changes. During each cycle of temperature changes the targeted section of DNA under investigation, which is flanked by the primers, is copied, doubling the quantity of the target DNA sequence. After 20 cycles of PCR it should have been amplified 220 = 1 million-fold. The whole process would usually take only 1–2 h.

The essential components necessary for a PCR reaction are:

DNA, a set of specific targeted primers, an enzyme needed for DNA to replicate (DNA polymerase); a supply of nucleotides which will make the DNA molecules (A, G, C and T bases); a suitable solution (buffer solution) and appropriate temperature cycles.

PCR is the first step in many techniques used in diagnostic laboratories to identify alterations in DNA sequences that may be the pathogenic cause of a genetic condition.

Prenatal Diagnosis for Marfan Syndrome

Prenatal diagnosis is available if the causative familial mutation in the FBN1 gene is known.

Another technique called QF-PCR (quantitative fluorescence polymerase chain reaction) is mainly used as an additional rapid prenatal test for common chromosomal trisomies (i.e. where there are three copies of one particular chromosome) and this is usually offered at the same time as targeted mutation detection with results available within 5 days. This provides added reassurance that the foetus is normal.

Small sections of DNA are copied, typically 3–5 sections from chromosomes 13, 18, 21 and each sex chromosome. Primers used to copy each section of DNA are labelled with different coloured fluorescent tags of varying sizes. This allows molecular geneticists to determine which parts of the chromosomes are represented by each result and the amount of DNA can be measured.

The amount of fluorescence and size of the DNA that has been copied is measured, and ratios are presented on a graph. The number and height of each peak shows the number of copies of alleles at that region on the chromosome in the patient's DNA sample i.e. how many copies of the chromosomes are present.

Possible Outcomes from the QF-PCR Analysis

If two copies of the chromosomes are present there will either be two peaks of equal size or one peak.

If there are three copies of the chromosome (trisomy) there will be either three peaks or two peaks in a 2:1 ratio. If just one single large peak is seen it is not possible to tell if that single peak is indicating the presence of one chromosome, or two or three identical chromosomes.

The results are compared to maternal cells that act as a control sample.

There are risks associated with this procedure and they would be discussed prior to consenting. An experienced obstetrician would perform this procedure.

RISKS Associated with CVS [1]

Miscarriage

Overall, chorionic villus sampling carries between 1 and 2 % risk of pregnancy loss. The risk of miscarriage appears to be slightly higher when the tissue sample is taken through the cervix (trans-cervical) rather than the abdominal wall (trans-abdominal). There is also a slight increase in miscarriage risk if the foetus is smaller than normal for his or her gestational age.

Rh Sensitization

Chorionic villus sampling might cause some of the baby's blood cells to enter the mother's bloodstream. If the mother has Rh-negative blood and has not developed antibodies to Rh-positive blood, medication in the form of Rh immunoglobulin may be administered after the CVS test to prevent the mother from producing antibodies against the baby's blood cells. This can be monitored through a simple blood test which can detect if the mother begins to produce antibodies.

Infection

Chorionic villus sampling may trigger a uterine infection, although this is extremely rare.

Chorionic villus sampling is typically offered when the test results might have a significant impact on the management of a pregnancy. Ultimately, the decision to have chorionic villus sampling is up to the individual and couple and it is important to have full discussions with a specialist and genetic counsellor who can help explain the outcomes and offer support during the decision-making pre- and post-testing.

Amniocentesis

This test is carried out between 14 and 20 weeks of gestation (Fig. 23.3). Guided by ultrasound to locate the foetus, a thin needle is inserted through the abdomen into the amniotic sac and a small quantity (10 ml) of amniotic fluid is removed. Foetal cells are then isolated from the fluid and cultured for cytogenetic or molecular analysis. Routinely biochemical analysis involves testing levels of alpha foetal protein (AFP) produced by the liver. High levels indicate there may be hole or "leak" indicative of a neural tube defect or abdominal wall defect. Cell culture for cytogenetic chromosome ploidy analysis routinely takes approximately 2 weeks. Increasingly, molecular analysis for chromosome ploidy is the diagnostic test favoured by most laboratories as the results are accurate and cell culture is not so critical in this instance. Molecular analysis by qf-PCR can detect the major chromosomes. Molecular analysis of DNA and detection of the familial or known FBN1 mutation for Marfan syndrome can be determined at this stage.

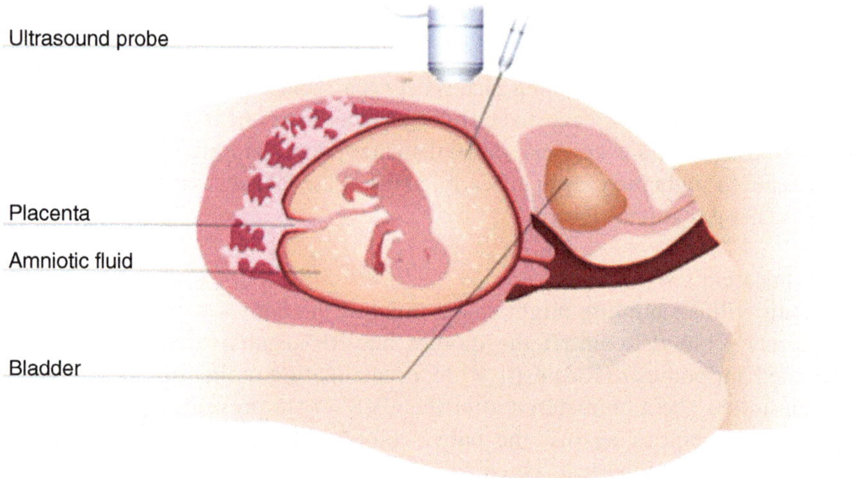

Fig. 23.3 Amniocentesis

RISKS Associated with Amniocentesis

Most women experience amniocentesis as painless, others may feel cramping when the needle enters the uterus, others describe a pressure when the amniotic fluid is extracted. The miscarriage rate is approximately 0.5–1 %, slightly lower than the CVS procedure. Some may experience cramping and spotting, and will be advised to rest and avoid intense activity for a day after. Serious complications are rare.

Choosing to have an amniocentesis is a measured and personal decision. It is important that individuals and couples are fully informed and understand the maternal age-related risk of chromosomal abnormality, and that an amniocentesis will reveal this in addition to the genetic mutation on FBN1 for Marfan syndrome. A discussion of the risk of maternal trisomies should take place pre-procedure, and support offered for decisions post procedure should be in place. Important decision-making regarding continuing or terminating a pregnancy at this stage would need to be carefully considered.

Preparing for the outcome of the test is important, and it is helpful to discuss this with a genetic counsellor or specialist health care practitioner. If the decision is made to proceed with the pregnancy, preparing for special needs, medication and support that the baby may need would be encouraged, to help parents plan for the birth.

Couples, individuals and families are encouraged to find out as much as possible about the types of prenatal testing that are available. Understanding the results, interpreting and supporting decision-making are essential, and health care professionals are available to facilitate this.

Next Generation Sequencing (NGS)

Next generation sequencing (NGS) is often referred to as massively parallel DNA sequencing, which means that millions of small fragments of DNA can be sequenced at the same time, creating a massive pool of data equivalent of one billion (1,000,000,000) base pairs of DNA. I n comparison, previous methods could sequence one DNA fragment at a time, perhaps generating 500–1000 base pairs of DNA in a single reaction.

Rapid sequencing of a whole gene or group of genes is now available and panels and assays have been developed for diagnostic use. Prenatal testing however is usually targeted as the mutation is known. NGS testing prenatally is currently not available in the UK but the guidelines are changing and this may be in use in the future. Seventy to ninety three percent of mutations in the FBN1 gene can be detected by NGS full gene sequencing so it is envisaged that confirmation of pathogenicity will increase.

Genetic laboratories are in the early stages of introducing NGS into service. The potential uses for this technology are far-reaching and need careful consideration. Traditional genetic testing involved the sequence analysis of a number of genes in a step-wise manner to try to identify where a genetic alteration might be. An example of this could be the genetic testing involved in cases of Marfan syndrome where FBN1 would be sequenced in the laboratory to look for genetic alterations in affected patients. Now panels are being developed to search for mutations in a number of aortic aneurysm genes.

NGS and Prenatal Diagnosis

This service is currently under development in the NHS in England with Great Ormond Street Hospital, London evaluating the procedure. A number of large teaching hospitals are in partnership with external diagnostic laboratories with a view to introducing the service into routine clinical practice.

Non-invasive Genetic Testing/Diagnosis (NIPT/NIPD)

A third option for diagnosing genetic conditions is non-invasive testing based on analysis of a maternal blood sample in the 10th week of pregnancy. At the time of writing NIPT is commercially available for aneuploidy screening in the private sector. NIPT and NIPD have been extensively evaluated by the prenatal diagnostic team at Great Ormond Street Hospital, London working on the RAPID project funded by the National Institute of Health Research (NIHR) for rollout into routine antenatal care across the NHS.

http://www.rapid.nhs.uk/about-rapid/background/

<u>NIPT/NIPD is available for</u>

1. Aneuploidy detection for chromosomes 21, 18 and 13, X and Y.
2. Foetal Sexing: at 10 weeks for pregnancies at risk of an X-linked serious genetic condition affecting boys.

3. Rhesus D factor
4. Foetal Genotyping e.g. Human Platelet Antibodies (HPA) and the Kell antigen blood group.
5. Single Gene Disorders: specifically mutations inherited from the father or certain *de novo* mutations e.g. fibroblast growth factor genes (FGFR) 1 and 2 mutations leading to skeletal dysplasias and Apert syndrome. The list of conditions currently tested is increasing.

How Does NIPT Work?

DNA cell fragments are always present in maternal blood, and during pregnancy approximately 10 % of these fragments are from the foetus arising as a result of apoptosis (cell death) from placental cells. This fraction is known as cell free foetal DNA (cffDNA) compared to the maternal fraction cfmDNA. The fragments are between 143 and 160 DNA base pairs in length. Amplification of these fragments using NGS or qfPCR and counting the number mapping to DNA sequences on a particular chromosome it is possible to detect when the amount of chromosome material is greater than expected. Increased amount of chromosome 21 would lead to a diagnosis of Down Syndrome. Accuracy levels vary depending on the test provider. Reported data indicates accuracy detection rates of 99 % for Downs and between 98 and 90 % for chromosomes 18 and 13 with a lower rate approximately 88 % for the X and Y aneuploidies. If a positive result is reported, a follow up amniocentesis is recommended to rule out confined placental mosaicism.

At the time of writing, testing is not currently available routinely for Marfan syndrome since there are no common mutations in the FBN1 gene. However if the FBN1 familial mutation is known it is possible to develop a unique prenatal test for NIPD. This work time up is approximately 8 weeks, so it is essential that the test is prepared prior to pregnancy (personal communication with Great Ormond Street, molecular diagnostics laboratory). Once the test is available, the turnaround time for a diagnostic result at 10 weeks of pregnancy is 5 days.

What is Required for NIPT/NIPD

An ultrasound scan is needed to confirm the exact number of weeks gestation, ensure the pregnancy is viable and whether it is a singleton or multiple pregnancy and 10–20 ml of maternal blood from a routine blood draw by a trained phlebotomist.

Benefits of NIPT/NIPD

The advantage of this option is that a definitive diagnosis can be made at an earlier stage in the pregnancy to facilitate decision-making. Women would have detailed counselling and discussions prior to testing and supported through the decision-making process post testing as for invasive prenatal testing. One of major advantages of NIPT/NIPD is the reduction of miscarriage risk.

The main limitation of NIPT/NIPD is that it is currently *not* possible to distinguish between DNA fragments in multiple pregnancies. There are reports in the literature that aneuploidy can be detected in twin pregnancies but this is not available through the NHS Rapid project. Follow up screening by CVS and/or amniocentesis would be recommended.

Depending on the local, regional and national restrictions in countries, the legal limit on termination of affected pregnancies would need to be observed. For some couples, termination of an affected pregnancy is not an option due to religious and culture beliefs. An alternative to prenatal diagnosis can be considered.

Preimplantation Genetic Diagnosis (PGD)

Preimplantation genetic diagnosis (PGD) [2] is often regarded as an alternative to prenatal diagnosis and the procedure is clinically well established. In the UK, the Human Fertilization and Embryology Authority (HFEA) is the government authority responsible for licensing, monitoring and regulating clinics performing In Vitro Fertilisation (IVF) and PGD. In order to perform PGD a licence must be granted by the HFEA and a licence allowing PGD for Marfan syndrome has been in place in the UK since 2010. The purpose of the PGD licence is to confirm that testing is appropriate and to ensure the service and test provided by the clinics and diagnostic laboratories are accurate and reliable.

PGD is performed by combining IVF treatment with genetic analysis on single cells removed from embryos to test for the presence of the specific genetic alteration prior to embryo transfer and implantation (Figs. 23.4 and 23.5). The aim of PGD is to reduce the risk of having a child with a genetic condition and prevent the condition being passed on in the family line. In the case of MFS, an autosomal dominant condition, the risk of transmission is reduced from 50 to <2 %. The oocytes (eggs) are retrieved following ovarian stimulation and are fertilised in the laboratory using either IVF or ICSI. Single cells are removed (biopsied) from each embryo at the cleavage stage (day 3 of embryo development) (Fig. 23.6). Increasingly, multiple cells (2 or 3) are biopsied at the blastocyst stage (day 5 or 6 of embryo development) Fig. 23.7. DNA from the biopsied cells are processed and analysed. Embryos diagnosed as unaffected and predicted to be free of MFS are transferred into the uterus (womb). Embryos diagnosed as affected are, with the couple's consent, humanely discarded.

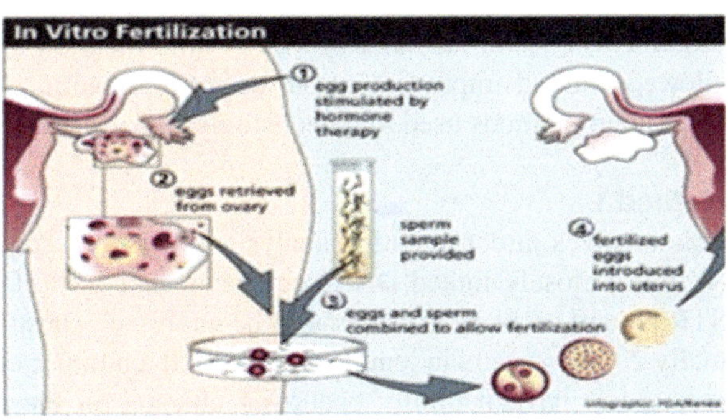

Fig. 23.4 IVF schematic. Four stages in IVF: (1) Superovulation, (2) egg retrieval, (3) fertilization/insemination, and (4) embryo transfer

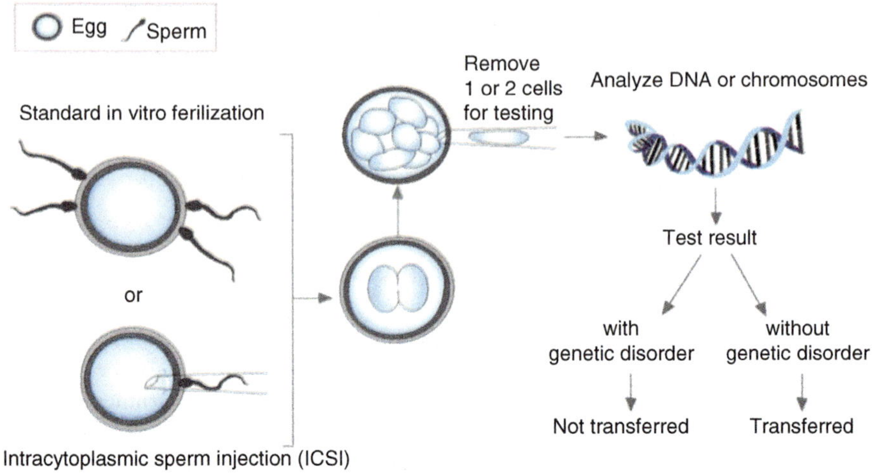

Fig. 23.5 PGD schematic

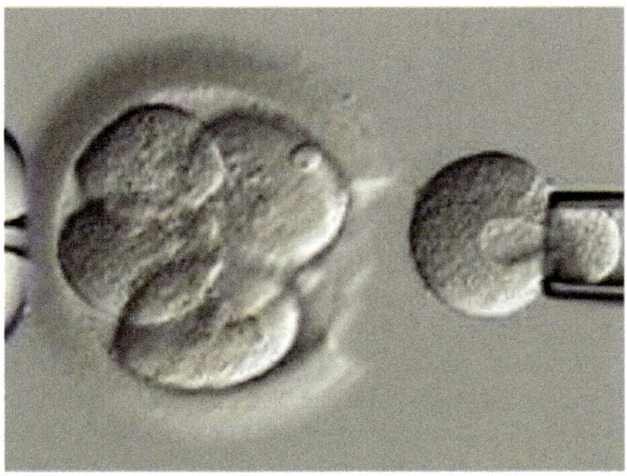

Fig. 23.6 Cleavage stage biopsy (day 3)
Single cell
Blastomeres
Fresh embryo transfer possible

Molecular Analysis Methods Used for PGD

Molecular techniques used to perform PGD have evolved since the first birth was described in 1990. Advances in DNA amplification and genetic sequencing have allowed marked improvements in detecting genetic changes. There are currently three main methods used to detect single gene disorders.

Method 1

This involves direct mutation analysis with fluorescent polymerase chain reaction (PCR) of closely linked DNA sequences called Short Tandem Repeat markers or STRs found on or near the gene to be analysed. These sequences of DNA are normally 2–5 base pairs in length and repeated a number of times. Within populations, individuals have naturally occurring changes in these STR sequences due to a

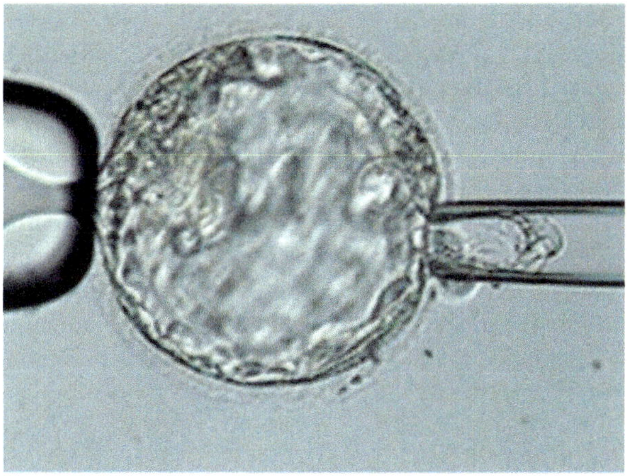

Fig. 23.7 Blastocyst biopsy (day 5 or 6) [3] Multiple cells Trophectoderm samples Embryo is vitrified post biopsy. Frozen embryo transfer

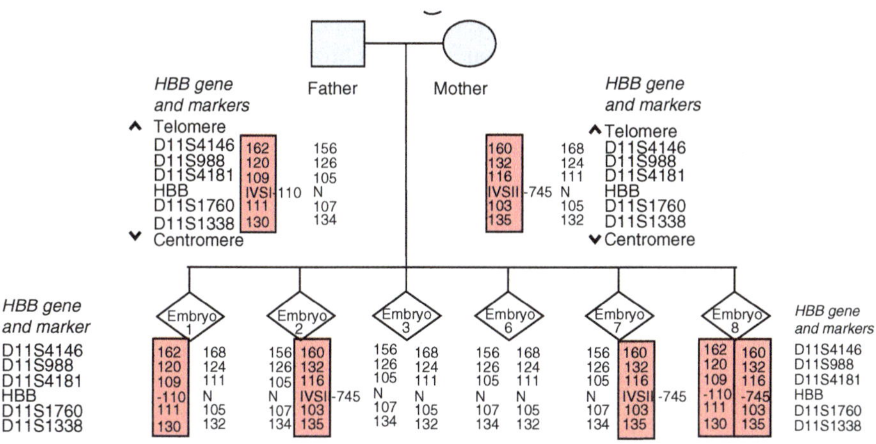

Fig. 23.8 Showing linked STRs to the HBB gene in an autosomal recessive inherited condition. Embryo 6 has inherited the mutation and the linked markers from the parents and is considered affected. Embryos 3 and 6 are mutation free and are unaffected and available for embryo transfer. Embryos 1, 2 and 7 are carriers like the parents and would also be available for embryo transfer

different number of copies of the repeat bases. These are known as naturally occurring "polymorphisms". By searching for specific STRs linked to the genetic mutation, the accuracy of detection of the mutation and therefore the diagnosis can be improved. The linked markers reduce the risk of misdiagnosis caused by a phenomenon known as allele dropout (ADO). ADO refers to the failed amplification of one of the two alleles (genes) which can potentially lead to a misdiagnosis. Figure 23.8 is a schematic of a number of linked markers linked to the HBB gene in a case of beta thalassemia, an autosomal recessive condition. Each parent is a carrier and has a different mutation on the gene. The homozygous affected embryo can be detected by analysing all the DNA sequences.

Method 2

Targeted haplotyping by multiplex PCR of STRs is a method involving linkage of genes [4]. The haplotype is created using a set of genetic markers near the gene and along the length of a chromosome. A haplotype can be visualised as sections along a chromosome with genes that are linked and therefore inherited together from one parent. The term "haplotype" can also refer to the inheritance of a cluster of single nucleotide polymorphisms (SNPs) that are variations at single positions in the DNA sequence among individuals. Developing a haplotype of genetic markers that have statistical associations to a target disease gene rather than identifying the mutation provides a diagnostic technique for analysing the inheritance of a mutated gene. This method is known as preimplantation genetic haplotyping (PGH).

Method 3

It is possible to perform genome wide individual haplotyping using high-density single nucleotide polymorphism (SNP) genotyping. Karyomapping [5] can be described as an extended form of haplotyping using SNP genotyping analysis to include the gene under investigation and all chromosomes in a biopsied cell. Karyomapping as a diagnostic technique can be considered a comprehensive method for linkage-based diagnosis of any single gene disorder. Genotyping of the parents and a close relative of known genetic disease status can be used to establish informative SNP loci and eliminates the need for lengthy customised PGD test development. The extensive coverage enabled by using SNPs across the whole genome and the complete set of chromosomes in a shorter time gives this technique greater diagnostic power for detecting the inheritance of specific altered genes and expands the test to include chromosomal aneuploidy.

All PGD tests are unique and specifically created for couples and can be time-consuming and labour intensive. The targeted approach using direct mutation analysis and haplotyping provides limited information on chromosome aneuploidy. This is clinically recognised to be a major cause of IVF failure and pregnancy loss. PGD by karyomapping or any enhanced SNP analysis is now becoming increasingly used by many clinics in the US and Europe offering PGD for single gene disorders.

How Does Karyomapping Work for Marfan Syndrome?

A blood sample is taken from the prospective parents (one of whom has a mutation in FBN1) and another relative who may or may not be affected by the condition and thus may or may not have a FNB1 mutation. In many cases the relative tested is a couple's child or another first degree relative of the affected parent. The relative is referred to as the "reference." If the mutation is de-novo in the parent, the reference can either be a parent or sibling of the affected individual and direct mutation analysis can be combined with genome wide SNP analysis to improve the accuracy of detection in the embryos. If there are no relatives available for reference DNA, embryos produced in the PGD cycle, can be used as the reference. Freezing embryos after biopsy will extend the analysis time in these cases.

By analysing SNPS on the chromosomes from biopsied cells and comparing the karyomaps with those of the parents and the reference case at approximately 300,000 different points it is possible to detect the key inheritance of the linked SNPS on the chromosome which carries the altered gene [6]. The karyomap can be described as a unique genetic profile. By developing this profile it is possible to test embryos. If detected it means the embryo has inherited the chromosome carrying the defective gene and in the case of Marfan syndrome would not be available for embryo transfer. Conversely, if the profile is *not* detected, it can be inferred that the embryo has inherited the unchanged copies of FBN1 and is predicted to be free of the disorder; these embryos are suitable for transfer. Figure 23.9 shows a complete karyomap profile.

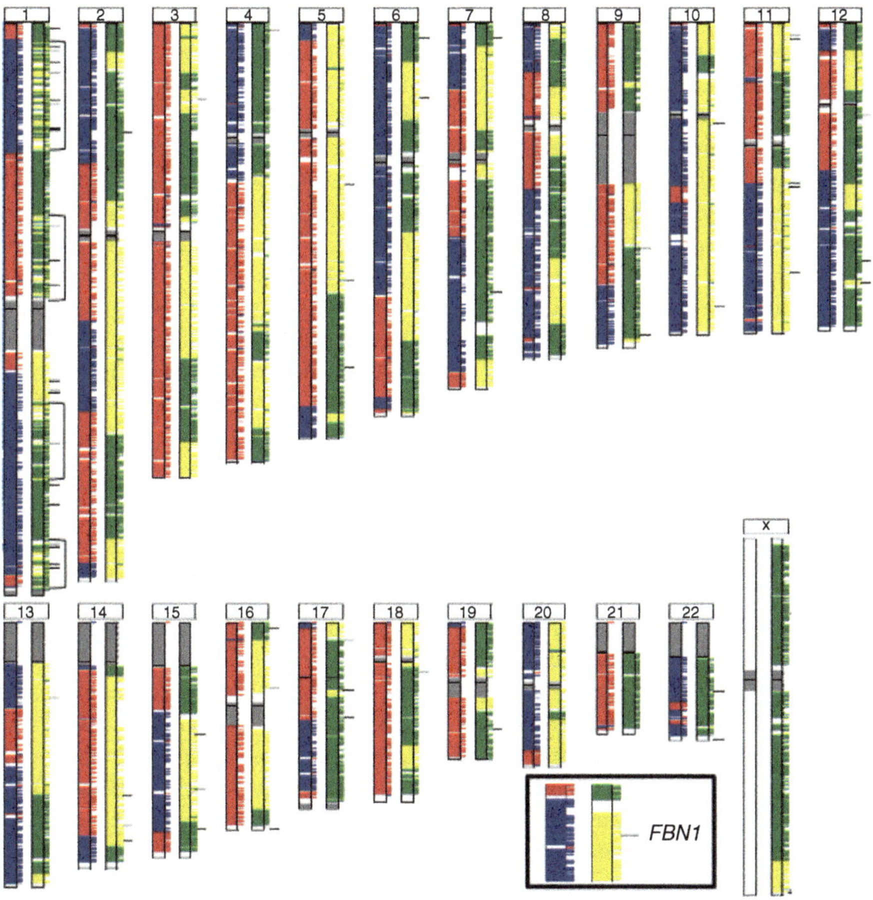

Fig. 23.9 Karyomap analysis one embryo. The *blue* and *red* chromosomes are paternal, the *green* and *yellow* chromosomes are maternal. The sample is showing a euploid karyomap, for a male (the Y chromosome is not evident in the image). The *grey images* are where the SNP amplification is scant. The *inset* is showing the FBN1 gene section on chromosome 15 [7]

Karyomapping Detect Chromosome Aneuploidies

Many embryos produced during IVF treatments are aneuploid. These embryos may succeed in implanting, but the pregnancy can often result in a miscarriage. More rarely, embryos with an abnormal number of chromosomes can lead to children affected by genetic conditions such as Down syndrome or the conditions associated with live birth. Karyomapping can detect most (although currently not all) aneuploid embryos, and can help select the embryo likely to result in a healthy pregnancy unaffected by MFS and aneuploidy. Transferring euploid unaffected embryos to the uterus reduces the chance of miscarriage and Down syndrome. This risk cannot be entirely eliminated hence prenatal diagnosis in addition for any pregnancy achieved by PGD is highly recommended for patients. This is an important consideration for couples prior to opting for this treatment as some may have very strong objections to PND and have opted for PGD accordingly.

Benefits of Karyomapping and Extended SNP Genotyping

SNP analysis decreases the time to develop a PGD test for a couple with a genetic mutation. Since the analysis is based on the inheritance of sections of DNA segregating with the altered gene, rather than the targeted mutation testing, the profile work up time is rapid and PGD tests can be ready within 2 weeks of DNA receipt. This compares favourably to standard direct mutation and linkage which take time to optimise and takes many months of labour intensive work before the test is released. Karyomapping can be used for single or multiple gene disorders. For example it is possible to test for the Human Leucocyte Antigen (HLA) panel in anaemias, especially sickle cell disease and beta thalassemias to detect a HLA matched unaffected embryo for use in sibling-to-sibling cord blood transfusions or bone marrow transplants to cure an affected child. Karyomapping is often referred to as a universal PGD test and increasingly many diagnostic laboratories are moving to these technologies in preference to the older techniques. There is flexibility to use direct mutation analysis with extensive SNP coverage so this diagnostic method is widely deployed.

Accuracy of PGD and the Need for Prenatal Testing PND

Whatever the diagnostic technique used for PGD, the test is performed on a single or couple of cells from an embryo. Any test carried out on such a small amount of material can never be 100 % accurate. In most cases, the chance of karyomapping successfully detecting an embryo affected by a specific inherited disorder is greater than 98 %, which is comparable to the other methods used for PGD. Because there is a small chance of an incorrect diagnosis after PGD, it is strongly recommended that prenatal testing (for example amniocentesis or chorionic villus sampling CVS) is used to confirm that any pregnancy achieved is unaffected. Amniocentesis and CVS techniques collect and culture thousands of cells from the foetus and can therefore provide an accurate result when checking for the FBN1 mutation and aneuploidy. It is foreseen that the option of mutation analysis at 10 weeks by NIPD will be recommended to reduce the miscarriage risk following PGD [7]. Like all tests involving analysis of embryos, PGD should be considered a risk-reducing method of avoiding an affected pregnancy, but not providing complete risk elimination [8]. The accuracy of karyomapping for the detection of chromosome abnormalities is not yet known, but it is thought the majority of aneuploidies are successfully detected and are currently being reported in clinical validation studies. At the time of writing, several ongoing trials validating karyomapping for aneuploidy detection are underway.

PGD can be stressful for some couples as there are many stages in the process and there are no guarantees that the treatment will result in a pregnancy. Couples are counselled and supported throughout the process by a team of professionals engaged in their treatment. Patients undergoing PGD treatment usually have no underlying infertility issues, hence the success rates are slightly higher for PGD compared to IVF treatment quoted for similar maternal ages.

Summary

To summarise, PGD is available for Marfan syndrome. The diagnostic method used to analyse embryos will depend on the number of DNA samples available and the service provided by the laboratory. For consanguineous cases, the number of informative STR markers can be limited, but with extensive coverage provided by SNP analysis, this is envisaged to provide a more accurate diagnostic technique. In summary the techniques described have evolved to provide improved SNP coverage, improved accuracy and shorter development time.

The following table compares the main PGD technologies

Analysis extent	Traditional mutation and STR	Haplotyping	Karyomapping
Number of linked markers	Min 3 to max 25 per locus	Min 3 to max 25 per locus	280 K genome wide coverage (130–600 for majority of Single Gene Disorders)
Number of Loci analysed	Single locus limit per STR set	Single locus with SNPS on single chromosomes or section	Multiple loci in parallel
Workup time	3–6 months	3–6 months	2–4 weeks
Linkage analysis	Manual	Manual	Software, bioinformatics assisted
Aneuploidy detection	Not part of analysis	Not part of analysis	Possible and validation underway

Haplotyping developed in-house is offered by Guy's and St Thomas' Hospital, London, UK, a major teaching hospital performing the majority of NHS PGD cases in the UK. Direct mutation analysis with linkage and karyomapping protocols are increasingly offered in the private sector performing PGD. The PGD consortium does not specify a preferred diagnostic method. The laboratories offering PGD must be CPA accredited (HFEA) in the UK. The ESHRE PGD Consortium regularly reviews and publishes guidelines for IVF centres and diagnostic laboratories offering this service

Natural Conception

Spontaneous pregnancy is an option available to all fertile couples. The decision whether to check the pregnancy for Marfan syndrome prior to birth is highly personal and depends on the individual or couple's cultural and religious beliefs. Some couples and families may have strong objections to terminating a pregnancy and may wish to proceed to term. Discussions with health care professionals would be encouraged to prepare for the outcome of a child with Marfan syndrome. Routine antenatal care and ultrasonography can be performed to check the development of the foetus and foetal heart in the first and second trimester. Due to the variability of the condition, it would not be possible to predict the severity of the condition in an affected pregnancy (although the parent's condition will give some indication). With this option, genetic testing is NOT offered during pregnancy.

Ultrasonography can detect the extremely rare congenital Marfan syndrome. In the event of a pregnancy being affected, the mother can prepare for the outcome with the relevant referrals to the specialist paediatric services so that monitoring and surveillance can be implemented shortly after birth following a clinical diagnosis. Support can be offered to these families through national Marfan syndrome support groups in their countries.

http://www.marfanworld.org/members.htm (and see Appendix 1).

Gamete (Egg or Sperm) Donation

http://www.dcnetwork.org/home

Deciding to use a gamete donor is a very personal decision and often reached after speaking with many health care professionals and agencies involved in providing gamete donation programmes.

The donor conception network in the UK has a wealth of information for prospective recipients and is recommended for any patient considering this option. One of the major changes in the last few years is the introduction of non-anonymity for donors in the UK, such that a donor-conceived child at the age of 18 can contact their genetic parent. The register is maintained by HFEA.

A couple may choose to use a known or anonymous egg or sperm donor. Gamete donors are routinely screened and offered appropriate genetic testing and screening. For information on gamete donation see:

1. National Gamete Donation Trust
   http://www.ngdt.co.uk.
2. Human Fertilisation Embryology Association (HFEA)
   http://www.hfea.gov.uk/egg-and-sperm-donors.html
3. Donor Conception Network UK: supporting families
   http://www.dcnetwork.org

Individual countries will have legislation and regulations in place if gamete donation is offered. Specific recommendations are made. This is a list of recommendations in Europe and America and emerging initiatives in Australia. Where gamete donation is not allowed, this can promote the trend of reproductive tourism, where individuals and couples will travel for treatment.

American Society of Reproductive Medicine (ASRM)
https://www.asrm.org/
European Society of Human Reproduction and Embryology
http://www.eshre.eu
Australia: an example of emerging regulations in New South Wales
http://www.health.nsw.gov.au/art/pages/default.aspx

Adoption

Adoption is a way of providing a permanent home and family to a child who is unable to be raised by their birth family. It is an alternative method of parenting. Today, the majority of adoptions in the UK involve older children, sibling groups and children with disabilities, who have been taken into care. Adoption can help to transform the lives of some of the most vulnerable children in society. The following aspects should be taken into consideration:

Parents with a genetic condition wishing to adopt a child: The adoption agency is responsible for making an assessment in the best interests of a child, therefore the genetic condition, prognosis, effect on the long term health of the parent(s) should all be factored into the decision on both sides. It is important that the prospective parent understands that they will be assessed for their suitability as adoptees in the light of the information about their condition. This can be difficult for parents who have decided on adoption as they are not willing to have a child at risk of a serious genetic condition, only to feel they are disadvantaged again in terms of the possibility of being rejected.

Adopting a child with a genetic condition: The parents must be given full, accurate and appropriate information about the effects of the condition and the prognosis for the child in order to ensure that adequate provision is made for the child.

The following links are available:

Government
https://www.gov.uk/child-adoption
Adoption UK
http://www.adoptionuk.org

Adoption and Fostering
http://www.baaf.org.uk/info/adoption
Inter-country adoption
http://pactcharity.org/adoption/intercountry-adoption

Each country will have legislation and regulations governing adoption so it is important to thoroughly research this option with independent agencies.

References

1. Clarke A, editor. Genetic Counselling: Practice and Principles. Routledge ISBN 0-415-08258-7
2. Handyside AH, Kontogianni EH, Hardy K, Winston RML. Pregnancies from biopsied human preimplantation embryos sexed by Y-specific DNA amplification. Nature. 1990;344:768–70.
3. Fiorentino F, Kahraman S, Karadayi H, et al. Short tandem repeats haplotyping of the HLA region in preimplantation HLA matching. Eur J Hum Genet. 2005;13:953–8.
4. Renwick P, Trussler J, Lashwood A, et al. Preimplantation genetic haplotyping: 127 diagnostic cycles demonstrating a robust, efficient alternative to direct mutation testing on single cells. Reprod Biomed Online. 2010;20:470–6.
5. Handyside AH, Thornhill AR, Ottolini C, Sage K, et al. Live birth by preimplantation genetic diagnosis following validation of a universal approach (Karyomapping) for simultaneous detection of monogenic and chromosomal disorders. Reprod Biomed Online. 2014. http://dx.doi.org/10.1016/j.rbmo.2014.07.007.
6. Thornhill AR, Handyside AH, Ottolini C, Taylor J, Sage K, et al. Comparison of targeted haplotype and mutation analysis with SNP genotyping and karyomapping in single cells for preimplantation genetic diagnosis of Marfan syndrome. J Assist Reprod Genet. 2015;32:347–56. doi:10.1007/s10815-014-0405-y.
7. Bustamante-Aragones A, Perlado-Marina S, Trujillo-Tiebas MJ, et al. Non-invasive prenatal diagnosis in the management of preimplantation genetic diagnosis pregnancies. J Clin Med. 2014;3:913–22. doi:10.3390/jcm3030913.
8. Harton GL, De Rycke M, Fiorentino F, et al. European Society for Human Reproduction and Embryology (ESHRE) PGD Consortium best practice guidelines for amplification-based PGD. Hum Reprod. 2011;26(1):33–40. doi:10.1093/humrep/deq231. Epub 2010.

Exercise in Marfan Syndrome

24

Bethan Davies and Anne H. Child

Introduction

For people with Marfan syndrome, certain activities are thought to increase the risk of some of the serious complications ([1]–[3]). In addition, some of the physical manifestations of Marfan syndrome may limit the person's ability to fully participate in exercise [4]. For example, those with eye problems such as dislocated lenses or severe myopia, may have difficulty playing sports involving hand-eye coordination, such as racquet sports. People with Marfan syndrome are affected in different ways, so what is suitable for one person may not be for another.

Diagnosis

Diagnosis is made after careful physical examination and echocardiography [5, 6], demonstrating classical features in two out of three major systems (eyes, heart, skeleton), supported by a family history in 75 % of cases [7]. There are many genes which can cause familial thoracic aortic aneurysm and dissection (FTAAD) [8]. If no genetic cause can be found, and aortic measurements are just outside the normal upper limits and are non-progressive, the athlete may be allowed to continue sporting activity with continual echo surveillance.

B. Davies, MBBS
Royal Sussex County Hospital, Brighton, UK
e-mail: bethanldavies@doctors.org.uk

A.H. Child, MD, FRCP (✉)
Cardiovascular and Cell Sciences Research Institute, St George's, University of London, London, UK
e-mail: achild@sgul.ac.uk

© Springer-Verlag London 2016

A.H. Child (ed.), *Diagnosis and Management of Marfan Syndrome*,
DOI 10.1007/978-1-4471-5442-6_24

Mutations can be found in the fibrillin-1 gene in 97 % of Marfan syndrome patients, assisting with screening of family members, and pregnancies [9].

Cardiac Problems

The most serious problems occur in the heart and blood vessels [10]. The aorta is usually wider than expected for a given body surface area and is more fragile due to deficiency in the amount of fibrillin-1 present. The dilatation tends to be progressive leading to aortic dissection with or without aortic regurgitation. Surgical repair is recommended when the aortic root becomes widened to 4.8 cm, or earlier in cases with a family history of early dissection. Beta-blocker therapy can delay dilatation. Mitral valve prolapse is also often present. Antibiotic prophylaxis is recommended for dental procedures involving bleeding, if a heart valve is leaking sufficiently to produce an audible heart murmur, or if a heart valve has been replaced.

Guidelines

In general, most people living with Marfan syndrome should exercise regularly through low-intensity, low-impact activities adapted to meet their specific needs. They should avoid contact sports because of the risk of damaging the aorta or loose ligaments and joints [13], and injuring the eyes [14]. Strenuous activities, such as competitive sports and weightlifting, also should be avoided because of the stress placed on the aorta.

The Marfan Association (UK) www.marfan.org.uk and the National Marfan Foundation (USA) www.marfan.org provide guidelines on what exercise is suitable for people with Marfan syndrome, and which activities are best avoided [15]. There is currently very limited evidence base for how exercise affects people with Marfan syndrome ([16], [17]) and therefore the advice given should be based on the guidelines issued by the Marfan Association and the National Marfan Foundation.

Recommended:- (Not high level competition)		
Archery	Cycling (on the level)	Hockey
Shotput	Badminton	Discus
Javelin	Skating	Bowls
Fencing	Netball	Swimming
Canoeing	Football (no heading)	Racketball
Table tennis	Cricket	Golf
Sailing	Tennis	Yoga
Walking/jog-walking	Dancing	Light weight-lifting

Please remember each patient is affected differently and our general recommendations need to be discussed with the patient's own medical attendants and parents. Children should be allowed to stop when tired.

Contraindicated- (To prevent damage to: E=Eye; H=Heart; J=Joints; L=Lungs)			
Boxing	(E)	High altitude mountaineering	(L)
Rugby	(H, J)	Trampolining	(J)
Deep sea diving	(L)	High diving	(E)
Rowing	(H, J)	Weight-lifting	(H, J)
Distance running	(H, J)	Karate/judo	(H, J)
Sky-diving	(L)	Wrestling	(H, J)
Hang gliding	(L)	*Squash	(E, H)

*See below

Heavy lifting is not advised (**H**).

- Basketball should be discussed with patient's doctor. If played as a contact sport, it can lead to repeated falls (**H**).
- Horse riding on a quiet horse is best. Jumping may cause falls (**H**, **J**).
- Squash (**E**, **H**) – For those who do not have heart problems, squash can be played wearing goggles, to protect the eyes.
- Participating in **Aerobics** (**H**, **J**) and **Abseiling** (**J**) should be governed by the patient's limitations.
- Prolonged exertion at peak capacity should be avoided. In the gym; short stints in a number of activities is recommended.

For children, alternative activities could include swimming in the school pool, to be undertaken at the same time as the peer group is performing more stressful PE activities. If that is impossible then the child should be given a task, with the necessary instruction to enable the child to complete it competently, such as refereeing which gives them a position of importance without being involved in the physical activity. Some children are given an individual fitness routine to work through in the corner of the gym.

Medication Impact on Physical Activity

Many people with Marfan syndrome take a beta-blocker medication to reduce stress on the aorta. This medication lowers the pulse at rest and during exercise and makes it somewhat more difficult to achieve a given level of physical fitness for the amount of physical work performed. They do not, however, enable a person with Marfan syndrome or other aortic aneurysm syndrome to perform very strenuous exercises or play contact sports. Some patients with Marfan syndrome take medications called angiotensin blockers (like losartan) or angiotensin converting enzyme inhibitors. These medications do not protect the aorta from strenuous exercise.

People who have artificial heart valves usually take an anticoagulant medication, warfarin (Coumadin ®). This medication interferes with blood clotting and increases the chances of bruising and internal haemorrhages. People taking this medication should avoid contact sports and any activity with a moderate risk of a blow to the head or abdomen.

FINAL ADVICE SHOULD COME FROM THE PATIENT'S OWN DOCTOR.

The Problems Encountered by Patients

In a survey of the exercise habits of 70 UK patients aged between 18 and 65 with Marfan syndrome, the following results emerged:-

- 72 % said that their exercise habits had been affected by having Marfan syndrome.
- The reasons for this were (most common first) joint pain, shortness of breath, medical advice, fatigue, palpitations, dislike of exercise, and overheating.
- By far the most popular exercise activity was walking, followed by gym, swimming, jogging, cycling and yoga/pilates. Only a handful of people participated in activities that are considered to be unsuitable (long distance running, heavy weight-lifting).
- Only 44 % of people had received information about exercise.
- Of these, the most common source of information was hospital consultant, followed by the Marfan Association, family physician, the internet and occupational therapists/physiotherapists.
- The advice given seems to have corresponded with the published guidelines.
- 17 % said that they had received conflicting advice.
- Of the 25 people who had cardiac surgery, only 13 had been offered subsequent rehabilitation. Of these, 9 took up the offer and in only 4 cases was the person in charge of the programme definitely aware of Marfan syndrome.
- A number of those engaging in rehabilitation programmes found that it was not tailored to their needs, but to the needs of an older population with different conditions (e.g. coronary artery disease).
- Many people commented that although they had been given general exercise advice, they were still unclear about what is actually meant in practice. In addition, they often found that doctors, other healthcare professionals and employees of gyms/fitness centres were not able to give accurate and appropriate advice.
- Worryingly, 2 people had been turned away from gyms once they disclosed that they had Marfan syndrome. A letter from the doctor to the gym instructor indicating suitable sports is therefore recommended.

- Some found the exercise advice frustrating and demoralising; for those who were keen to improve their fitness, positive suggestions on how to achieve this were limited – much of the advice focussed on what not to do.
- A number of people commented on their negative experiences of sport at school and the distress at being told that they could no longer do their favourite sport or compete. Tapering unsuitable sports such as long distance running, and gradually replacing them with more suitable sports such as jog-walking is recommended.

Who Should Be Aware

Hospital doctors, family physicians, physiotherapists, physical education teachers, sports coaches and those working in the fitness industry should be aware of the nature of Marfan syndrome and how it relates to exercise ability. A letter from the hospital doctor to a physical education teacher or other supervisor of exercise programme is helpful.

What Advice Is Needed

- A system should be in place to ensure that all people with Marfan syndrome receive information about exercise as soon as possible after diagnosis.
- Patients should be encouraged to exercise as much as possible within their capabilities in order to improve and maintain their general health.
- When giving advice to patients, the advice should be tailored to the needs of the individual, taking into account how they are affected by Marfan syndrome, their age and their general health.
- Patients need more than a couple of activity suggestions (such as walking and swimming). They need to know what level they should exercise at, how long and how often to exercise and, especially for those keen to maximise their fitness, practical suggestions on how this can be achieved. Where possible, the patient's own preferences of sporting and exercise activities should be accommodated.
- For those who are involved in exercise considered to be a risk to their health, the advice should be to taper down the activity over a period of time, rather than stopping it suddenly. This is more acceptable to the patient and gives time to develop an interest in an alternative sport.
- As a general rule, the patient should be able to converse while exercising.

After Surgery

Following heart surgery, the patient should be offered a cardiac rehabilitation programme suitable to their needs and age.

Other Aortopathies

The younger a patient is at the time of discovery of ascending aortic aneurysm or actual dissection, the more likely it is that there is an underlying genetic predisposition. Also, a positive family history for TAAD signals an increased risk. Each offspring of an affected parent has up to 50 % risk of also developing an aortic aneurysm, at approximately the same age. There are many predisposing dominantly inherited genes reported [8] and the list is growing annually. Some have associated phenotypic features; many do not (see Table 24.1).

Table 24.1 Genotype-phenotype correlation of selected genetic mutations involved in FTAAD

Gene (protein)	Phenotypic characteristics	Pathway
Extracellular matrix protein		
FBN1 (fibrillin-1)	MFS; highly penetrant ascending aortic aneurysm; ectopia lentis; scoliosis; dolichostenomelia (marfanoid habitus)	TGF-β
COL 3 A1[collagen α-1(III)]	EDS type 4; arterial dissection with infrequent aneurysm; thin skin; large eyes; beaked nose; thin lips, lobeless ears; acrogeria (aged appearance extremities)	Collagen Metabolism
Transmembrane protein		
TGFBR1 (TGF-β receptor type 1)	LDS; TAAD with other arterial involvement (cerebral, carotid, abdominal) marfanoid but no ocular disease; early age of onset (30s). bifid uvula; hypertelorism; craniosynostosis; congenital heart defects; mental retardation	TGF-β
TGFBR2 (TGF-β receptor type 2)	LDS; TAAD with marfanoid appearance; cerebral artery involvement; onset 40s; dissection at low aortic root diameter. Operate by 4.5 cm	TGF-β
Cytoplasmic protein		
SMAD3 (SMAD family member 3)	LDS; TAAD with osteoarthritis (AOS). Risk of involvement of cerebral arteries, entire aorta extending into iliac arteries	TGF-β

Table 24.1 (continued)

Gene (protein)	Phenotypic characteristics	Pathway
ACTA2 (α-smooth muscle actin)	Association with PDA, BAV, early coronary artery disease and stroke; livedo reticularis, iris flocculi. smooth muscle cell dysfunction leads to gut immobility, pulmonary hypertension	IGF-1, Ang II
MYH11 (smooth muscle myosin)	Association with PDA	IGF-1, Ang II

FTAAD familial thoracic aortic aneurysm and dissection, *TGF-β* transforming growth factor beta, *EDS* Ehlers-Danlos syndrome, *TGFBR1* transforming growth factor beta receptor type 1, *LDS* Loeys-Dietz syndrome, *TGFBR2* transforming growth factor beta receptor type 2, *SMAD3* Mothers against decapentaplegic homolog 3, *ACTA2* alpha-smooth muscle actin, *PDA* patent ductus arteriosus, *BAV* bicuspid aortic valve, *IGF-1* insulin-like growth factor 1, *Ang II* angiotensin II, *MYH11* myosin heavy chain 11

An athlete with ascending aortic dimension equal to or greater than 4.0 cm, no matter how tall should be referred to a cardiovascular genetic screening clinic, where family history will be taken, snapshots of affected family members reviewed for phenotypic features such as height, body build, factual features, joint hypermobility, and careful past medical history taken and physical examination performed. If increased risk is confirmed, a 5 ml EDTA blood sample should be taken for TAAD gene screen or exome sequencing to study reported causative genes, and search for unidentified genes. The athlete should have three consecutive annual echocardiograms to assess progression. If this is shown, the patient should be placed on medication such as beta-blocker or irbesartan, and referred for elective aortic root surgery between aortic root diameters 4.5 and 4.8 cm, depending on the gene and the family history.

First degree relatives (siblings, parents and offspring) should also be screened by echocardiogram. Such athletes should not be allowed to compete at high level, and advised to limit sporting activities to moderate exercise in order to keep fit.

An affected patient should be counselled that there may be up to 50 % risk of genetic predisposition to aortic aneurysm, for each offspring, regardless of sex.

Summary

Each patient with Marfan syndrome or other genetic aortopathy is unique, and the systems affected are determined by how the genotype (gene mutation) affects the phenotype (body build). Frank dialogue between physician, patient and coach will determine what level of suitable sporting activity will maintain fitness without jeopardising future health. Competitive sport at high level involving prolonged exertion at peak capacity should be discouraged unless the individual is mildly affected and is kept under careful, regular echocardiographic surveillance.

References

1. Abid N, Davies K, Grahame R, Woo P, Murray KJ. Joint hypermobility syndrome in childhood. A not so benign multisystem disorder? Rheumatology (Oxford). 2005;44(6):744–50. Epub 2005 Feb 22.
2. Yim ES. Aortic root disease in athletes: aortic root dilation, anomalous coronary artery, bicuspid aortic valve, and Marfan's syndrome. Sports Med. 2013;43(8):721–32. doi:10.1007/s40279-013-0057-6.
3. Maron BJ, Chaitman BR, Ackerman MJ, Bayés de Luna A, Corrado D, Crosson JE, Deal BJ, Driscoll DJ, Estes 3rd NA, Araújo CG, Liang DH, Mitten MJ, Myerburg RJ, Pelliccia A, Thompson PD, Towbin JA, Van Camp SP, Working Groups of the American Heart Association Committee on Exercise, Cardiac Rehabilitation, and Prevention, Councils on Clinical Cardiology and Cardiovascular Disease in the Young. Recommendations for physical activity and recreational sports participation for young patients with genetic cardiovascular diseases. Circulation. 2004;109(22):2807–16. Review.
4. Crilley JG, Bendahan D, Boehm EA, Styles P, Rajagopalan B, Wordsworth P, Clarke K. Investigation of muscle bioenergetics in the Marfan syndrome indicates reduced metabolic efficiency. J Cardiovasc Magn Reson. 2007;9(4):709–17.
5. Dean JC. Marfan syndrome: clinical diagnosis and management. Eur J Hum Genet. 2007;15(7):724–33. Epub 2007 May 9. Review.
6. Stout M. The Marfan syndrome: implications for athletes and their echocardiographic assessment. Echocardiography. 2009;26(9):1075–81. doi:10.1111/j.1540-8175.2009.00945.x. Review.
7. Loeys BL, Dietz HC, Braverman AC, Callewaert BL, De Backer J, Devereux RB, Hilhorst-Hofstee Y, Jondeau G, Faivre L, Milewicz DM, Pyeritz RE, Sponseller PD, Wordsworth P, De Paepe AM. The revised Ghent nosology for the Marfan syndrome. J Med Genet. 2010;47(7):476–85. doi:10.1136/jmg.2009.072785.
8. Milewicz DM. In: Regalado E, Pagon RA, Adam MP, Ardinger HH, Bird TD, Dolan CR, Fong CT, Smith RJH, Stephens K, editors. GeneReviews® [Internet]. Thoracic aortic aneurysms and aortic dissections. Seattle: University of Washington; 1993–2014. 2003 [updated 2012 Jan 12]. www.ncbi.nlm.nih.gov/books/NBK1120/
9. Faivre L, Collod-Beroud G, Child AH, Callewaert B, Loeys BL, Binquet C, Gautier E, Arbustini E, Mayer K, Arslan-Kirchner M, Stheneur C, Kiotsekoglou A, Comeglio P, Marziliano N, Halliday D, Beroud C, Bonithon-Kopp C, Claustres M, Plauchu H, Robinson PN, Ades L, De Backer J, Coucke P, Francke U, De Paepe A, Boileau C, Jondeau G. Contribution of molecular analyses in diagnosing Marfan syndrome and type I fibrillinopathies: an international study of 1009 probands. J Med Genet. 2008;45(6):383–90.
10. Dietz HC. In: Pagon RA, Adam MP, Ardinger HH, Bird TD, Dolan CR, Fong CT, Smith RJH, Stephens K, editors. GeneReviews® [Internet]. Marfan syndrome. Seattle: University of Washington; 1993–2014. 2001 [updated 2014 June 12]. www.ncbi.nlm.nih.gov/books/NBK1335/
11. Crosher R, Holmes A. Marfan syndrome: dental problems and management. Dent Update. 1988;15(3):120–2.
12. Braverman AC. Exercise and the Marfan syndrome. Med Sci Sports Exerc. 1998;30(10 Suppl):S387–95. Review.
13. Jones KB, Sponsellor PD, Erkula G, Sakai L, Ramirez F, Dietz 3rd HC, Kost-Byerly S, Bridwell KH, Sandell L. Symposium on the musculoskeletal aspects of Marfan syndrome: meeting report and state of the science. J Orthop Res. 2007;25(3):413–22.
14. Loewenstein A, Barquet IS, De Juan Jr E, Maumenee IH. Retinal detachment in Marfan syndrome. Retina. 2000;20(4):358–63.
15. Boodhwani M, Andelfinger G, Leipsic J, Lindsay T, McMurthy MS, Therrien J, Siu SC. Canadian Cardiovascular Society position statement on the management of thoracic aortic

disease. Canadian Cardiovascular Society. Can J Cardiol. 2014;30(6):577–89. doi:10.1016/j.cjca.2014.02.018. Epub 2014 Feb 28. Review.
16. Peres P, Bernardelli GF, Mendes CC, Fischer SS, Servantes DM, Medeiros WM, Carvalho AC. Immediate effects of submaximal effort on pulse wave velocity in patients with Marfan syndrome. Braz J Med Biol Res. 2010;43(4):397–402. doi:10.1590/S0100-879X2010007500021. Epub 2010 Mar 19.
17. Giske L, Stanghelle JK, Rand-Hendrikssen S, Strøm V, Wilhelmsen JE, Røe C. Pulmonary function, working capacity and strength in young adults with Marfan syndrome. J Rehabil Med. 2003;35(5):221–8.

Ageing in Marfan Syndrome 25

Ali Hasan, J. Poloniecki, and Anne H. Child

Prior to the use of life-saving cardiac surgery in the mid-twentieth century, Marfan syndrome (MFS) with cardiac involvement resulted in a shortened life span, with an average age of death of 32 years and a median probability of 48 years [1]. More recently, surveys have been aimed at describing the complications, including those affecting the eyes, heart, and musculoskeletal system, faced by older survivors.

UK Survey

All 2500 patient records from the national Marfan syndrome clinical database were reviewed to identify suitable participants aged 50 or over. Of 156 postal questionnaires 60 were returned, comprised of 28 female patients and 32 male patients with a median age of 57 years. Control data were provided from a second questionnaire sent to each participant, to be completed by an age and sex matched unrelated subject. Fifty-six eligible controls were recruited. Results revealed that these patients provide an early aging model, specifically with a higher risk than previously reported for retinal detachment and arrhythmia. Interestingly, cataract was reported by 27 %.

A. Hasan, MBBS, FRCS
FRCS Clinical Operations Director, Vitality UK, London, UK

J. Poloniecki, MSc, DPhil
Population Health Research Institute, St George's, University of London, London, UK
e-mail: sggp300@sgul.ac.uk

A.H. Child, MD, FRCP (✉)
Cardiovascular and Cell Sciences Research Institute, St George's, University of London, London, UK
e-mail: achild@sgul.ac.uk

© Springer-Verlag London 2016

A.H. Child (ed.), *Diagnosis and Management of Marfan Syndrome*,
DOI 10.1007/978-1-4471-5442-6_25

Life Expectancy

Murdoch et al. 1972 [1] and Silverman et al. 1995 [2] stated the median probabilities of survival were 47 and 72 years respectively. Modern medicine and surgery have significantly increased the life span of patients with Marfan syndrome [2]. Gray et al. 1998 performed a study in Wales and Scotland and found the median survival to be 53 for male patients and 72 years for female patients [3]. For patients who have had one aortic aneurysm repair, Finkbohner et al. quoted a median life expectancy of 61 years [4]. These figures are still noticeably lower than the average life expectancy of 76 years in men and 81 years in women in the UK [5].

Ocular Features

We found that only 27 % of the MFS responders did not suffer eye problems, as opposed to 80 % of controls (significantly different $P < 0.0000001$). Thirteen MFS patients (22 %) experienced both retinal detachment and dislocated lenses in their lifetimes. Cataract was reported by 27 % of MFS patients, significantly higher than the incidence in controls (9 %) ($P = 0.015$).

Cardiac Features

Forty-six percent of patients had aortic surgery, and of those 20 % had aortic root repair and 25 % had aortic valve and root replacement. These differences were all highly significantly different from the control population, however the figures for mitral valve repair (3 %) and mitral valve replacement (5 %) were not significantly different from the control population. Fifty-three percent of patients reported arrhythmia as opposed to 21 % of controls ($P = 0.00053$) with 26 % of the patient group taking medication for arrhythmia as opposed to 5 % in the control group ($P = 0.025$).

Musculoskeletal Symptoms

Women with MFS reported painful joints more frequently than men (64 % vs. 34 %; significantly different, $P = 0.02$). The incidence of scoliosis/kyphosis was 29 % which is somewhat lower than other studies in the literatures (see Table 25.1). There were significant differences between MFS patients and controls in prevalence of pectus excavatum (18 % in MFS, $P = 0.017$), Pectus carinatum (29 %, $P = 0.000004$) and scoliosis/kyphosis ($P = 0.000004$). Thirty percent (18 out of 60) of patients with MFS were affected by either rheumatoid arthritis or osteoarthritis.

Table 25.1 Prevalence of spinal and chest wall abnormalities reported by patients with MFS and controls, compared with other groups' findings

	Our Study Population	Our Controls	Pyeritz and McKusick (1979) [6]	Roman et al. (1989) [7]	Finkbohner et al. (1995) [4]	Grahame and Pyeritz (1995) [8]	Rossi-Foulkes 1999 [9]	Joseph et al. (1992) [10]	Hobbs et al. (1997)[a] [11]	Lipscomb et al. (1997) [12]
Population	50 selected from UK National MFS database	57 as described above	50 consecutive patients seen in the USA with MFS (Age not available)	59 patients with MFS already recruited into other prospective studies in the USA (age 7–68 years; mean age 29 years)	192 patients having aortic aneurysm repair in the USA (age unavailable)	27 children (age 2–17 years; median age 9 years) and 48 adults (age 18–76 years; median age of 36) randomly selected from outpatients In the USA	53 children of average age 9.4 years	36 paediatric patients including 18 definite, nine probable MFS and nine marfanoid (multiple minor signs)	104 unselected patients at genetic appointment follow-up	40 children from a regional register of MFS, UK
Scoliosis/kyphosis	29 %	0 %	44 %	61 % (scoliosis alone)	49 %	78 % of children 47 % of adults	55 %	'Almost all'	See below	68 %
Pectus carinatum	29 %	0 %	68 % reported to have either type	24 %	58 % reported to have either type	N/A	38 %	N/A	N/A	43 %
Pectus excavatum	18 %	4 %		49 %		N/A	40 %	N/A	N/A	35 %

[a]Hobbs et al. (1997) found 16 % of patients had focal cervical kyphosis, with 90 % having a cervical kyphosis above 20°

Other Features

Varicose veins were more common in female patients with MFS than male patients with MFS (82 % vs. 25 %, $P < 0.01$). Hernia was more common in male patients than female patients (44 % vs 11 %, $P < 0.01$).

Genitourinary Features

Urinary frequency and nocturia, symptoms commonly occurring with age, are reported significantly more frequently in patients with MFS than controls.

Mental Health

Twenty percent of patients with MFS reported suffering depression, with onset commencing from puberty to 53 years. Depression was reported in 2 males (6 % of all males) and 6 females (21 % of all females). None were currently on anti-depressant medication. Of these patients, two had counselling, one had psychotherapy and one, medication for anxiety. Two controls, both male, noted depression commencing at age 61. The difference in prevalence of depression was significantly greater in female subjects with MFS, compared with controls ($P = 0.024$).

Medication

Eighty-two percent of MFS respondents were on regular medication. Of these, 65 % were on three of more regular medications. Fifty-eight percent were taking anti-hypertensive medication. Sixty-three percent of controls were on regular medication, with 26 % on three or more (significantly different from the MFS group, $P = 0.00004$). Twenty-nine percent of control subjects were on anti-hypertensive medication.

Alternative Therapy

Twenty-two percent of patients with MFS reported using at least one type of alternative therapy, e.g. acupuncture or homeopathy. In comparison, 13 % of controls reported use of alternative therapy.

Discussion

This study had a response rate of 35 %, however further studies of a similar nature should refine our findings.

Musculoskeletal Features

Musculoskeletal problems are extremely common in Marfan syndrome and can be very detrimental to patient quality of life. Only 23 % of patients did not suffer musculoskeletal symptoms. A high proportion of MFS patients suffer from muscle weakness and easy fatigability, from a relatively young age. In a MFS patient group investigated by Grahame and Pyeritz, only 2 out of 48 adults aged 18–76 had never experienced locomotive symptoms. This study mentioned that 69 % reported spine pain, and 58 % had arthralgia [8].

There is a high prevalence of claw toes/hammer toes (more common in MFS men in outpatient population) and flat feet in patients with MFS when compared with controls. Joseph et al. also described a variety of foot problems in MFS [10]. Grahame and Pyeritz found that 44 % of 48 MFS patients had experienced ligament injury: 19 % of our respondents reported torn ligaments or tendons, three times more than our controls, ($P = 0.044$).

Employment, Rehabilitation and Exercise Recommendations

Those with MFS should avoid lifting heavy weights, and great physical exertion at peak capacity, which may have deleterious effects on their cardiovascular and musculoskeletal systems.

Physiotherapists and others must be warned not to be aggressive in their management of this patient group. Gentle, light sports, particularly swimming and walking, are recommended to maintain muscle tone and keep the patient active.

Psychological

The psychological problems of self-image which affect adolescents, may in middle age become compounded by problems of increasingly failing health. Van Tongerloo and De Paepe [13] reported from interviews of 17 patients between 16 and 35 years, that patients were significantly burdened by their disease in terms of its effects on day to day life, schooling and career opportunities. During childhood, most of them had experienced teasing because of their typical phenotypic traits. The female cohort expressed concern regarding potential problems of childbirth, and as in the general population, female patients experienced higher rates of depression than male patients. All patients found psychological support helpful.

Conclusion

In summary, one may look at MFS as a model of premature old-age, with patients suffering from many problems that the general population encounter, but at younger ages and higher frequencies. More research needs to be conducted, and especially interesting will be the correlation of genotype with phenotype in predicting health problems throughout life so that these may be anticipated and prevented [14]. Meanwhile, the available information should help practitioners to manage mature MFS patients [15].

Conditions of old age must be treated appropriately, and not dismissed as a complication of MFS.

References

1. Murdoch JL, Walker BA, Halpern BL, Kuzma JW, McKusick VA. Life expectancy and causes of death in the Marfan syndrome. N Engl J Med. 1972;286:804–8.
2. Silverman DI, Burton KJ, Gray J, et al. Life expectancy in the Marfan syndrome. Am J Cardiol. 1995;75:157–60.
3. Gray JR, Bridges AB, West RR, et al. Life expectancy in British Marfan syndrome populations. Clin Genet. 1998;54:124–8.
4. Finkbohner R, Johnston D, Crawford ES, Coselli J, Milewicz DM. Marfan syndrome. Long-term survival and complications after aortic aneurysm repair. Circulation. 1995;91:728–33.
5. National statistics data on life expectancy. http://www.statistics.gov.uk/CCi/nugget.asp?ID-881&pos=1ColRank=2&Rank=1000(checked11/05/05).
6. Pyeritz RE, McKusick VA. The Marfan syndrome: diagnosis and management. N Engl J Med. 1979;300:772–7.
7. Roman MJ, Devereux RB, Kramer-Fox R, Spitzer MC. Comparison of cardiovascular and skeletal features of primary mitral valve prolapse and Marfan syndrome. Am J Cardiol. 1989;63:317–21.
8. Grahame R, Pyeritz RE. The Marfan syndrome: joint and skin manifestations are prevelant and correlated. Br J Rheumatol. 1995;34:126–31.
9. Rossi-Foulkers R, Roman MJ, Rosen SE, et al. Phenotypic features and impact of beta blocker or calcium antagonist therapy on aortic lumen size in the Marfan syndrome. Am J Cardiol. 1999;83:1364–8.
10. Joseph KN, Kane HA, Milner RS, Steg NL, Williamson Jr MB, Bowen JR. Orthopedic aspects of the Marfan phenotype. Clin Orthop. 1992;277:251–61.
11. Hobbs WE, Sponseller PD, Weiss AP, Pyeritz RE. The cervical spine in Marfan syndrome. Spine. 1997;22:983–9.
12. Lipscomb KJ, Clayton-Smith J, Harris R. Evolving phenotype of Marfan's syndrome. Arch Ophthalmol. 1995;113:103–9.
13. Van Tongerloo A, de Paepe A. Psychosocial adaptation in adolescents and young adults with Marfan syndrome: an exploratory study. J Med Genet. 1998;35(5):405–9.
14. Faivre L, Collod-Beroud G, Loeys B, Child A, et al. Effects of mutation type and location on clinical outcome in 1057 probands with Marfan Syndrome or related phenotypes with FBN1 mutation: an International Study.). Am J Hum Genet. 2007;81(3):454–66.
15. Hasan A, Poloniecki J, Child AH. Ageing in Marfan syndrome. Int J Clin Pract. 2007;61(8):1308–20.

Psychosocial Aspects of Marfan Syndrome

26

Anne H. Child and Joanna Rowntree

The diagnosis of a genetic disorder such as Marfan syndrome affects the entire family. Each member must adjust to the diagnosis, making allowances for it, while maintaining their individual self-fulfilment. Couples may experience a temporary strain in their relationship when they first learn that their child has Marfan syndrome. It is important to communicate to each other and to grandparents, aunts and uncles of the child, their hopes and fears. Common reactions include dismay, worry regarding the future, a tendency to blame oneself, one's partner, or the doctors for the infant's condition. Grieving for the loss of perfect health in the child must also be experienced. The whole family should offer support to the parents. Prolonged discussion as to the prognosis for the child, and a plan for medical and psychological support and contact with another family who have older Marfan syndrome children, should be arranged at interview with the doctor in charge of the child's care.

Treatment is available for every aspect of Marfan syndrome, and the child should lead as normal a life as possible.

Childhood and Puberty

The affected child, up to the age of 5, appears to have few worries about the condition. If regular hospital visits are required, these may be explained as check-ups to make sure that nothing is changing. After each visit, the child should be reassured that they are well, if possible. From age 5–11, children realise they are different, and may report teasing and bullying due to increased height, poor eyesight, thin body build and slight clumsiness due to lax ligaments and long limbs. The child may

A.H. Child, MD, FRCP (✉) • J. Rowntree
Cardiovascular and Cell Sciences Research Institute, St George's, University of London, London, UK
e-mail: achild@sgul.ac.uk

© Springer-Verlag London 2016

A.H. Child (ed.), *Diagnosis and Management of Marfan Syndrome*,
DOI 10.1007/978-1-4471-5442-6_26

fatigue easily. Limitation of sporting activities may lead to feelings of isolation which must be actively combated by encouraging a special friend to play with the child and to stand by them at school if teasing occurs. A sense of humour with regard to teasing should be fostered; bullying should be reported to the teacher, for whom a book is available [1], and parental insistence on playground supervision is important. The child's special talents should be discovered and encouraged. Musical talent may lead to group activities. Computer studies or other sedentary activities and handicrafts should be encouraged, and may actually lead to a suitable career choice. The child should keep fit by participating in non-contact sports.

The child should be kept in a normal school if possible, with expert advice regarding visual and other teaching aids, and statementing to provide extra one-to-one teaching time, if necessary. Children should not be overprotected which leads to resentment, and delays normal psychological development. Mild depression may appear due to resentment at being different, and can often be dispelled by a quiet talk between the child and parent, who can point out the skills and talents which the child does possess. Accomplishments should be praised.

During the pubertal growth spurt, from age 10 to 20, features of Marfan syndrome may appear or worsen. A *Booklet for Teenagers* [2] is available to help youngsters through this difficult period. The child may have difficulty with body image, and referral to a psychologist may prevent negative feelings from developing. Purchasing clothing and shoes to fit may be a problem.

Close friends may be informed of the nature of the condition. Genetic advice should be offered to a couple when the affected young person has a serious girl or boyfriend, and is contemplating a lasting relationship. A counselling session together, and individually if a partner has extra questions and anxiety, is indicated.

Family Survey by Questionnaire

Background

Children with long term physical disorders have an increased risk of psychological problems, because they look and feel different, they have restrictions imposed because of their physical problems (eyes, hear, skeleton in Marfan syndrome), and because they may have frequent school absence due to hospital visits. In addition, the family history of members experiencing sudden death may be a worry.

A previous study by Hofman and colleagues [3], of 30 school children with Marfan syndrome, showed average intellectual development, but half of the children had problems, with learning disability (13 %), short attention span (17 %), and better results on verbal intelligence testing that performance testing due to loose joints, clumsiness and short sightedness (30 %).

Schneider and colleagues [4] studied 22 adolescents with Marfan syndrome and pointed out that puberty is the peak time for psychological problems. Because physical features may appear or worsen during puberty, youngsters have difficult with their body image, they realise they are different from their peers, they find easy fatigability limiting, and may have a prolonged dependence period on their parents. At interview, they said their lives would be significantly better without Marfan syndrome, especially with regard to physical activity and self-image.

Aims

The aims of our study were to determine the rate of common behavioural and psychological problems in young people with Marfan syndrome, compared to an unaffected control group. We also determined the prevalence of bullying. One hundred and one children aged 4–16 years (60 males and 41 females) were recruited from Dr. Child's Marfan syndrome outpatient clinic, the regional genetic centre, and volunteer members of the Marfan Association U.K. We are grateful to all families for participating. For children aged 5–7, the parents filled out the questionnaires, and all parents were asked to fill out the child behaviour check list (CBCL). Children aged 8–12, and 13–16 were asked to fill out a children's depression inventory (CDI), a perceived competence scale (Harter) and a bullying questionnaire.

Results

Parents

Parents reported that the Marfan syndrome children had more time off school, more operations, more medication, were more likely to have seen a psychologist or a psychiatrist, less likely to be in a single sex school, and more likely to be statemented, and to attend remedial or special classes. Parents also filled out the child behaviour check list (CBCL) and 15 children with Marfan syndrome had a high score indicating that they needed medical attention for behavioural problems, while only 3 controls had a high score. Parents reported that Marfan syndrome children tended to internalise (keep to themselves) their worries, resulting in withdrawn children with attention problems, physical complaints, anxiety and depression. Interestingly, they were not more likely to be aggressive or antisocial (externalising their worries). Significantly more common in the Marfan syndrome group were the following comments, ticked by their parents: cannot concentrate; cannot pay attention for long; is disobedient at home; is accident-prone; gets teased a lot; feels dizzy; has aches and pains (not headaches); is poorly coordinated or clumsy; sees things that are not there; has speech problems; is underactive and lacks energy.

The Children Speak

Depressive Tendency

Answers to the **child depression inventory** showed a significant difference between responses from the 75 children with Marfan syndrome as compared with 90 control children. Twenty-one Marfan syndrome children had a score higher than 11, whereas only 8 controls had a score higher than 11. The key differentiating questions were as follows (the children have to tick which one applies most correctly to their own situation):

- I HATE MYSELF/I DO NOT LIKE MYSELF/I LIKE MYSELF
- I HAVE PLENTY OF FRIENDS/I HAVE SOME FRIENDS BUT WISH I HAD MORE/I DO NOT HAVE ANY FRIENDS

Poor Self-Esteem

The **Harter self-esteem questionnaire** was answered by 63 children with Marfan syndrome and 76 controls. Marfan syndrome children had a lower opinion of themselves with respect to social and physical competence, and feelings of general self-worth. Marfan children saw themselves as not being sure of themselves, not being liked by others, not being happy in their present school, not being sure they were doing the right thing, and not being good enough at sports.

Bullying

The results from 74 subjects and 90 controls reveal that children with Marfan syndrome were bullied more often, chiefly by being called nasty names, having children tell nasty stories about them, and having their belongings taken away from them (theft). Marfan syndrome children were more likely to be bullied by several children, usually from a different class and often a higher year, were more likely to tell a teacher and a parent, and had fewer friends, thus being more often on their own in the playground.

Summary

Affected children are vulnerable to emotional and behavioural problems. Early identification and prompt intervention may reduce suffering. Advice regarding schooling is to stay in mainstream schooling wherever possible, to request extra help in the classroom, including statementing, and to establish a good parent-teacher relationship. Special attention should be given to seating to take account of short sightedness, extra height, and poor concentration, and visual aids such as large print text, and computers to speed up written tasks. Loose joints may be supported by splints, and extra time to rest the hands should be requested during long written examinations.

Time off school should be minimised by asking for hospital appointments and operations to be arranged wherever possible during school holidays. The child may feel too tired or unwell to go to school occasionally, and should be helped to catch up immediately or will become anxious that they have missed out, and do not fit in with the peer group.

Bullying is highly stressful and results in low self-esteem, and emotional and behavioural problems. To counteract this problem, parents should liaise with teachers, encourage special friends to act as allies, and help the child develop special interests and skills to improve self-image (e.g. music, swimming, archery, pets, art and handicrafts).

Lastly, professional psychological counselling may help with self-image at any age, and improve social interactions with peers.

Siblings

Unaffected brothers and sisters also need support, as they may feel guilty that they are unaffected, or fearful that they may still become affected or have children who are affected. They may resent the special attention the affected child receives. Parents should spend special time talking to children about their feelings, as they need reassurance that parents are as interested in them as in their affected sibling. Once the situation is explained, children usually become very protective of, and helpful to, the affected sibling. They may wonder what to tell their friends or partner, and individual counselling with an interested physician will be helpful.

Adulthood

Affected young adults may react by trying to prove they are normal, taking part in dangerous or highly competitive sports, avoiding medication, or travelling around the world. The threat of early death, present in those with serious cardiac involvement, may make them adult before their time. Some react by marrying early, and having children quickly, often without genetic advice. Pregnancy in the young female with Marfan syndrome may be contraindicated due to heart and aorta involvement. Pregnancy should be supervised closely by a cardiologist and obstetrician. A booklet, *Before and After Birth* [5], may be helpful.

Careers

Career choice should be decided after advice from specialist physicians caring for the young adult. Education should be pursued as far as possible, so that a sedentary occupation may be chosen. Young adults diagnosed mid-training may have to change their career, or choose a quiet branch which is not physically taxing. Heavy lifting should be avoided, and occupations where repetitive joint strain is a feature, for example, physical education and the armed forces, are unsuitable. Being tall is an advantage in seeking a responsible position, or promotion, as employers usually look upon tall individuals as being older and more responsible than their shorter peers. Easy fatigability is a feature of Marfan syndrome, and regular working hours in an office close to home are recommended. Extra-curricular activities may have to be pursued only on weekends.

Insurance and Pensions

Life insurance may be difficult to obtain. Pension schemes should be carefully studied if the working life may be foreshortened due to illness. Early retirement on grounds of ill health usually provides full pension rights.

Reproduction

Some affected patients avoid or postpone a permanent relationship, feeling that it is not fair to a potential spouse, or that they do not want to have affected children. However, the vast majority of patients do establish happy relationships, providing genetic counselling includes the intended partner. It is difficult for the unaffected partner to accept a diagnosis after the partnership is established, especially if affected children have been born.

The decision to have children will be taken by the couple, with expert advice from a genetic counsellor. The 50/50 risk of passing the gene on to each offspring is always applicable, but predicted severity of systems involved may be modified in the light of the family history. If the couple can accept the manifestations of the disease in all affected family members, then they can accept the diagnosis in their child. Prenatal diagnosis may be available, or the baby may be screened for the family mutation after birth. If the husband is affected, artificial insemination by donor is possible, and if the wife is affected, ovum donation is a possibility. This allows the affected parent to be the environmental parent without the concern of being the genetic parent. Once a gene mutation is discovered, pre-implantation genetic diagnosis is available either through the NHS, or privately.

Partner's Response

The unaffected partner may have to worry about the affected partner and also affected children. Counselling should be given to the couple, as well as the unaffected partner alone. In this way, temporary rejection in the unaffected partner may soon become total acceptance and support. Each of us has a number of genes which are not normal; moreover we are not responsible for our genes, nor do we request them. The patient's positive self-image, and the attitude of the partner, should not be dependent on one's genetic inheritance.

Coming to Terms with Marfan Syndrome

Accepting loss is part of the family adjustment to Marfan syndrome – loss of health, self-image, loss of a job or job opportunities – the psychological stresses similar to that of any long term disorder with variable age of onset. Patients should be encouraged to accept what they cannot change, and to make the most of their abilities.

There is a danger of patients becoming cardiac hypochondriacs, but sudden catastrophic events normally only occur if the situation is not being monitored. The patient is a member of a team caring for him or her, and returning for annual echocardiograms is the part he or she must play to participate in the decision-making process of whether, and when, elective cardiac surgery is required. The surgery bears small mortality risk, and prolongs life. Medication can buy time, during which medical and surgical treatment are constantly improving.

Further Support

Support is available from many directions, including peer group counselling, especially pre- and post- cardiac surgery. In the UK, the Marfan Association offers information, resources, referrals, meetings and support to those who are interested. In addition, it has close contact with similar organisations around the world, which is especially encouraging for the travelling patient. Active research is being undertaken internationally, and any advances will be instantly communicated to those affected. This offers hope for improved quality of life and a normal lifespan for both the patient and their descendants.

All the following publications (excluding 5 & 6) are available from the Marfan Association UK, Rochester House, 5, Aldershot Road, Fleet, Hampshire, GU52 8NG. Tel: 01252810472

References

1. Child AH, Rust DL. A booklet for teachers. Marfan Association UK. 1993.
2. Bernhardt A, Haul P, Weiner J, Weiss J. A booklet for teenagers. Courtesy of NMF USA. Marfan Association UK. 2005
3. Hofman KJ, Bernhard BA, Pyeritz RE. Marfan syndrome: neuropsychological aspects. Am J Med Genet. 1988;31(2):331–8.
4. Schneider MB, Davis JG, Boxer RA, et al. Marfan syndrome in adolescents and young adults: psychosocial functioning and knowledge. J Dev Behav Pediatr. 1990;11:122–7.
5. Rust DL, Howard FM. Before and after birth. Marfan Association UK. 1998.

Patient Support

27

Diane L. Rust

It is some years since my husband, Mr Robin Rust, FISOB, FIMIT and MIFM, and the late Dr Martin J Briggs, MB BS DFPHM, worked very hard together with Dr Anne Child, MD FRCP, and the authors of the previous "The Marfan Syndrome – A Clinical Guide Revised edition 2002" and we will always be extremely grateful to the British Heart Foundation for publishing that vital guide. Much headway has been achieved by us all and it has been wonderful to work with so many eminent Marfan syndrome professionals over the years.

"Yes Together We Can!"

When a diagnosis of Marfan syndrome is suspected, many families react in the same way as they did in the past – worried, confused, angry, fearful, guilty, full of despair and concerned for the future. What a difference time has made. Early diagnosis is vital to enable an appropriate Medical Care Programme to be put together for the individual patient, since Marfan syndrome is extremely variable in its nature. Sadly, some people are very seriously affected, thus vigilant care is essential.

Patients can now search for help on the internet. Many general practitioners are now more aware of this condition and should be able to point patients in the right direction for appointments to specialists concerning eyes, skeleton, heart and lungs, which eventually should provide the diagnosis of, or rule out, Marfan syndrome. By now the patient will be aware that this disorder of the connective tissue is thought to be hereditary in 75 % of cases and spontaneous in 25 %. Some patients are mildly affected, but for some it may sadly be life-threatening.

D.L. Rust, MJF, LCIF
Chairman, Marfan Association UK, 70 Greenways, Courtmoor, Fleet Hants, UK
e-mail: chairman@marfan-association.org.uk

© Springer-Verlag London 2016

A.H. Child (ed.), *Diagnosis and Management of Marfan Syndrome*,
DOI 10.1007/978-1-4471-5442-6_27

Patients find it very helpful to speak to non-medical people, so please don't forget to tell your patients that the Marfan Association UK is here for them.

Throughout the life of the Marfan Association UK, we have worked closely with our member patients, frequently undertaking studies in order that we stay close to how Marfan syndrome truly affects them, identifying any shortfalls that may exist in their care. This enables us to work more effectively with our medical colleagues. The revised Ghent criteria for diagnosis (2010) together with the Marfan care pathways and numerous Marfan research studies around the world are huge steps forward in gaining an improved understanding of the condition, whereby it is now possible that some patients with Marfan syndrome can live a "normal lifespan." However, we are all aware that this condition is variable and each patient requires individual ongoing assessment, an appropriate care plan and timely surgical intervention if indicated. In any hereditary disorder, family screening should be initiated and any necessary action taken.

We provide support for the patient and their family members, often working together with their medical specialists, and we recognise that many of our members need extra support and understanding at certain times in their lives.

We continually create awareness and publish educational literature both for the medical profession and for the patients.

We undertake research amongst our membership on the various aspects of this perplexing disorder, which enables us "to better understand the patients that we serve". We can then help and support them in a more purposeful way, continually amending our 'Five Year Plan' whilst working closely with our "Marfan Medical and Scientific Advisory Team."

Robin and I co-founded the European Marfan Support Network in 1990 (EMSN) and co-ordinated this for the first 10 years, making many valuable contacts who remain in touch with us. We are also on the founding committee of the International Federation of Marfan Syndrome Organizations (IFMSO), and it is with great joy that we witness the growth of Support organizations across the world. This is helping Marfan patients worldwide, and joint Marfan research projects provide a widening knowledge of Marfan syndrome.

"Support for Today with Tomorrow in Mind"

Marfan "In Touch" Magazine

Members of the Marfan Association UK and medical professionals worldwide receive a Marfan "In Touch" magazine twice yearly.

Annual Marfan Association UK Information Day

These meetings are always well attended and much welcomed by the patients and doctors who attend. Our medical speakers are always happy to participate in a "Questions and Answers Session". Being bombarded with questions is not an easy task, but much is learned by patients and medical specialists alike.

Marfan Association UK Support Network

We operate this Network in order to provide local support for patients. Many of them also fundraise to enable us to continue our vital work of Support, Education and Research. Some of them participate in local medical meetings.

Representing Marfan Syndrome Across the UK

Robin, Diane and trained staff have been invited to schools to inform the teachers, school nurses and pupils about Marfan syndrome. Doctors may be required to assist the parents of the child to obtain the appropriate help required during their school years.

We participate in medical meetings around the country. Recently we have held and participated in meetings in Glasgow, London, Birmingham, Manchester, Cardiff, Southampton and Dorking, amongst others.

These have included meetings in the House of Commons, speaking to Lions Groups, Ladies meetings, fundraising events and participation in International Marfan Research Meetings. This enables us to meet up with medical colleagues with whom we have been in touch for many years. It is good to share information with one another.

Publications

We have recently published our new Marfan Fact Sheet and have already received good feedback on this helpful aid. This helps patients to go equipped to their many medical appointments and is indeed "a must" for every doctor's library.

Marfan Mascot

Our mascot, "Marf", accompanies us to many meetings, having been chosen due to the eye, skeletal and heart problems also encountered by the giraffes.....and they have such beautiful eyes!

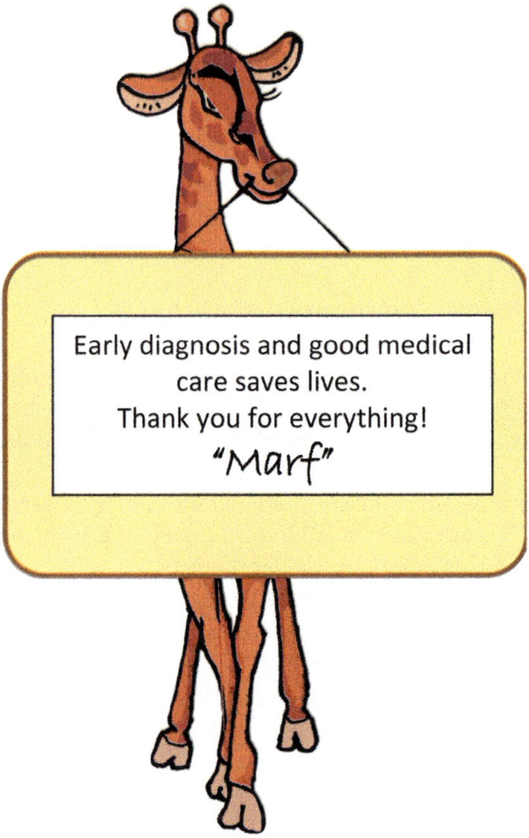
Early diagnosis and good medical care saves lives.
Thank you for everything!
"Marf"

Appendix

MARFAN WORLDWIDE
IFMSO

Member Organizations

Argentina
Mario del Frade, Chairman
Marfan Argentina
Charcas 33913er piso office 32
Buenos Aires, Republic Argentina
www.marfan.org.ar
e-mail: Marfan@argentina.com

Australia
Queensland, Australia
Susanne Hemphill
Marfan Association, Queensland Branch
P.O. Box 294
Sumner Park, Queensland 4074
Australia
Telephone: ++61 7 3376 6160
Fax: ++61 7 3279 1927
e-mail: marfanaustralia@hotmail.com

Victoria, Australia
Marfan Association Victoria Inc.
Sally Ferguson, President
PO Box 42
Sunbury, Victoria. 3429
Australia
Telephone: ++61 3 5784 1357
Fax: ++61 3 5784 1357
www.marfanvic.org.au
e-mail: yvette1@bigpond.com

New South Wales, Australia
Marfan Support Group
Trudy Whaite
mail@marfan.net.au
www.marfan.net.au

Belgium
Yvonne Flemal - Jousten
Association Belge du Syndrome de Marfan
27A, rue Residence Air Pur
B 4623 - Magnee
Belgium
Telephone: ++32 4 355 13 59
e-mail: yvonne.jousten@easynet.be
www.marfan.be

Brazil
Brazilian Marfan Association (Marfan Brasil)
Flavia Gioia, President
e-mail: flavia.gioia@br.abnamro.com
www.marfan.com.br

Contact:
Adriano Rodrigues
Rua dos Juritis - Quadra 07 - Apt.403 - Ed. Mirela
Jardim Renascença
Sao Luis, MA, Brazil
CEP 65075-240
Tel: 55 98 3236 0455
Cell phone: 8129 9224
e-mail: adrianocostarodrigues@yahoo.com

Canada
"Making A Difference"
"Le Pouvoir de changer les choses"

Eva Theofilopoulos, Executive Manager
Josipa Paska, Director
Central Plaza Postal Outlet
128 Queen St. S., P.O. Box 42257
Mississauga Ontario L5M 4Z0
Canada
Telephone: (905) 826–3223; FAX: (905) 826-2125
e-mail: josipa.paska@aak.com
info@marfan.ca
website: www.marfan.ca

China
Lydia Chen
e-mail: lcsnoopy@21cn.com

Costa Rica
Michelle Gómez
Tel: (506) 817- 0001
e-mail: mich_go19@hotmail.com

Cuba
Carolina Douglas
Cuban Association of Marfan Syndrome
Calle 34 No. 310, apto2
entre 3ra y 5ta, Miramar
Ciudad de La Habana 11300
Cuba
Fax: ++337 330145

Denmark
Ms. Bodil Davidsen
Danish Marfan Association
Frederikshave 34 st. th.
DK-3400 Hillerod
Denmark
Tel. ++45 4826 3652
Fax ++45 4826 3752
e-mail: msdk@get2net.dk
www.marfan.dk

Finland
Leila Raninen
Finnish Marfan Association
PO Box 1328 SF-00101
Helsinki, Finland
Telephone: ++35894171727
e-mail: iinfo@marfan.fi
www.marfan.fi

France
Annette Belloncle
Association Syndrome de Marfan Amis d'Antoine (A.S.M.A.A.)
B.P. 63
F-95160 - Montmorency
France
Telephone/Fax: ++33 139 64 56 12
e-mail: jtihierr@free.fr

Paulette Morin
Association Française du Syndrome de Marfan (A.F.S.M.)
13, Allee des Terasses
F-77200 Torcy
France
Tel. ++33 164620375
Fax ++33 160 057 910
e-mail: vivremarfan@caramail.com
www.vivremarfan.org

Germany
Marfan Hilfe (Deutschland) e.V.
Post Box 0145
D-23691 Eutin
Germany
Tel: ++49 4521 8305035
Fax: ++49 4521 8305034
e-mail: kontakt@marfan.de
www.marfan.de

Greece
Xanthi Zafiris
Greek Association of the Marfan Syndrome
tel/fax 0030 210-2793075
Athens
e-mail: marfansyndromegr@yahoo.com

Guatemala
Evelyn Oliva Barrios
Guatemala, City
e-mail: marfanguatemala@hotmail.com

India
Chirarnjib Nath
South Hazarapar,
Tezpur, Assam
India 784001
e-mail: sc.nath@gmail.com and ck.nath15@yahoo.com

Ireland
Mary O'Driscoll
Marfan Syndrome Support Group Ireland, Ltd
78 Whitehorn Drive
Palmerstown, Dublin 20
Ireland
e-mail: Marfan@eircom.net
http://www.marfan.ie

Italy

Silvia Salice
Associazione Vittorio
Strada alla Villa d'Agliè 23/3
I-10132 Torino
Italy
Telephone/Fax: ++39 11898 0995
e-mail: michaela.tarantini@marfan.info
www.marfan.info

Japan

Marfan Network Japan (MNJ)
President, Yoko Shimozaki
Fukuike 1-17-1, Tenpaku-ku
Nagoya-city, Aichi-ken,
Japan 468-0049
e-mail: yoko-shimo@gf6.so-net.ne.jp
info@marfan.gr.jp (MNJ)
website: www.marfan.gr.jp (Japanese only)

Japan Marfan Association (JAMAA)
Keiko Inoi, Representative Director
c/o Aichi Japan Intractable Diseases Information Center
N105 COMBi Honjin, 1–24 Matsubara-cho, Nakamura-ku, Nagoya, Aichi 453-0021
Telephone: ++050-5532-6503
FAX: ++053-454-6764
e-mail: info@marfan.jp
website: http://www.marfan.jp
http://www.marfan.jp/modules/jamaa/index.php?content_id=57

Mexico

Marcos and Geraldine Duran
Sindrome de Marfan de Mexico A.C.
Paseo de Lilas #92
Loc. 58, Suite 143
Bosques de Las Lomas
Mexico D.F. C.P. 05120
Mexico
Tel/Fax: ++52-452260
e-mail: admin@marfan.org.mx
www.marfan.org.mx

Netherlands

Contactgroep Marfan Nederland
Postbus 1809
3800 BV Amersfoort

The Netherlands
Phone +31 (0)33 422 65 46
website: www.marfansyndroom.nl
e-mail: contact@marfansyndroom.nl

New Zealand
No current contacts

Norway
Wenche Snekkevik
Marfanforeningen co/FFO
PB 4568
0404 Oslo, Norway
Tel. 47–46 66 00 06
e-mail: info@marfan.no
wenche@marfan.no
http://www.marfan.no

Peru
Contáctenos a:
La Asociación Peruana del Síndrome de Marfan (APSIM)
Cecilia Delgado Tello
Calle Carlos Aguirre 189 – 301.
Urb Prolongación Benavides. Santiago de Surco.
Lima. Perú
Telefono: (511) 2743767
e-mail: marfanperu@marfanperu.org
website: http://www.marfanperu.org

Poland
Polish Marfan Association
Swietojanska 49/17
PI-81-391 Gdynia
Poland
Telephone: ++48 601286245
Fax: ++48 58 629 4425
e-mail: marfan@marfan.pl
marfan@gdansk.sprint.pl
www.marfan.pl

Portugal
Telf: + 351 225 431 080 / +351 210 970 766
Fax: +351 225 431 089
e-mail: marfan.pt@gmail.com

Singapore
Willie Loh Chung Wei
Blk 471 Ang Mo Kio Ave 10 #11-774 SE 560471
Republic of Singapore
Telephone: + 65 9145 5708
e-mail: Lchungwe@yahoo.com

Singapore Marfan Support
www.marfansingapore.org
e-mail: support@marfansingapore.org

Slovakia
Post address: AMS, Lukovicova Betty
Vajnorska 54, 831 04 Bratislava, Slovakia
Tel: 00421 2 44257904, mobile phone: 00421 903 74 74 24
e-mail: marfan.sk@mail.t-com.sk
e-mail: lukovicova@stonline.sk
website: http://marfan.szm.sk/

South Africa
South African Marfan Syndrome Organisation
(Suid-Afrikaanse Marfansindroom Ondersteuningsgroep)
P O Box 12895
Queenswood 0121
Telephone: +27 12 333 3894
e-mail: info@marfan.org.za
http://www.marfan.org.za

Online Marfan Syndrome diagnosis tool:
http://www.marfan.org.za/diagnosis.html

Spain
SIMA Asociación de Afectados Síndrome de Marfan
Oficinas Centrales
C/ Pardo Jimeno n° 55, entlo. C
E - 03007 Alicante
Teléfono: + 34 965 11 11 02 - +34 619 19 61 65
e-mail: Info@marfan.es
www.marfan.es

Sweden
Karin Olsson
Svenska Marfanföreningen
c/o Ulla Frick
St. Eriksgatan 50 A
112 34 Stockholm
Sweden
Tel: +46 8 651 3609
e-mail: bertil.frick@swipnet.se
karin.olsson@vansterpartiet.se
www.marfanforeningen.se

Switzerland
Marfan Stiftung Schweiz
Marktgasse 31
CH-3011 Bern
Switzerland
Telephone: 41 31 312 11 22

Fax: 41 31 312 11 20
e-mail: info@marfan.ch
www.marfan.ch

Syria

Mohammad Mouchli
Tel:00963-11-6664647
Tel:00963-11-6662864
P.O.Box:16428 Damascus -Syria
e-mail: Marfan@Shuf.Com

Ukraine

Contact Person: Sergii Demchenko
Ukrainian Marfan Care Centre (UMCC)
P.B. #213
Odessa-23 65023 UKRAINE
Tel. + 380-(66)-7-700-710
e-mail Address: info@marfan.in.ua
website Address: http://www.marfan.in.ua

United Kingdom

Diane Rust
Marfan Association UK
Rochester House
5, Aldershot Road
Fleet, Hampshire GU51 3NG
United Kingdom
Telephone: ++44 1252 810472
Fax: ++44 1252 810473
e-mail: contactus@marfan-association.org.uk
www.marfan-association.org.uk

United States

Carolyn Levering
National Marfan Foundation
22 Manhasset Avenue
Port Washington, New York 11050
USA
Telephone: ++ 516-883-8712
++800-862-7326
Fax: ++516-883-8040
e-mail: staff@marfan.org
www.marfan.org

World Organizations:

Beatruce Preston
Chairman

European Marfan Support Network (EMSN)
Römerweg 4
CH-4410 Liestal
Switzerland
+41 61 921 91 89
e-mail: preston5@bluewin.ch

Priscilla Ciccariello
President
International Federation of Marfan Syndrome Organizations (IFMSO)
c/o National Marfan Foundation
22 Manhasset Avenue
Port Washington, NY 11050
e-mail: Cilla71@aol.com
www.marfanworld.org
http://www.marfanworld.org/members.htm

Index

© Springer-Verlag London 2016
A.H. Child (ed.), *Diagnosis and Management of Marfan Syndrome*,
DOI 10.1007/978-1-4471-5442-6

Printed by Printforce, the Netherlands